Occupational and Environmental Medicine
Self-Assessment Review

SECOND EDITION

Occupational and Environmental Medicine
Self-Assessment Review
SECOND EDITION

Editor-in-Chief
Robert J. McCunney, M.D., M.P.H., M.S.
Research Scientist
Department of Biological Engineering
Massachusetts Institute of Technology
Cambridge, Massachusetts
Clinical Associate
Pulmonary Unit
Massachusetts General Hospital
Harvard Medical School
Boston, Massachusetts
Past President
American College of Occupational and Environmental Medicine

Editor
Paul P. Rountree, M.D.
Professor and Vice-Chairman
Occupational and Environmental Medicine
University of Texas at Tyler
Tyler, Texas

Associate Editors

Debra Cherry, M.D., M.S.   J. Torey Nalbone, M.S., C.I.H.
Sharon Hall Davis, M.D., M.P.H.   Barbara Pinson, M.D., M.S.
Jeffrey L. Levin, M.D., M.S.P.H.   Ellen Remenchik, M.D., M.P.H.
Larry K. Lowry, Ph.D.

Occupational Health Sciences
University of Texas Health Center at Tyler
Tyler, Texas

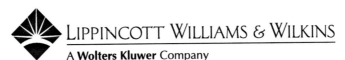

LIPPINCOTT WILLIAMS & WILKINS
A **Wolters Kluwer** Company
Philadelphia · Baltimore · New York · London
Buenos Aires · Hong Kong · Sydney · Tokyo

Acquisitions Editor: Danette Somers
Developmental Editor: Stacey L. Baze
Production Editor: Emily Lerman
Manufacturing Manager: Colin J. Warnock
Cover Designer: Patricia Gast
Compositor: Lippincott Williams & Wilkins Desktop Division

© 2004 by LIPPINCOTT WILLIAMS & WILKINS
530 Walnut Street
Philadelphia, PA 19106 USA
LWW.com

Printed in the USA

Library of Congress Cataloging-in-Publication Data

Occupational and environmental medicine : self-assessment review / editors, Robert J. McCunney, Paul P. Rountree.—2nd ed.
  p. ; cm.
  Includes bibliographical references and index.
  ISBN 0-7817-5292-2 (alk. paper)
  1. Medicine, Industrial—Examinations, questions, etc. 2. Environmental
health—Examinations, questions, etc. I. McCunney, Robert J. II. Rountree, Paul P.
  [DNLM: 1. Occpational Medicine—Examination Questions. 2. Environmental
Medicine—Examination Questions. WA 18.2 O147 2004]
  RC963.3.M23 2004
  616.9′803′076—dc22

                                                        2003058921

Care has been taken to confirm the accuracy of the information presented and to describe generally accepted practices. However, the authors, editors, and publisher are not responsible for errors or omissions or for any consequences from application of the information in this book and make no warranty, expressed or implied, with respect to the currency, completeness, or accuracy of the contents of the publication. Application of this information in a particular situation remains the professional responsibility of the practitioner.

The authors, editors, and publisher have exerted every effort to ensure that drug selection and dosage set forth in this text are in accordance with current recommendations and practice at the time of publication. However, in view of ongoing research, changes in government regulations, and the constant flow of information relating to drug therapy and drug reactions, the reader is urged to check the package insert for each drug for any change in indications and dosage and for added warnings and precautions. This is particularly important when the recommended agent is a new or infrequently employed drug.

Some drugs and medical devices presented in this publication have Food and Drug Administration (FDA) clearance for limited use in restricted research settings. It is the responsibility of the health care provider to ascertain the FDA status of each drug or device planned for use in their clinical practice.

Contents

Preface

The idea for the *Occupational and Environmental Medicine: Self-Assessment Review*, or OMSAR, was first conceived by the American College of Occupational and Environmental Medicine (ACOEM) Committee for Enduring Materials and Distance Learning in 1996, and rigorously promoted by the editor of this text, Paul P. Rountree, M.D. The first edition was published in 1998. This project was intended to respond to a voiced need for materials that would allow physicians to obtain CME credit while studying at home about occupational and environmental health issues.

The majority of patients who see primary care physicians have concerns about the relationship between disease and workplace or environmental exposures. Unfortunately, most primary care physicians have little training in occupational and environmental medicine. Such information is still absent from the curriculum in most medical schools.

This review book is based on material from the popular textbook *A Practical Approach to Occupational and Environmental Medicine, Third Edition*. The editors have outlined the material in the book chapters, attempted to identify the key points, and developed a series of questions based on the text. It is our hope that the review book, when used in conjunction with the text, will lead to an enhanced understanding of occupational and environmental medicine for both the generalist and those with intensive exposure to the field.

This book reached completion through the energy, enthusiasm, and direction of my friend, Paul Rountree. Like the first edition, this book was rigorously peer-reviewed. The first edition was also approved by the American Board of Preventive Medicine as a study guide.

Robert J. McCunney, M.D., M.P.H., M.S.

Acknowledgments

The material in this edition was scrutinized by an *ad hoc* committee at a special session in Chicago, Illinois. Members of the peer-review session included Robert Dedmon, John Gibbs, John D. Meyer, Kevin O'Shea, and Tufail Q. Shaikh. In addition, we are grateful for assistance from Barbara Choyke, Sandy Piszkiewicz, and Marianne Dreger. Mark A. Roberts, as Chairman of the Committee on Enduring Materials and Distance Learning, also played a key role in this publication.

Associate Editors

(CHAPTERS 33, 40, 48, 52)
Debra Cherry, M.D, M.S. *Assistant Professor, Occupational Health Sciences, University of Texas Health Center at Tyler, Tyler, Texas*

(CHAPTERS 5, 9, 13, 27, 55, 56)
Sharon Hall Davis, M.D., M.P.H. *Assistant Professor, Occupational Health Sciences, University of Texas Health Center at Tyler, Tyler, Texas*

(CHAPTERS 7, 10, 14, 18, 20, 49, 59)
Jeffrey L. Levin, M.D., M.S.P.H. *Professor and Chairman, Occupational Health Sciences, University of Texas Health Center at Tyler, Tyler, Texas*

(CHAPTERS 16, 35, 39, 47, 50, 53, 60)
Larry K. Lowry, Ph.D. *Associate Professor, Occupational Health Sciences, University of Texas Health Center at Tyler, Tyler, Texas*

(CHAPTERS 3, 26, 37, 38, 42, 43, 46, 57, 58)
J. Torey Nalbone, M.S., C.I.H. *Assistant Professor, Occupational Health Sciences, University of Texas Health Center at Tyler, Tyler, Texas*

(CHAPTERS 4, 11, 19, 25, 44, 45)
Barbara Pinson, M.D., M.S. *Assistant Professor, Occupational Health Sciences, University of Texas Health Center at Tyler, Tyler, Texas*

(CHAPTERS 2, 22, 23, 29, 41)
Ellen Remenchik, M.D., M.P.H. *Assistant Professor, Occupational Health Sciences, University of Texas Health Center at Tyler, Tyler, Texas*

(CHAPTERS 1, 6, 8, 12, 15, 17, 21, 24, 28, 30–32, 34, 36, 51, 54)
Paul P. Rountree, M.D. *Professor, Occupational Health Sciences, University of Texas Health Center at Tyler, Tyler, Texas*

Special Thanks

This review book directly extracts material from chapters in *A Practical Approach to Occupational and Environmental Medicine, Third Edition*. For this reason, we believe that the contributors to the various chapters must be recognized in this new text. The editors have chosen not to include references, which are available in that text. Contributors to the various chapters include:

Chapter	Contributor(s)
1	Robert J. McCunney
2	Junius C. McElveen, Jr.
3	James A. Hathaway
4	William B. Patterson
5	Kent W. Peterson and D. Gary Rischitelli
6	Bonnie Rogers
7	Christopher R. Brigham, William Boucher, and Alan L. Engleberg
8	Frank H. Leone
9	Kent W. Peterson
10	Dennis Schultz
11	Dee W. Eddington and Wayne N. Burton
12	Molly J. McCauley and Robert J. McCunney
13	Jeffrey G. Jones, Donald S. Herip, and David O. Freedman
14	Jeffrey S. Harris
15	David J. Tollerud and Edward A. Emmett
16	Kent W. Peterson, Todd D. Kissam, and Barry A. Cooper
17	William B. Bunn and Sadhna Paralkar
18	Jeffrey S. Harris
19	Melissa D. Tonn
20	Rose H. Goldman
21	Ian A. Greaves
22	Reid T. Boswell and Robert J. McCunney
23	Arthur Frank
24	Daniel E. Forman, Paul P. Rountree, and Larry M. Starr
25	Robert G. Feldman and Chang-Ming Joseph Chern
26	John D. Meyer
27	Edward A. Emmett
28	Stuart Gitlow and Peter J. Holland
29	Jack E. Farnham and Donald Accetta
30	Nortin M. Hadler
31	Alain Couturier
32	Ross M. Myerson

Chapter	Contributor(s)
33	William E. Wright
34	Bernard R. Blais, Thomas J. Tredici, and John Williams, Sr.
35	Peter G. Shields
36	Amy J. Behrman and Judith Green-McKenzie
37	J. Torey Nalbone and James P. McCunney
38	Myron C. Harrison
39	Jonathan B. Borak and Richard C. Pleus
40	Joseph K. McLaughlin and Loren Lipworth
41	Philip Harber, Craig Colon, and Robert J. McCunney
42	John Whysner and Kenneth H. Chase
43	Stacy R. Rose, Erin K. Walline, J. Steven Moore, and Jonathan B. Borak
44	Marilyn V. Howarth and Mark Russi
45	Natalie P. Hartenbaum
46	Jean Spencer Felton
47	Victor S. Roth, David H. Garabrant, and Craig F. Turet
48	William W. Greaves and Kevin Soden
49	Tee L. Guidoti and Weimin Song
50	William B. Bunn, Claudia O'Brien, and Jack Shih
51	William B. Bunn and Jessica Herzstein
52	Alan M. Ducatman
53	Robert K. McLellan
54	Jonathan B. Borak
55	L. Kristian Arnold
56	L. Kristian Arnold
57	Ridgway M. Hall, Jr., William B. Bunn, and Thomas J. Slavin
58	Roger O. McClellan and William B. Bunn
59	Peter A. Valberg
60	David M. Gute

User Instructions for CME Credit

Congratulations on your purchase of *Occupational and Environmental Medicine: Self-Assessment Review, Second Edition* by Robert J. McCunney, M.D., M.P.H., M.S. and Paul P. Rountree, M.D., which is designed to be used with *A Practical Approach to Occupational and Environmental Medicine, Third Edition.* Please check your book to ensure that all of the following program materials have been included in your copy of *Occupational and Environmental Medicine: Self-Assessment Review, Second Edition*:

- **Answer sheets for Parts 1, 2, 3, and 4**
- **An evaluation form**
- **CME credit request forms**

TWO WAYS TO USE THE PROGRAM

1. *Beginning to end...* You can read *A Practical Approach to Occupational and Environmental Medicine, Third Edition* from cover-to-cover, and complete all the test questions from *Occupational and Environmental Medicine: Self-Assessment Review, Second Edition* at one time for the entire **90 category 1 credits toward the AMA Physician's Recognition Award.**

2. *Review...* You can concentrate on the chapters in *A Practical Approach to Occupational and Environmental Medicine, Third Edition* that are most relevant to your practice, and return the answer sheets for the units completed in *Occupational and Environmental Medicine: Self-Assessment Review, Second Edition* for **22.5 credits per unit.**

LEARNING OBJECTIVES

After completing this entire review, the user will understand the following as it relates to occupational medicine:

- scope of practice
- legal and ethical issues
- role of regulatory agencies
- development of worksite occupational health programs and centers
- clinical assessments
- accreditation for health centers
- health and productivity
- diseases and disorders common in the workforce
- toxicology
- epidemiology and surveillance
- ergonomics
- environmental health

PROGRAM INFORMATION

- Target audience: Persons preparing for the Boards; persons desiring to update and check their knowledge base
- Estimated time to complete this entire CME program: **90** hours
- Method of physician participation: Reading *A Practical Approach to Occupational and Environmental Medicine, Third Edition*, and answering questions found in *Occupational and Environmental Medicine: Self-Assessment Review, Second Edition*
- Evaluation methods: Participants will complete, self-correct, and return self-assessment examination forms with the completed *Self-Assessment Review Evaluation.*

Educational Credit

The American College of Occupational and Environmental Medicine (ACOEM) is accredited by the Accreditation Council for Continuing Medical Education to provide continuing medical education for physicians.

The American College of Occupational and Environmental Medicine designates this educational activity for a maximum of **90** category 1 credits toward the AMA Physician's Recognition Award. Each physician should claim only those credits that he or she actually spent in the activity.

Date of Original Release: July 1998

Date of Release, Second Edition: December 2003

Accreditation Expires: January 2007

Each of the four *Occupational and Environmental Medicine: Self Assessment Review, Second Edition* Parts has a maximum of 22.5 category 1 credits. Participants may request credits in increments of one Part for 22.5 credits. Completion of all four Parts or completion of the Units in a particular order is not required to earn credits.

Continuing medical education credit can be earned on a one-time-only basis for each section of the *Occupational and Environmental Medicine: Self-Assessment Review, Second Edition.*

The CME credit for each part requires the following:

1. Completion of reading all chapters of the relevant Unit in *A Practical Approach to Occupational and Environmental Medicine, Third Edition.*
2. Completion of reading the objectives, the outlines, and the key points related to each of the chapters of the relevant Unit of *Occupational and Environmental Medicine: Self-Assessment Review, Second Edition.*
3. Completion of all questions related to each chapter in *Occupational and Environmental Medicine: Self-Assessment Review, Second Edition.*
4. Self-scoring of all questions cited above with the scores reported.
5. Review of the answer explanations. It is suggested that the answers to all questions are read in their entirety to maximize learning and that the references are reread.

6. Completion of the appropriate forms included in *Occupational and Environmental Medicine: Self-Assessment Review, Second Edition.* Please note that one form must be completed per part of the *Review.*

7. The mailing of that form (those forms) and the answer sheet(s) plus **payment** in the amount of **$250.00 for each Part** or **$850.00** for all **four Parts** in *Occupational and Environmental Medicine: Self Assessment Review, Second Edition* to the following address:

> Education Department
> CME Coordinator
> The American College of Occupational and Environmental Medicine
> 1114 North Arlington Heights Road
> Arlington Heights, IL 60004-4770

Your letter awarding your CME credits should arrive within four (4) weeks.
For questions or concerns, contact the ACOEM Education Department.

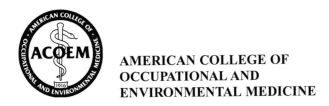

**AMERICAN COLLEGE OF
OCCUPATIONAL AND
ENVIRONMENTAL MEDICINE**

CME Registration for Part 1

Occupational and Environmental Medicine: Self-Assessment Review, Second Edition

COMPLETE BOTH SIDES OF THIS FORM - PLEASE <u>PRINT</u> CLEARLY

Name _____   Medical Degree _____

Address _____   City _____   State _____   Zip Code _____

Phone _____   Fax _____   E-mail _____

Total **Part 1** Answers: Correct _____   Incorrect _____

<table>
<tr><td>

<u>**METHOD OF PAYMENT**</u>

☐ Check
☐ American
   Express
☐ Diners Club

☐ Visa
☐ MasterCard

</td><td>

<u>**Attestation Statement**</u>

I certify that I have completed this activity as designed and claim 22.5 category 1 credits toward the AMA PRA.

_____

_____
Attestation Statement Signature

</td></tr>
</table>

Instructions

To earn 22.5 category 1 credits toward the AMA Physicians' Recognition Award for the study of parts in *A Practical Approach to Occupational and Environmental Medicine, Third Edition*, and *Occupational Medicine Self-Assessment Review, Second Edition*, complete the following requirements:

- Study the Part(s) in *A Practical Approach to Occupational and Environmental Medicine, Third Edition.*
- Study all of the materials in *Occupational and Environmental Medicine: Self-Assessment Review* for the corresponding Part.
- Complete the self-test for the corresponding Part.
- Evaluate your responses by using the key at the bottom of the answer sheet. Note your score on the form.
- Complete the CME registration form, including your attestation signature, and mail it with a $250.00 fee per OMSAR Part or $850.00 fee when submitting all four OMSAR parts at once to:

Education Department, American College of Occupational and Environmental Medicine
1114 North Arlington Heights Road
Arlington Heights, IL 60004-4770

Occupational and Environmental Medicine Self-Assessment Review
Evaluation – Part 1

Please check all that apply:

☐ Resident ☐ Fellow ☐ Attending
☐ Private Practice ☐ Corporate

Years in Practice _____ **Specialty** _____

	Strongly Agree				Strongly Disagree
1. The stated objectives were successfully met.	⑤	④	③	②	①
2. Overall, the quality of the instructional process met my expectations.	⑤	④	③	②	①
3. OMSAR was successful in developing or enhancing my competencies in a variety of areas in OEM.	⑤	④	③	②	①
4. I will apply the knowledge/information gained from OMSAR to improve my practice.	⑤	④	③	②	①

5. Did you observe any commercial bias? ○ Yes ○ No

6. Please tell us about your education needs and interests.

Topic Areas	Greatly Interested		Not Interested		
Disability management and work fitness	⑤	④	③	②	①
Public health surveillance	⑤	④	③	②	①
Hazard recognition, evaluation, and control	⑤	④	③	②	①
Cardiology	⑤	④	③	②	①
Dermatology	⑤	④	③	②	①
Emergency medicine	⑤	④	③	②	①
Ear, nose, throat, and hearing	⑤	④	③	②	①
Hematology/oncology	⑤	④	③	②	①
Infectious diseases	⑤	④	③	②	①
Neurology	⑤	④	③	②	①
Ophthalmology	⑤	④	③	②	①
Musculoskeletal	⑤	④	③	②	①
Mental health	⑤	④	③	②	①
Respiratory, allergy, and immunology	⑤	④	③	②	①
Reproductive medicine	⑤	④	③	②	①
Toxicology	⑤	④	③	②	①
Regulations and government agencies	⑤	④	③	②	①
Research in OEM	⑤	④	③	②	①
Environmental health and risk assessment	⑤	④	③	②	①
Management and administration in OEM	⑤	④	③	②	①
Medical/legal issues	⑤	④	③	②	①
Professionalism/personal development	⑤	④	③	②	①
Other	⑤	④	③	②	①

CME Registration for Part 2

Occupational and Environmental Medicine: Self-Assessment Review, Second Edition

COMPLETE BOTH SIDES OF THIS FORM - PLEASE <u>PRINT</u> CLEARLY

Name _____   Medical Degree _____

Address _____   City _____   State _____   Zip Code _____

Phone _____   Fax _____   E-mail _____

Total **Part 2** Answers: Correct _____   Incorrect _____

<u>**METHOD OF PAYMENT**</u>

☐ Check
☐ American Express
☐ Diners Club

☐ Visa
☐ MasterCard

<u>Attestation Statement</u>

I certify that I have completed this activity as designed and claim 22.5 category 1 credits toward the AMA PRA.

_____

_____
Attestation Statement Signature

Instructions

To earn 22.5 category 1 credits toward the AMA Physicians' Recognition Award for the study of parts in *A Practical Approach to Occupational and Environmental Medicine, Third Edition*, and *Occupational Medicine Self-Assessment Review, Second Edition*, complete the following requirements:

- Study the Part(s) in *A Practical Approach to Occupational and Environmental Medicine, Third Edition*.
- Study all of the materials in *Occupational and Environmental Medicine: Self-Assessment Review* for the corresponding Part.
- Complete the self-test for the corresponding Part.
- Evaluate your responses by using the key at the bottom of the answer sheet. Note your score on the form.
- Complete the CME registration form, including your attestation signature, and mail it with a $250.00 fee per OMSAR Part or $850.00 fee when submitting all four OMSAR parts at once to:

**Education Department, American College of Occupational and Environmental Medicine
1114 North Arlington Heights Road
Arlington Heights, IL 60004-4770**

Occupational and Environmental Medicine Self-Assessment Review
Evaluation – Part 2

Please check all that apply:

☐ Resident   ☐ Fellow   ☐ Attending

☐ Private Practice   ☐ Corporate

Years in Practice   **Specialty**

	Strongly Agree				Strongly Disagree
1. The stated objectives were successfully met.	⑤	④	③	②	①
2. Overall, the quality of the instructional process met my expectations.	⑤	④	③	②	①
3. OMSAR was successful in developing or enhancing my competencies in a variety of areas in OEM.	⑤	④	③	②	①
4. I will apply the knowledge/information gained from OMSAR to improve my practice.	⑤	④	③	②	①

5. Did you observe any commercial bias?   ○ Yes   ○ No

6. Please tell us about your education needs and interests.

Topic Areas	Greatly Interested		Not Interested		
Disability management and work fitness	⑤	④	③	②	①
Public health surveillance	⑤	④	③	②	①
Hazard recognition, evaluation, and control	⑤	④	③	②	①
Cardiology	⑤	④	③	②	①
Dermatology	⑤	④	③	②	①
Emergency medicine	⑤	④	③	②	①
Ear, nose, throat, and hearing	⑤	④	③	②	①
Hematology/oncology	⑤	④	③	②	①
Infectious diseases	⑤	④	③	②	①
Neurology	⑤	④	③	②	①
Ophthalmology	⑤	④	③	②	①
Musculoskeletal	⑤	④	③	②	①
Mental health	⑤	④	③	②	①
Respiratory, allergy, and immunology	⑤	④	③	②	①
Reproductive medicine	⑤	④	③	②	①
Toxicology	⑤	④	③	②	①
Regulations and government agencies	⑤	④	③	②	①
Research in OEM	⑤	④	③	②	①
Environmental health and risk assessment	⑤	④	③	②	①
Management and administration in OEM	⑤	④	③	②	①
Medical/legal issues	⑤	④	③	②	①
Professionalism/personal development	⑤	④	③	②	①
Other	⑤	④	③	②	①

CME Registration for Part 3

Occupational and Environmental Medicine: Self-Assessment Review, Second Edition

COMPLETE BOTH SIDES OF THIS FORM - PLEASE <u>PRINT</u> CLEARLY

Name   Medical Degree

Address   City   State   Zip Code

Phone   Fax   E-mail

Total **Part 3** Answers: Correct   Incorrect

METHOD OF PAYMENT

☐ Check
☐ American Express
☐ Diners Club

☐ Visa
☐ MasterCard

Attestation Statement

I certify that I have completed this activity as designed and claim 22.5 category 1 credits toward the AMA PRA.

Attestation Statement Signature

Instructions

To earn 22.5 category 1 credits toward the AMA Physicians' Recognition Award for the study of parts in
A Practical Approach to Occupational and Environmental Medicine, Third Edition, and *Occupational Medicine Self-Assessment Review, Second Edition,* complete the following requirements:

- Study the Part(s) in *A Practical Approach to Occupational and Environmental Medicine, Third Edition.*
- Study all of the materials in *Occupational and Environmental Medicine: Self-Assessment Review* for the corresponding Part.
- Complete the self-test for the corresponding Part.
- Evaluate your responses by using the key at the bottom of the answer sheet. Note your score on the form.
- Complete the CME registration form, including your attestation signature, and mail it with a $250.00 fee per OMSAR Part or $850.00 fee when submitting all four OMSAR parts at once to:

Education Department, American College of Occupational and Environmental Medicine
1114 North Arlington Heights Road
Arlington Heights, IL 60004-4770

Occupational and Environmental Medicine Self-Assessment Review
Evaluation – Part 3

Please check all that apply:

☐ Resident   ☐ Fellow   ☐ Attending
☐ Private Practice   ☐ Corporate

Years in Practice _____   **Specialty** _____

	Strongly Agree				Strongly Disagree
1. The stated objectives were successfully met.	⑤	④	③	②	①
2. Overall, the quality of the instructional process met my expectations.	⑤	④	③	②	①
3. OMSAR was successful in developing or enhancing my competencies in a variety of areas in OEM.	⑤	④	③	②	①
4. I will apply the knowledge/information gained from OMSAR to improve my practice.	⑤	④	③	②	①

5. Did you observe any commercial bias?   ○ Yes   ○ No

6. Please tell us about your education needs and interests.

Topic Areas	Greatly Interested				Not Interested
Disability management and work fitness	⑤	④	③	②	①
Public health surveillance	⑤	④	③	②	①
Hazard recognition, evaluation, and control	⑤	④	③	②	①
Cardiology	⑤	④	③	②	①
Dermatology	⑤	④	③	②	①
Emergency medicine	⑤	④	③	②	①
Ear, nose, throat, and hearing	⑤	④	③	②	①
Hematology/oncology	⑤	④	③	②	①
Infectious diseases	⑤	④	③	②	①
Neurology	⑤	④	③	②	①
Ophthalmology	⑤	④	③	②	①
Musculoskeletal	⑤	④	③	②	①
Mental health	⑤	④	③	②	①
Respiratory, allergy, and immunology	⑤	④	③	②	①
Reproductive medicine	⑤	④	③	②	①
Toxicology	⑤	④	③	②	①
Regulations and government agencies	⑤	④	③	②	①
Research in OEM	⑤	④	③	②	①
Environmental health and risk assessment	⑤	④	③	②	①
Management and administration in OEM	⑤	④	③	②	①
Medical/legal issues	⑤	④	③	②	①
Professionalism/personal development	⑤	④	③	②	①
Other	⑤	④	③	②	①

CME Registration for Part 4

Occupational and Environmental Medicine: Self-Assessment Review, Second Edition

COMPLETE BOTH SIDES OF THIS FORM - PLEASE <u>PRINT</u> CLEARLY

Name _____   Medical Degree _____

Address _____   City _____   State _____   Zip Code _____

Phone _____   Fax _____   E-mail _____

Total **Part 4** Answers: Correct _____   Incorrect _____

<table>
<tr><td>

<u>METHOD OF PAYMENT</u>

☐ Check
☐ American
  Express
☐ Diners Club

☐ Visa
☐ MasterCard

</td><td>

Attestation Statement

I certify that I have completed this activity as designed and claim 22.5 category 1 credits toward the AMA PRA.

_____

_____

Attestation Statement Signature

</td></tr>
</table>

Instructions

To earn 22.5 category 1 credits toward the AMA Physicians' Recognition Award for the study of parts in
A Practical Approach to Occupational and Environmental Medicine, Third Edition, and *Occupational Medicine Self-Assessment Review, Second Edition*, complete the following requirements:

- Study the Part(s) in *A Practical Approach to Occupational and Environmental Medicine, Third Edition.*
- Study all of the materials in *Occupational and Environmental Medicine: Self-Assessment Review* for the corresponding Part.
- Complete the self-test for the corresponding Part.
- Evaluate your responses by using the key at the bottom of the answer sheet. Note your score on the form.
- Complete the CME registration form, including your attestation signature, and mail it with a $250.00 fee per OMSAR Part or $850.00 fee when submitting all four OMSAR parts at once to:

**Education Department, American College of Occupational and Environmental Medicine
1114 North Arlington Heights Road
Arlington Heights, IL 60004-4770**

Occupational and Environmental Medicine Self-Assessment Review
Evaluation – Part 4

Please check all that apply:

☐ Resident   ☐ Fellow   ☐ Attending

☐ Private Practice   ☐ Corporate

Years in Practice _____   **Specialty** _____

	Strongly Agree				Strongly Disagree
1. The stated objectives were successfully met.	⑤	④	③	②	①
2. Overall, the quality of the instructional process met my expectations.	⑤	④	③	②	①
3. OMSAR was successful in developing or enhancing my competencies in a variety of areas in OEM.	⑤	④	③	②	①
4. I will apply the knowledge/information gained from OMSAR to improve my practice.	⑤	④	③	②	①

5. Did you observe any commercial bias?   ○ Yes   ○ No

6. Please tell us about your education needs and interests.

Topic Areas	Greatly Interested		Not Interested		
Disability management and work fitness	⑤	④	③	②	①
Public health surveillance	⑤	④	③	②	①
Hazard recognition, evaluation, and control	⑤	④	③	②	①
Cardiology	⑤	④	③	②	①
Dermatology	⑤	④	③	②	①
Emergency medicine	⑤	④	③	②	①
Ear, nose, throat, and hearing	⑤	④	③	②	①
Hematology/oncology	⑤	④	③	②	①
Infectious diseases	⑤	④	③	②	①
Neurology	⑤	④	③	②	①
Ophthalmology	⑤	④	③	②	①
Musculoskeletal	⑤	④	③	②	①
Mental health	⑤	④	③	②	①
Respiratory, allergy, and immunology	⑤	④	③	②	①
Reproductive medicine	⑤	④	③	②	①
Toxicology	⑤	④	③	②	①
Regulations and government agencies	⑤	④	③	②	①
Research in OEM	⑤	④	③	②	①
Environmental health and risk assessment	⑤	④	③	②	①
Management and administration in OEM	⑤	④	③	②	①
Medical/legal issues	⑤	④	③	②	①
Professionalism/personal development	⑤	④	③	②	①
Other	⑤	④	③	②	①

ANSWER SHEET FORM

for Part 1 in *Occupational and Environmental Medicine: Self-Assessment Review, Second Edition*
(Return for CME Credit Hours)

Chapter 1
Question 1 _____
Question 2 _____
Question 3 _____
Question 4 _____
Question 5 _____

Chapter 2
Question 1 _____
Question 2 _____
Question 3 _____
Question 4 _____
Question 5 _____
Question 6 _____

Chapter 3
Question 1 _____
Question 2 _____
Question 3 _____
Question 4 _____
Question 5 _____
Question 6 _____

Chapter 4
Question 1 _____
Question 2 _____
Question 3 _____
Question 4 _____

Chapter 5
Question 1 _____
Question 2 _____
Question 3 _____
Question 4 _____
Question 5 _____
Question 6 _____

Chapter 6
Question 1 _____
Question 2 _____

Chapter 7
Question 1 _____
Question 2 _____
Question 3 _____
Question 4 _____
Question 5 _____
Question 6 _____

Chapter 8
Question 1 _____
Question 2 _____
Question 3 _____
Question 4 _____
Question 5 _____

Chapter 9
Question 1 _____
Question 2 _____
Question 3 _____
Question 4 _____
Question 5 _____
Question 6 _____

Chapter 10
Question 1 _____
Question 2 _____
Question 3 _____
Question 4 _____
Question 5 _____

Chapter 11
Question 1   _____
Question 2   _____
Question 3   _____
Question 4   _____
Question 5   _____

Chapter 12
Question 1   _____
Question 2   _____
Question 3   _____
Question 4   _____
Question 5   _____

Chapter 13
Question 1   _____
Question 2   _____
Question 3   _____
Question 4   _____
Question 5   _____
Question 6   _____

Chapter 14
Question 1   _____
Question 2   _____
Question 3   _____
Question 4   _____
Question 5   _____
Question 6   _____
Question 7   _____

Chapter 15
Question 1   _____
Question 2   _____
Question 3   _____
Question 4   _____
Question 5   _____

Chapter 16
Question 1   _____
Question 2   _____
Question 3   _____
Question 4   _____

Chapter 17
Question 1   _____
Question 2   _____
Question 3   _____
Question 4   _____

Chapter 18
Question 1   _____
Question 2   _____
Question 3   _____
Question 4   _____
Question 5   _____
Question 6   _____
Question 7   _____
Question 8   _____

Chapter 19
Question 1   _____
Question 2   _____
Question 3   _____
Question 4   _____
Question 5   _____

ANSWER SHEET FORM

for Part 2 in *Occupational and Environmental Medicine: Self-Assessment Review, Second Edition*
(Return for CME Credit Hours)

Chapter 20
Question 1 _____
Question 2 _____
Question 3 _____
Question 4 _____
Question 5 _____
Question 6 _____
Question 7 _____
Question 8 _____

Chapter 21
Question 1 _____
Question 2 _____
Question 3 _____
Question 4 _____
Question 5 _____
Question 6 _____

Chapter 22
Question 1 _____
Question 2 _____
Question 3 _____
Question 4 _____

Chapter 23
Question 1 _____
Question 2 _____
Question 3 _____
Question 4 _____
Question 5 _____

Chapter 24
Question 1 _____
Question 2 _____
Question 3 _____
Question 4 _____

Chapter 25
Question 1 _____
Question 2 _____
Question 3 _____
Question 4 _____
Question 5 _____

Chapter 26
Question 1 _____
Question 2 _____
Question 3 _____
Question 4 _____

Chapter 27
Question 1 _____
Question 2 _____
Question 3 _____
Question 4 _____
Question 5 _____
Question 6 _____

Chapter 28
Question 1 _____
Question 2 _____
Question 3 _____
Question 4 _____
Question 5 _____
Question 6 _____
Question 7 _____
Question 8 _____

Chapter 29
Question 1 _____
Question 2 _____
Question 3 _____
Question 4 _____
Question 5 _____

Chapter 30

Question 1   _____

Question 2   _____

Question 3   _____

Question 4   _____

Chapter 31

Question 1   _____

Question 2   _____

Question 3   _____

Question 4   _____

Question 5   _____

Question 6   _____

Question 7   _____

Question 8   _____

Question 9   _____

Chapter 32

Question 1   _____

Question 2   _____

Question 3   _____

Question 4   _____

Question 5   _____

Question 6   _____

Chapter 33

Question 1   _____

Question 2   _____

Question 3   _____

Question 4   _____

Chapter 34

Question 1   _____

Question 2   _____

Question 3   _____

Question 4   _____

Question 5   _____

Question 6   _____

Question 7   _____

Chapter 35

Question 1   _____

Question 2   _____

Question 3   _____

Question 4   _____

Chapter 36

Question 1   _____

Question 2   _____

Question 3   _____

Question 4   _____

Question 5   _____

ANSWER SHEET FORM

for Part 3 in *Occupational and Environmental Medicine: Self-Assessment Review,*
Second Edition
(Return for CME Credit Hours)

Chapter 37
Question 1 _____
Question 2 _____
Question 3 _____
Question 4 _____
Question 5 _____
Question 6 _____
Question 7 _____
Question 8 _____
Question 9 _____
Question 10 _____

Chapter 38
Question 1 _____
Question 2 _____
Question 3 _____
Question 4 _____
Question 5 _____
Question 6 _____
Question 7 _____

Chapter 39
Question 1 _____
Question 2 _____
Question 3 _____
Question 4 _____
Question 5 _____

Chapter 40
Question 1 _____
Question 2 _____
Question 3 _____
Question 4 _____
Question 5 _____
Question 6 _____

Chapter 41
Question 1 _____
Question 2 _____
Question 3 _____
Question 4 _____
Question 5 _____

Chapter 42
Question 1 _____
Question 2 _____
Question 3 _____
Question 4 _____
Question 5 _____

Chapter 43
Question 1 _____
Question 2 _____
Question 3 _____
Question 4 _____
Question 5 _____

Chapter 44
Question 1 _____
Question 2 _____
Question 3 _____
Question 4 _____
Question 5 _____

Chapter 45
Question 1 _____
Question 2 _____
Question 3 _____
Question 4 _____
Question 5 _____

ANSWER SHEET FORM

Chapter 46
Question 1 _____
Question 2 _____
Question 3 _____
Question 4 _____
Question 5 _____

Chapter 47
Question 1 _____
Question 2 _____
Question 3 _____
Question 4 _____

Chapter 48
Question 1 _____
Question 2 _____
Question 3 _____
Question 4 _____
Question 5 _____
Question 6 _____
Question 7 _____
Question 8 _____

ANSWER SHEET FORM

for Part 4 in *Occupational and Environmental Medicine: Self-Assessment Review, Second Edition*
(Return for CME Credit Hours)

Chapter 49
Question 1 _____
Question 2 _____
Question 3 _____
Question 4 _____
Question 5 _____
Question 6 _____
Question 7 _____

Chapter 50
Question 1 _____
Question 2 _____
Question 3 _____
Question 4 _____
Question 5 _____

Chapter 51
Question 1 _____
Question 2 _____
Question 3 _____
Question 4 _____

Chapter 52
Question 1 _____
Question 2 _____
Question 3 _____
Question 4 _____

Chapter 53
Question 1 _____
Question 2 _____
Question 3 _____
Question 4 _____

Chapter 54
Question 1 _____
Question 2 _____
Question 3 _____
Question 4 _____
Question 5 _____

Chapter 55
Question 1 _____
Question 2 _____
Question 3 _____
Question 4 _____
Question 5 _____

Chapter 56
Question 1 _____
Question 2 _____
Question 3 _____
Question 4 _____
Question 5 _____

Chapter 57
Question 1 _____
Question 2 _____
Question 3 _____
Question 4 _____
Question 5 _____

Chapter 58
Question 1 _____
Question 2 _____
Question 3 _____
Question 4 _____
Question 5 _____

Chapter 59

Question 1	_____
Question 2	_____
Question 3	_____
Question 4	_____
Question 5	_____
Question 6	_____
Question 7	_____
Question 8	_____

Chapter 60

Question 1	_____
Question 2	_____
Question 3	_____
Question 4	_____

Learning and Performance Strategies for the Occupational Medicine Certification Examination

Linda M. Roth, Ph.D.

Certification and recertification processes are intended to ensure that practitioners maintain their competence. When you take the occupational medicine board examination, you are evaluating your clinical knowledge and comparing yourself with your peers. When you recertify, you are satisfying yourself, your colleagues, and your patients that you have continued to keep up-to-date. Because certification and recertification scores tend to be the strongest predictors of subsequent recertification scores (1,2), it is important to maximize your knowledge and your test-taking skills early in your career.

As a physician, you have achieved numerous academic milestones in your life. Successfully completing undergraduate education, medical school, and one or more postgraduate programs means that you have taken many formal examinations. In your early years of academic training, and perhaps during the academic portion of your residency training, examinations were frequent throughout courses. Although at the time you may not have looked at it this way, frequent tests are actually motivating and informative; they provide feedback concerning how well you are succeeding at mastering content, and they guide your future study. In your clinical practice years, it is typical that the only formal examinations you experience are the certification examinations for your specialty or specialties. Once certified in occupational medicine, you will sit for recertification in ten years.

When you experience long intervals between examinations, test-preparation and test-taking skills you once used automatically may no longer be immediately available to you. This section will acquaint you with information about effective approaches to learning in general, as well as some specific advice about preparing for and taking the occupational medicine certification examination. As you read, try to recall specific techniques that have worked well for you in the past. Jot down your ideas so that you can use them in your current preparation. You can also keep a record for future use.

ORGANIZING FOR LEARNING

Where do you currently work when you are studying? Do you have an organized area in which you keep resources and the written products you create as you learn? Committing or recommitting a place devoted exclusively to studying can enhance your learning sessions. To determine an appropriate selection of study materials, consult Meyer's list of resources in this volume, and the list of materials provided in the *Study guide materials/Exam content outlines* from the American Board of Preventive Medicine (3). In addition, for a recommended approach to reading to maintain competence in any medical specialty, see the chapter by Sackett et al., *Surveying the Medical Literature to Keep Up to Date in Clinical Epidemiology: A*

Basic Science for Clinical Medicine (4). The authors offer a comprehensive method for selecting and reviewing pertinent literature.

According to studies of experts and novices in fields such as physics and medicine, not only do experts have more knowledge than novices, but their knowledge is also better organized and developed (5). As you study, notice the categories of information that are easy for you to remember as opposed to those that take more effort. It's likely that easy-to-recall information is well learned and well organized in your memory. You will need to work at learning (often relearning) more difficult information and organizing it for rapid recall. You will probably need to spend more time and effort on these latter categories.

Because learning tasks are not all of the same difficulty level, you will want to choose times at which you have the greatest ability to focus to perform the most demanding work. Reading and taking notes requires intense concentration, so you can target times at which you're most alert and unlikely to be distracted for such tasks. To get the most from these intensive sessions, (a) review what you mastered in your most recent study session; (b) create a written product as you learn new material, in your own words or design (such as an outline, matrix or diagram); and (c) decide what and when you will study next.

The less demanding tasks of reviewing and practicing what you've mastered in your intensive sessions can be fit in at other times. On breaks at work or at home, or perhaps while you're walking, riding in a car, or waiting in line at a bank or store, challenge yourself to reproduce information, rather than passively reviewing it. Discussing study topics with colleagues, residents, or students, informally or as part of a structured study group (for example, a journal club), can also reinforce your learning.

PREPARING FOR THE EXAMINATION

Educational researchers have investigated a number of approaches to preparing for examinations, and recommend an approach consisting of assessing your current capacity to perform on the examination, acquiring new material, encoding new material and developing cues for retention, reviewing, and maintaining motivation (6).

Assess Your Current Capacity to Perform on the Exam

To effectively plan and use study time, familiarize yourself with the content and the format of the occupational medicine certification examination. A content outline is provided in the pamphlet *Study guide materials/Exam content outlines* provided by the American Board of Preventive Medicine (3). Knowing your current level of knowledge in each content area can help you determine how best to schedule your learning sessions—the frequency and duration of study times you'll need. For example, use the self-test in this book to determine which subjects need the most effort, and then apportion the time for studying accordingly. Because we know that goal-setting facilitates learning, it will benefit you to write out a master study schedule with a specific topic or topics designated for each study period. Do this in pencil so that you can make adjustments as needed. After all, once you delve into a subject you may learn that you know more or less than you estimated.

Of course, your experience in the clinic also informs you about your current knowledge level. When in your daily work you find yourself needing to look up information or consult with a colleague, you have an insight into an area on which you may need to focus in a study session. Try jotting down questions that arise during the day, and then follow-up by writing out the answers you find and adding this information to your existing study materials.

In addition to familiarizing yourself with exam content, you will want to know what to expect with respect to test format. The American Board of Preventive Medicine pamphlet mentioned above provides a description of the test, as well as sample questions. Because answering examination questions methodically and efficiently increases feelings of confidence and control during the exam, be sure to practice answering questions during each of your study sessions, or at least once or twice a week. Practice makes the process seem automatic, so answering questions will demand less mental energy and time during the actual test.

Some physicians find it worthwhile to create and take one or more mock examinations that are representative of the certification exam. Simulating the actual exam setting and time allotment, or even giving yourself less time than you will have to complete the test, can inform you about your ability to progress through the actual test. The purpose of such rehearsal is to make the certification examination seem like a familiar experience.

Acquire New Material

Reading is the most common method for acquiring new information. Because reading can be both effortful and time-consuming, it's important to use this skill strategically. This means carefully pinpointing exactly which material needs to be processed in depth versus that which can be skimmed or skipped entirely. Too often, we revert to the habit of starting with the first word in a chapter or article and reading every word until we reach the end or until we find that we have lost concentration. Use your reading time efficiently. "Shop" for precisely the information you need and no more. Ask yourself, "Exactly what do I want to be able to say or write when I've finished reading this?" Then search for that information.

When using study guides in which pre-tests and post-tests are provided, use the questions at the beginning of each unit to target your reading, then select only the information that needs attention. On the post-test, skip questions unrelated to your reading. Use the table of contents and index of a book to help you determine exactly which chapters, and which sections within them, to read. Once you've selected what to read, get a structural overview by glancing at the introductory material, scanning through headings and boldfaced or italicized words, and noting any summaries that are provided. For some topics, this approach alone will provide everything you need to know. Journal articles can be approached in the same way. Ask yourself what new information you wish to gain by reading the article. Scan the article to determine its structure and then read only the sections that contribute new knowledge or understanding to your current knowledge.

Encode New Material and Develop Cues for Retention

Once you've identified and understood information to add to your knowledge base, you want to ensure that you'll retain it. Too often, after the hard work of reading and understanding, we simply shelve reading material and trust that we'll be able to remember what we read. As time goes by, memory fades, and we eventually find ourselves looking for the same information again.

Note-taking allows you to structure and save information that you want to store both in your long-term memory and in your external memory—your written files and note-cards, for example. With some articles or other printed matter that you intend to keep on file, underlining or highlighting information may be sufficient. However, be aware that these activities are simply recognition techniques. In other words, you've designated the data that you want to know, but often you haven't processed it enough to master it.

For information you want to make your own, you need to do more than underline or high-light. You might write a summary sentence or notes at the top of an article or on the first page of a chapter you're saving. However, to truly integrate and own new knowledge, you may need to produce separate cards or pages on which you create written or graphical memory aids. Sackett et al. recommend encoding an article's key details on a 3 in. x 5 in. card and keeping it in your pocket until you have committed the new knowledge to memory (4). Another method is to create flash cards with a term, concept, or question on one side and the answer or explanation on the reverse. Some learners create a split-page note-taking system that mimics flash cards: they write the term or question on the left-hand side of a page and record the explanation on the right. They then can lay pages of notes atop one another, with only the question columns showing, and quiz themselves. Flash cards or split-page note-taking allows you to actively test yourself on recently mastered material to make sure you are retaining it. These methods force you to ask yourself questions about what you've studied, rather than simply "re-viewing" notes on a written page—a passive and often ineffective study method.

More complex memory devices include outlines, summaries, matrices, diagrams, algorithms, and concept maps. All of these but the last are familiar memory aids. A concept map is a newer idea and is a graphical method of demonstrating both the elements of information in a conceptual network and the relationships among them (7). While concept maps deal with cognitive information, the fact that they represent it visually takes advantage of the fact that concrete visual information is usually remembered better than abstract or conceptual information (5). A concept map has been included at the end of this section.

Just as concept maps help us to remember because of their visual presentation, mnemonic devices assist us in remembering because they provide cues for retrieval of information that we wish to remember. For example, the acronym PINES assists one to remember the differential diagnosis for a chest x-ray with a reticulonodular pattern: pneumoconiosis, infection (e.g., miliary tuberculosis), neoplasm (e.g., alveolar cell cancer), eosinophilic granuloma, and sarcoidosis. Similarly, two mnemonics are used in remembering symptoms of organophosphate poisoning. DUMBELS refers to the muscarinic effects of defecation, urination, miosis, bronchospasm/bradycardia, emesis, lacrimation, and salivation/sweating. Nicotinic effects are remembered using MATCH—muscle weakness/fasciculations, adrenal medulla activity, tachycardia, cramping of skeletal muscles, and hypertension.

Review

Taking the steps outlined above in order to locate, understand, and organize knowledge is usually quite a thought- and labor-intensive process. In order to ensure that this hard work pays off in practice and on the Board examination, an additional step is required. Once you have mastered information, spaced review is necessary to promote recall in the future.

Memory researchers have found that memory performance improves with repeated attempts at recall. On a regular basis, challenge yourself to reproduce information that you have previously learned. To enhance memory, elaborate in more than one way on the information you're refreshing (8). For example, draw a concept map or create a diagram in addition to stating aloud or writing the targeted information. A weekly review of newly mastered knowledge is recommended, followed by intermittent reviews.

An additional memory-enhancing principle is overlearning, which is continued learning beyond the point of simple mastery. Education researchers have demonstrated that overlearning strengthens learning and improves retrieval speed.

Maintain Motivation

Occupational physicians are motivated to pass the certification examination for many reasons. Being certified is a key career goal which leads to job opportunity and to personal and professional satisfaction. For many physicians, the examination process is an emotional experience. Wlodkowski, who has written extensively on adults' motivation, points out that because adult learning often deals with success and failure in achievement and accomplishment activities, learners often react quite emotionally to their progress or lack of it. He emphasizes that an adult's emotional state is a significant influence on learning. Wlodkowski further notes that emotions not only influence behavior, but may affect thinking as well. Therefore, he recommends that adults work to maintain a positive attitude toward learning, which can, in turn, assist them to persist at learning and also deepen their interest in the material that they are studying (9).

Reminding yourself of your professional goals and how your knowledge mastery and subsequent certification and/or recertification fits in with your lifetime career plans can be motivating. For example, Meyer (this volume) suggests that physicians reflect upon and appreciate the satisfaction that comes from completing an organized review of one's field, the confidence that results from knowing that knowledge gaps have been addressed, and the improvement in teaching that can accompany content mastery. It is also likely that you will note a positive impact on your clinical practice from your studying, and this can be a source of regular reinforcement for your efforts.

The learning processes suggested in this chapter are recommended by education researchers and learning specialists to be effective in helping you to reach your goals of keeping up-to-date and becoming Board certified or recertified. However, these processes are also complex and time-consuming. To help you to persist, Wlodkowski recommends that you consider including some of the following features in your study program: using a variety of materials from which to study; keeping your study materials in an organized, orderly fashion; breaking large topics into small, manageable chunks; and spending some time in group study (9).

Wlodkowski notes that a sense of competence occurs when an adult realizes that he or she has achieved personal mastery. While the end goal of the certification process is to obtain the professional recognition of mastery, you can create a sense of personal mastery in the interim by tracking your performance throughout your study sessions. Once you have determined the subject matters you need to focus on, consider creating a graph, chart, or narrative journal through which you document your progress. Log the nature and amount of reading you do, for example, and count the number of note cards or note pages you produce. Examining this documentation and reflecting upon your learning strategies can provide insights about those techniques that are paying off and should be retained, and those that are inefficient and could be altered or abandoned. When testing yourself, chart how many questions you attempt in a subject area and the percentage you answer correctly. You can increase both your confidence level and your motivation to persist by providing feedback for yourself that informs you about how well you are doing and allows you to make internal statements such as "I really understand this," or "I am doing proficiently" (9).

TAKING THE EXAMINATION

In this volume, Meyer provides comprehensive information about the occupational certification examination itself, and he suggests many practical strategies for approaching the trip to the exam site and the experience of taking the exam. His advice corresponds with that of many experienced test-takers who have found that having a game plan for the examination allows them to feel calmer and in better control. Some additional suggestions follow.

- At the examination itself, as soon as you are permitted to open your test booklet, open to a blank page and write out any information you think you may forget under the pressure of the examination, such as mnemonic devices, outlines, or other memory aids that you have developed in preparation for the test. Some physicians have found that even jotting down points that may seem easy to recall actually saves time later. This step can help you easily remember your memory devices so you do not have to take time to access them while you're focusing on test content. One occupational medicine physician wrote out formulas and sketched out blank two-by-two tables before starting the test. She noted that having them on hand was helpful because you can get caught up in the wording of the problem and won't think about what you're really looking at in tables, diagrams, etc.

- Next, read the directions and survey the test. Some of the most important reading you'll do is in the directions, rather than in the questions. Be certain that you understand directions thoroughly and follow them to the letter. To use time effectively, an important next step is to survey the test. This way you can find out where the lengthy or challenging problems are, and plan your time accordingly. You do not have to answer questions in the order in which they appear. Choose the most logical order for yourself. Some people prefer to answer easy questions first to gain confidence. Others find that difficult questions prey on their mind and distract them, so they address those first. When answering questions out of order, it is essential, of course, to be meticulous about answering each question in its appropriate location on the answer sheet.

- Some physicians find it helpful to sketch out a time schedule for the entire morning or afternoon session. They can judge their progress against this estimate in order be able to answer all of the questions and save time for checking that they have marked their answers correctly. Another helpful technique to pace yourself appropriately is to mark the half-way spot in the test booklet, and check the time at which you arrive there. You may find that you need to speed up in order to finish.

- As you answer questions, work at a quick, steady pace. Keep your place on your answer sheet with your pencil, and move it methodically as you advance through the test. For multiple choice questions, try reading only the "stem", or leading statement, of the question, think about what you know about the topic, and then predict the answer. This way you can look among the choices and find the answer you predicted, rather than being distracted by choices that may seem plausible as you consider them. If you can't predict an answer, examine the choices, eliminate those that you can, and guess. You may prefer to reserve your final choice until later. In either case, make a mark in the test margin so that you can return to the question. After more experience with the test, you may find the question easier to answer. Of course, since all answers are of equal value, you will want to avoid lingering on difficult questions, and you will want to answer every question.

- Narrative questions require careful, focused reading. A helpful approach is to scan the questions before reading the passage so that you can eliminate unnecessary information as you read—you might even draw a line through irrelevant facts so that you won't reread them. Some physicians like to underline key points or create an abstract or outline on the side of the passage so that they can collect facts as they read. They then refer only to these notes, without having to go back to the narrative.

• A final point is to continue to stay aware of the time as you progress through the test. You will want to save five to ten minutes at the end of each session to check to make sure that you have recorded your answers accurately.

Once the test is over, reflect upon your test-preparation and test-taking experience. Record insights about content that you knew well, as well as content that was more challenging than you expected. Note the examination-preparation and test-taking strategies that you found useful and will want to repeat, as well as those that should be revised. After all, if all goes as well as you expect, you will not be taking another certification examination for ten years, and at that time you may be grateful that you have a file that can guide you through another successful certification experience.

REFERENCES

1. Leigh TM, Johnson TP, Piscano NJ. Predictive validity of the American Board of Family Practice entraining examination. *Acad Med* 1990;65:454.
2. Waxman H, Braunstein G, Dantzker D, et al. Performance on the internal medicine second-year residency in-training examination predicts the outcome of the ABIM certifying examination. *J Gen Intern Med* 1994;9:692.
3. Study guide materials/Exam content outlines. American Board of Preventive Medicine, Inc.
4. Sackett DL, Haynes RB, Guyatt GH, Tugwell P. *Clinical epidemiology: a basic science for clinical medicine,* 2nd ed. Boston: Little Brown, 1991.
5. Pressley M, El-Dinary PB. Memory strategy instruction that promotes good information processing. In: Hermann DJ, Weingartner H, Searleman A, McEvoy C, eds. *Memory improvement: implications for memory theory.* New York: Springer-Verlag, 1992.
6. Flippo RF, Caverly DC, eds. Teaching reading and study strategies at the college level. Newark, DE: International Reading Association, 1991.
7. Glynn SM, Yeany RH, Britton BK, eds. *The psychology of learning science.* Hillsdale, NJ: Lawrence Erlbaum Associates, 1991.
8. Hermann DJ, Weingartner H, Searleman A, McEvoy C, eds. *Memory improvement: implications for memory theory.* New York: Springer-Verlag, 1992.
9. Wlodkowski RJ. *Enhancing adult motivation to learn: a guide to improving instruction and increasing learner achievement.* San Francisco: Jossey-Bass, 1991.

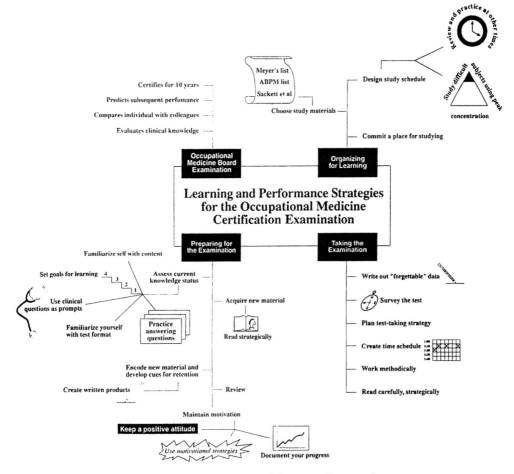

Figure 1. A concept map of the preceding section.

Taking the Board Exam in Occupational Medicine

John D. Meyer, M.D., Ph.D.

The American Board of Preventive Medicine (ABPM) offers certification in the specialties of Occupational Medicine, Aerospace Medicine, and General Preventive Medicine based on the results of an examination given in November of each year. Eligibility to sit for the examination is determined by criteria set forth by the Board, and is based upon residency training and practice in the field, or on several alternate pathways for those who graduated from medical school before widespread training in the field was available. Requirements for admission to the exam, as well as application forms, are available from the Board at its Web site and address, which are listed in the appendices at the end of this article. This chapter provides principles for review and study for the Board examination, and should be read in conjunction with Dr. Roth's earlier chapter on learning strategies. Familiarity with review strategies and the expected examination content will increase the likelihood of a passing score. Used in conjunction with the *Occupational and Environmental Medicine: Self-Assessment Review, Second Edition*, this section will give a prospective examinee a clearer picture of how to systematically acquire the knowledge base both for passing the certification exam and for subsequent practice in occupational medicine.

THE ABPM EXAM: SCOPE AND CONTENT

The ABPM examination is a full-day, seven-hour exam given in two parts. The core examination, which covers preventive medicine as a whole (including basic questions on each of the three specialty areas), consists of 225 multiple-choice questions. Four hours are allotted for completion of the morning core section. The afternoon is devoted to specialty exams in occupational, aerospace, and preventive medicine; three hours are given to complete this 150-question section. A passing score is required on both morning and afternoon sections of the exam for certification. The pass rate for the exam varies from year to year, and is based upon comparison of the year's exam scores with a benchmark derived from past exam results. In recent years, those passing the exam in occupational medicine compose slightly less than half of all those certified. According to statistics provided by the Board, the overall pass rate in 2001 was 67.5% for the ABPM examinations; 60.7% of examinees passed the occupational medicine boards. The failure rate on the exam is, therefore, substantial. Thorough preparation, beginning four to six months before the Boards, is required in order to have a chance at a passing score.

The material that appears on the core and specialty exams is outlined in a pamphlet prepared by the ABPM. An outline of the content is shown in Tables 1 and 2; additional detail is provided in the Board's publication entitled *Study Guide Materials and Exam Content Outlines*. The core section tests the examinee's knowledge of epidemiology, biostatistics, preventive health services, health care administration, environmental health, and behavioral factors

TABLE 1. *Exam content outline, core examination*

I. **Health Services Administration**
   A. Organization
   B. Services payment and financing
   C. Managed care
   D. Health care economics
   E. Bureaucracy characteristics
   F. Strategic planning and policy development
   G. Financial management
   H. Quality
   I. Organizational development
   J. Program assessment and evaluation
   K. Disaster planning and relief
   L. Legal and ethical issues

II. **Biostatistics**
   A. Design and methods
   B. Interpretation
   C. Vital statistics and demography

III. **Clinical Preventive Medicine**
   A. Acute
   B. Chronic
   C. Genetic
   D. Maternal and Child Health
   E. Occupational disease and injury
   F. Nontraditional types of care
   G. Nutrition
   H. Injury prevention
   I. International travel risk
   J. Aerospace
   K. Recreational

IV. **Epidemiology**
   A. Design and methods
   B. Interpretation
   C. Determinants of disease
   D. Prevention and control
   E. Legal and ethical aspects, IRB

V. **Behavioral**
   A. Health promotion
   B. Changing individual behavior
   C. Changing group/community behavior and social norms

VI. **Environment**
   A. Agents
   B. Community health
   C. Legal issues
   D. Risk Assessment
   E. Risk management
   F. Risk communication

in preventive medicine, as well as information fundamental to the three specialty areas. Although the content of the core section may change slightly every year, biostatistics and epidemiology are certain to be covered in detail, and a thorough grounding in these areas is essential to pass the morning session. The afternoon exam in occupational medicine covers material on clinical occupational medicine, occupational toxicology, hazard recognition and control, disability management and work fitness, workplace health and surveillance and occupational medical management and practice, and environmental health.

TABLE 2. *Exam content outline, occupational medicine*

I. Disability management and work fitness
  A. Disability prevention and management
  B. Americans with Disabilities Act
  C. Fitness for duty and return to work
	V. Occupational medical practice
	  A. Medical ethics and confidentiality
	  B. Regulation
	  C. Workers' compensation
	  D. Health promotion
	  E. Early intervention
	  F. Health care delivery systems
	  G. Medical quality management
	  H. Emergency planning

II. Workplace health and surveillance
  A. Injury and illness risk factors
  B. Medical surveillance programs
  C. Sentinel health effects
  D. Cluster analysis
  E. Interventions	

	VI. Environmental health and risk assessment
	  A. Risk assessment
	  B. Community "right-to-know"
	  C. Environmental monitoring
	  D. Human health effects
	  E. Environmental exposures

III. Hazard recognition, evaluation, and control
  A. Types
  B. Hazard characterization
  C. Interpretation of existing standards
  D. Ergonomics
  E. Chronobiology
  F. Physical hazards
  G. Hazard communications
  H. Industrial hygiene controls
  I. Medical programs
	VII. Industrial toxicology
	  A. Toxicokinetics
	  B. Carcinogenesis
	  C. Hydrocarbons and halohydrocarbons
	  D. Metals and metalloids
	  E. Gases
	  F. Dusts
	  G. Pesticides
	  H. Epoxy resins and polymer systems
	  I. Glycol ethers
	  J. Nitrogen compounds
	  K. Chemical warfare agents

IV. Clinical
  A. *General*
  B. Cardiology
  C. Dermatology
  D. Ear, nose, and throat
  E. Hematology/oncology
  F. Infectious diseases and biohazards
  G. Musculoskeletal
  H. Neurology
  I. Ophthalmology
  J. Psychiatry
  K. Pulmonary
  L. Reproductive medicine	

REVIEWING: WHAT TO STUDY

Clearly, no single source can provide all the material needed to prepare for and pass the Board exam in occupational medicine. In studying for the exam, plan to use a number of reference sources, each with its own particular strengths (full citations for each book are at the end of this chapter). For the core section of the Boards, the texts that have stood the tests of time and usefulness are the Maxcy-Rosenau-Last *Public Health and Preventive Medicine,* now in its 14th edition, and Brett Cassens' outline and study guide *Preventive Medicine and Public Health,* which, although still in its 1992 edition, remains one of the best outlines of the subject. These texts serve particularly well for review of environmental health, health care administration, and the public health aspects of chronic disease. For epidemiology and biostatistics, the review volume that has stood the test of time is the *Study Guide to Epidemiology and Biostatistics* by Morton, Hebel, and McCarter. The time taken to master the material and study questions in this small book will be rewarded by an understanding of the material sufficient to answer nearly any epi/biostats question the Board can ask. Finally, two standard public health texts that should be included in any review, and from which many exam questions appeared to be taken, are the *Guide to Clinical Preventive Services* of the U. S. Preventive Services Task Force, now in an updated 1996 edition, and the American Public Health Association's venerable *Control of Communicable Diseases Manual,* now in its 17th edition, which outlines the epidemiology and public health management of infectious diseases.

Prospective examinees should also begin to read the *Morbidity and Mortality Weekly Reports* (MMWR) published by the Centers for Disease Control and Prevention (CDC). Questions are frequently taken from articles in this bulletin that are at least a year old. In addition, the MMWR's Recommendations and Reports provide a summary of current knowledge and best practices in the field; the issues that cover areas such as immunizations, tuberculosis, and post-exposure prophylaxis should be read carefully. An added benefit of reading the MMWR is that many issues have accompanying continuing medicine education (CME) credits for an exam taken on-line; this will have the salutary effect of reinforcing your study of material on key public health topics.

Occupational medicine texts useful for Board review can be grouped into two categories: the comprehensive text used as an encyclopedic reference during training and practice, and the shorter guides to the range of occupational health problems and practice, which provide concise summaries valuable for review as study time becomes limited. In the first category, are the texts by Rom, Brooks, and Rosenstock and Cullen. At least one of these references should be read cover-to-cover during your training to gain a thorough grounding in clinical occupational medicine; these texts can be used in much the same way that Cecil or Harrison, for example, are used in internal medicine. The third edition of Rom's textbook, published in 1998, currently serves as the most comprehensive source of information in the field; Rosenstock and Cullen's textbook, while more clinically oriented, has also formed an indispensable part of many occupational medicine libraries, and is currently undergoing revision for a new edition. Brooks' *Environmental Medicine* provides an excellent general background in this related area. Among the shorter concise reviews are McCunney's *A Practical Approach to Occupational and Environmental Medicine, Third Edition*, LaDou's *Occupational Medicine*, and Levy and Wegman's *Occupational Health*. All highly readable and valuable as references as you continue to practice in occupational medicine, at least two of these sources should be used to integrate material presented from different aspects of occupational medicine practice. The *ATSDR Case Studies in Environmental Medicine*, published by the U. S. Public Health Service, provide concise outlines and study questions on common environmental toxicants; these are now beginning to appear in an Internet-based format. Finally, it is essential to review the management aspects of occupational health, although this information is rarely covered in clinical textbooks. The material in McCunney's text, supplemented by either Moser's or Felton's monographs on OEM management, will serve to cover the details of this area. A 1996 issue of the *Occupational Medicine State-of-the-Art Reviews*, entitled *Law and the Workplace*, has been exceptionally useful for review of legal and regulatory issues, covering especially areas such as the Americans with Disabilities Act.

Several study guides, which supplement and focus the material needed to review for the Boards, are available. This volume and the accompanying examination questions will help you to review and solidify the knowledge gained from McCunney's *Practical Approach* text. Additionally, the study guide by Vlachos available from the OEM press provides a nondirected but comprehensive review for both the core exam and all three specialty exams. Considerable effort is required to work through this guide, but for those whose mode of study is served by searching texts to answer a more general question, it can be well worth the effort. An alternative means of exam preparation is represented in Board Review courses given by several organizations. The American College of Preventive Medicine offers a week-long comprehensive review course targeted toward both the broader preventive medicine aspects of the exam as well as the specialty areas, while the ACOEM offering, a two-day course in conjunction with the American Occupational Health Conference, provides more detailed review for the occupational medicine exam. If your motivation to review is stimulated by didactic or lecture approaches, these materials can be worthwhile for those who can spare the travel and classroom time.

REVIEWING: HOW TO STUDY

Regardless of your style of study, a considerable investment of time is required to review for the exam. Preparation should begin four to six months before the scheduled exam date in early November. Little can be gained and much will be forgotten, or left uncovered, by late cramming close to the date of the exam. Time management can be difficult, particularly for those starting out in practice after residency and who are faced with a host of other demands on their attention. Nonetheless, remember the baseball manager's old saw that "games in May are just as important as those in September." Time spent preparing early, regularly and consistently, is likely to pay dividends as the Board exam draws closer. Your areas of weakness can be identified early, and attended to with less hurry, once the majority of material has been covered. Therefore, pick a time, even an hour or two, to review *daily*, beginning in June or earlier if possible, and stick to it religiously. Most helpful is to get into a routine when reviewing. If a particular time of day is most suitable (for example, the early morning hours before work or the evening just after the clinic has closed), make it a daily routine to read and review at that time. Early establishment of a daily study time and study routine will prove a good defense against procrastination, and ensure that there is always time carved out of the day to get the work done.

Now that I've covered what to study, the question arises: *How* do you study for the Boards? For most, this exam is the next in a long series of standardized exams dating back to the PSAT in high school, and interpreting the questions and filling in the ovals on the answer sheet may be second nature. More likely, the Board exam comes after at least several years spent in training and practice, and the exam skills learned earlier have long since atrophied. No one will pretend that it is not hard work to regain those skills, yet taking a positive mental attitude toward doing it can have its rewards. As a physician taking a board exam late in his career wrote:

> All in all, taking a subspecialty Board exam at the age of 54 was great fun. A systematic review of the literature is always worthwhile, and there is no stimulus like a formal examination to coerce a person into actually doing this. The day before the examination, I had a feeling of great mastery of a large body of knowledge, and frankly I felt as if I were 25 again (McNamara, p. 1795).

This leads to some basic principles that can be established to increase the effectiveness of studying for an exam: *concentration, integration,* and *problem-solving.* The contribution of each toward success in the ABPM examination can be outlined.

To effectively review the amount of material required, it will be important to develop the habit of *concentration*. The location in which you study should be comfortable and as free as possible from extraneous distractions. Most importantly, your mind should also be cleared of extraneous thoughts. Various meditative exercises can be useful in clearing your mind before study. Dr. Herbert Benson's famous series on the relaxation response describes one such technique aimed at a Western audience; students of yoga or Zen can utilize similar methods. Invariably, distracting thoughts arise when you set your mind to reading and studying. You may be wondering if you will pass the exam; you may be concerned about a patient or situation that you dealt with earlier in the day. It is important not to let these thoughts continue to deter you from your task by dwelling on them. Instead, acknowledge the thoughts that have come to you, if necessary make a note to yourself to deal with it later, and return to your study with a cleared mind. By emptying your mind of all that is extraneous to the subject in front of you at the moment, you will not only increase the power of your concentration, but you will also become less anxious about taking the examination itself.

Integration is the second principle that can be used to increase your ability to retain the material you need to learn. Different texts and different sources present and interpret material in varying ways. By being aware of differing points of view, by taking into account the alteration in viewpoint to different professionals (the clinician vs. the researcher vs. the administrator), and by asking yourself what might be missing from the treatment of the subject in one text that might be covered elsewhere, you can increase your understanding of the material by correlating two or three different sources. Integrate what you are learning from the variety of viewpoints and disciplines in occupational health. As you review, consider what the ramifications of exposure to a hazard are from the viewpoint of the clinician, the industrial hygienist, the health services manager, the epidemiologist, and the regulator. This approach will help you to cover the specified content areas outlined by the ABPM for the exam (Tables 1 and 2) for a given substance or hazard. By doing this, you will establish a multi-dimensional view of a topic, and this material will be retained longer because of a greater *understanding* of the subject. Creation of a system of file cards for most of the occupational hazards you review, including metals, solvents, and pesticides, is a method that works for many. As you read, abstract material from different sources and viewpoints onto the card until it gives you a complete picture of the hazard. For example, in reviewing lead toxicity, consider the clinical manifestations (anemia, peripheral neuropathy, central nervous system effects, and so forth); protective measures (exhaust ventilation, respirators); and regulatory mandates (medical removal at specified blood lead levels), and how each area contributes to the overall goal of managing the hazard. Similarly, many find it helpful to make overview cards correlating hazards and effects, for example listing the dermatologic effects of specific solvents. These cards can then be used for review without returning to the original texts later in the fall.

The best reinforcement for knowledge is direct practical experience. You should keep your eyes and ears open at all times in your training and practice, and follow-up on questions that are raised in the general run of the clinical and the occupational health service. How does knowledge of anatomy help you distinguish between an L5 radiculopathy and one involving the S1 root? Of what significance is a normal zinc protoporphyrin accompanying an elevated lead level? Many areas that I explored on an *ad hoc* basis in my practicum year because they presented a problem in diagnosis or management did show up in questions on the examination, although at the time they seemed of limited import outside of the particular question I was working on. It is likely you will have the same experience; always consider what you do daily in practice and training as preparation for the exam.

Problem-solving is the last of the three aids to study. To reiterate, direct, purposeful experience is the most powerful method by which we learn, while other forms of pedagogy make much less of an impression. We all have experienced this phenomenon in our training and practice; consider how much you learn from the responsibility for direct patient care during medical school, residency, and practice when you compare it with the didactic teaching (often not practically reinforced) of the first two years in medical school. This method of learning can have its limitations when the need to review for a comprehensive exam arises. No one can have seen all the patients or clinical situations presented on the Boards. However, in using a study guide such as this one, you can try to adopt a version of this experiential approach. Consider each question as a problem to be solved, and use the same texts, articles, and other authoritative sources that you would use when faced with a clinical or evaluative problem. Discuss the solution with peers or other knowledgeable sources if needed. Only then, once you have arrived at a solution to the problem, should you check the answer in the guide. Regular reading of periodicals, especially the *Morbidity and Mortality Weekly Reports*, will also help reinforce the principles of public health you are studying by demonstrating their application to current problems and situations. The odds are that by proceeding in this way you will explore the subject in greater depth than is provided by an answer key, and that you will retain it longer by having done so.

TAKING THE EXAM

Now that preparation for the Boards has been discussed, I would also like to offer some advice about taking the exam itself. Much depends on the individual habits and style of the examinee, but a few general points can be offered. First of all, recognize that travel can be a fatiguing process, especially when balanced with the demands of work and exam preparation. I advise arriving at the site of the examination (currently near Chicago) at least a day ahead of schedule to settle into a routine in the hotel. Make sure that you can be well rested for the day of the exam. Moderate exercise can be a good stress reliever (this advice applies outside of Board preparation as well!), and Chicago is a superb city to visit if you need a distraction from studying. Little can be gained by an attempt to study after you have arrived, and may serve only to increase your apprehension about taking the exam. If you feel the need to review, pick no more than one or two small subjects (epidemiologic rates and ratios is one such topic), where last-minute memorization of formulas would be advantageous. Then quit studying entirely.

Knowing that you have appropriately prepared with respect to the smaller details can help reduce the stresses of exam day itself. Wear casual comfortable clothes, since you will be sitting there for most of the day. Always make certain that your entrance ticket is with you, and that you have several pencils (I brought ten, used six) available. In recent years, the testers have provided individual pencil sharpeners, a small but important detail that made taking the exam easier. No food or other materials are permitted on the tabletop during the exam; however, I brought an energy bar and other small snacks to the exam to eat just before starting, and thereby staved off the drop in concentration that comes when I'm hungry. Finally, schedule your flight out for late in the day (or stay in Chicago overnight) so that time pressures of travel will not affect your performance in the afternoon section.

Keep in mind the time allotted for the examination. The morning section of the exam is the most pressured, with four hours given to answer 250 questions, which allows an average of less than a minute per question. Many examinees are unable to finish the morning section because of these time limitations. If, after you have spent a minute on a particular question, you are still unable to answer it, consider marking it and returning to it later. Not only will this reduce the time pressure that you might feel to complete the exam, but you may be presented with the same question in a different form later in the exam. This is likely to jog your memory for the correct answer of the earlier question. A subsequent question may also provide a definition or additional information that helps you with the earlier answer. Additionally, once you've reached the end of the exam, those questions you skipped can be reconsidered with time pressures reduced. The afternoon session allows more time (three hours for 150 questions, or nearly a minute-and-a-half per question) and, assuming proper preparation, should prove less stressful to complete.

Most importantly, you should practice the above-mentioned principle of concentration when taking the examination. Clear your mind of extraneous thoughts; the only thing that matters is the exam question in front of you. Distractions ("Am I going to pass?" "Will I have time to catch my flight?") should be acknowledged as such, and then put out of mind. The exam is most analogous to driving long distance: you need to be simultaneously concentrating on the task at hand in the moment (the question) and aware of the distance, route, and time course (the exam as a whole). If you do this, the core exam will appear both less onerous and less pressured; the exam will flow as a series of individual questions, each of which you have given your full concentration and attention.

A FINAL WORD

To restate the earlier quotation, studying for the Board exam does involve an attempt to master an ever-growing body of knowledge, and can often be a frustrating and lonely experience. However, successfully completing a review of the core material of preventive and occupational medicine is, in the long run, greater recompense for the frustrations. I found that I was able to focus on the entire field of occupational medicine in an organized and systematic fashion, and I filled in some of the blanks in my knowledge that lay in areas I had not sufficiently covered in the practicum. My practice in occupational medicine has benefited considerably from the broadening of knowledge that came with review and study for this exam, and this review has helped inform my teaching with students and residents in occupational medicine. Approaching the challenges of this exam with the advice offered above will, I hope, enable you to overcome them with the same positive attitude.

SELECTED REFERENCES
Core Examination

Centers for Disease Control and Prevention. *Morbidity and Mortality Weekly Reports* (MMWR). Available on-line at *http://www.cdc.gov/mmwr/*

Chin J. *Control of communicable disease manual*, 17th ed. Washington: American Public Health Association, 1995.

Cassens BJ. *Preventive medicine and public health*, 2nd ed. Baltimore: Williams & Wilkins, 1992.

Wallace RB, Doebbling BN. *Maxcy-Rosenau-Last public health and preventive medicine*, 14th ed. New York: McGraw-Hill Professional, 1998.

Morton RF, Hebel JR, McCarter RJ. *A study guide to epidemiology and biostatistics*, 5th ed. Rockville, MD: Aspen Publishing, 2001.

U.S. Preventive Services Task Force. *Guide to clinical preventive services*, 3rd ed. 2000–2002. Available on-line at *http://www.ahcpr.gov/clinic/uspstfix.htm*

Occupational Medicine Specialty Examination

Brooks SM. *Environmental medicine: concepts and practice*. St Louis: Mosby-Year Book, 1995

Felton JS. *Occupational medical management*. Boston: Little, Brown & Co, 1989.

LaDou J. *Occupational medicine*. Norwalk, CT: Appleton & Lange, 1996.

Levy BS, Wegman DH. *Occupational health: recognizing and preventing work-related disease*, 4th ed. Philadelphia: Lippincott Williams & Wilkins, 2000.

McCunney RJ. *A practical approach to occupational and environmental medicine*, 3rd ed. Philadelphia: Lippincott Williams & Wilkins, 2003.

Moser R. *Effective management of occupational and environmental health and safety programs*, 2nd ed. Beverly, MA: OEM Press, 1999.

Rom W. *Environmental and occupational medicine*, 3rd ed. Philadelphia: Lippincott-Raven, 1998.

Rosenstock L, Cullen MR. *Textbook of clinical occupational and environmental medicine*. Philadelphia: WB Saunders Co, 1994.

Snyder JW, Klees JE, eds. *Law and the workplace*. Occup. Med. State-of-the-Art Reviews. Vol. 11 (1) January–March, 1996. Philadelphia: Hanley & Belfus, 1996.

Other Useful Materials

Benson, H. *The relaxation response*. New York: Morrow, 1975.

McNamara JJ. On taking a board examination at the age of 54. *N Engl J Med* 1995;332:1794–1795

Vlachos NA, Parmet AJ, Chaulk CP. *Study guide for preventive medicine certification*. Beverly, MA: OEM Press, 1996.

Information on the *ATSDR Case Studies in Environmental Medicine* can be obtained from:

        Agency for Toxic Substances and Disease Registry
        Division of Health Education
        1600 Clifton Road, NE
        Atlanta, GA 30333

Several are now available on the Internet at *http://www.atsdr.cdc.gov/HEC/CSEM/*

Application materials and further information on the content of the ABPM examination are available at the following address:

        American Board of Preventive Medicine
        330 South Wells Street, Suite 1018
        Chicago, IL 60606-7106
        Telephone: (312) 939-ABPM [2276]
        Home page: *http://abprevmed.org/index.html*

The *Study Guide Materials and Exam Content Outlines* is available for download at: *http://abprevmed.org/public/studyguide.pdf*

Occupational and Environmental Medicine
Self-Assessment Review
SECOND EDITION

ACOEM DISCLOSURE

The ideas represented in this publication do not necessarily reflect the American College of Occupational and Environmental Medicine (ACOEM) positions. ACOEM disclaims responsibility or liability for all products, services or information presented in this book. ACOEM does not endorse any product or service, nor does it necessarily support the content contained in this educational offering.

DISCLOSURE POLICY

As a sponsor accredited by the ACCME, ACOEM must ensure balance, independence, objectivity, and scientific rigor in all of its educational activities. In accordance with the ACCME Essentials and Standards, all contributing authors have been asked to disclose any significant financial interest (e.g., grants or research support, employment, consultancy, major stock holder, member of a speaker's bureau, etc.) or other relationship with the manufacturer(s) of any commercial services discussed in their presentation(s). This disclosure is not intended to prevent a contributing author with a financial or other relationship from writing content for the book, but rather to provide readers with information in order to make their own judgments. It remains for the reader to determine whether the contributing author's interests or relationships may influence the book.

Contributing authors are expected to disclose the FDA-approval status of all medical devices and pharmaceuticals for the uses discussed or described in the book. Status of each contributing author's disclosure of interest (as of October 27, 2003) is indicated below.

Symbol Key

* This contributing author has not yet submitted a disclosure of interest statement as of October 27, 2003.

\+ This contributing author discloses no financial interests with any companies related to the content of the educational activity.

Debra Cherry, M.D., M.S.
University of Texas Health Center at Tyler, Tyler, Texas +

Sharon Hall Davis, M.D., M.P.H.
University of Texas Health Center at Tyler, Tyler, Texas *

Jeffrey L. Levin, M.D., M.S.P.H.
University of Texas Health Center at Tyler, Tyler, Texas *

Larry K. Lowry, Ph.D.
University of Texas Health Center at Tyler, Tyler, Texas +

Robert J. McCunney, M.D., M.P.H., M.S.
Massachusetts Institute of Technology, Cambridge, Massachusetts
Massachusetts General Hospital, Boston, Massachusetts +

J. Torey Nalbone, M.S., C.I.H.
University of Texas Health Center at Tyler, Tyler, Texas +

Barbara Pinson, M.D., M.S.
University of Texas Health Center at Tyler, Tyler, Texas +

Ellen Remenchik, M.D., M.P.H.
University of Texas Health Center at Tyler, Tyler, Texas +

Paul P. Rountree, M.D.
University of Texas Health Center at Tyler, Tyler, Texas +

1

Occupational Medical Services

OBJECTIVES

- Discuss the scope of occupational medicine practice
- Explain essential and elective components of such practice
- List the need for occupational medicine services
- Enumerate various methods of delivery of occupational medicine services

OUTLINE

I. History of occupational medicine
II. Occupational health services
    A. Table 1.1: Occupational and environmental health programs: essential components
    B. Table 1.2: Elective components of occupational and environmental health programs
    C. Clinical services
        1. Preplacement evaluation
        2. Work-related injuries
        3. Return-to-work evaluation
        4. Periodic examinations
        5. Health assessments
    D. Ancillary services
    E. Nonclinical activities
    F. Health promotion activities
    G. Referral patterns
        1. Occupational medicine physicians
        2. Local medical specialists
        3. Other professionals
III. The delivery of occupational medical services
    A. Determining the need for occupational medical services
        1. Table 1.3: Factors in establishing the need for occupational medical services for small businesses
    B. Corporate-sponsored health care delivery
    C. Union-sponsored occupational health care
        1. Table 1.4: Local union health and safety involvement
    D. Hospital-based occupational health programs
    E. University-based teaching centers
IV. Summary

KEY POINTS

- Knowledge about occupational exposure can be traced into antiquity, but it was not until the late seventeenth century that Ramazzini urged physicians to pay attention to diseases of the workplace. Occupational medicine has been a distinct discipline within the American Board of Preventive Medicine since 1954, but there continues to be a shortage of specialists. Most work-related problems are treated by primary care physicians.

- More than 90% of businesses in the United States and in the world have 100 or fewer employees, often making it economically difficult to provide onsite health care for workers.

- Occupational health services can include all forms of health care delivery to working populations. A variety of factors determine the types of services provided, but the American College of Occupational and Environmental Medicine (ACOEM) has published guidelines regarding essential and elective components (see Table 1.1 and Table 1.2 in the text).

- Clinical services such as preplacement and return-to-work evaluations, management of work-related injuries, periodic examinations, and other health assessments should include careful consideration of medical confidentiality. Decisions regarding work capabilities should always focus on the worker's health. Employees should be made aware of medical information reported to businesses with said information focusing on the ability to perform essential job functions. Arbitrary use of certain tests, such as random back x-rays to predict future injury, may be considered discriminatory and of limited medical utility.

- In the provision of occupational health services to small businesses, the following items are considered essential: an audiometric booth and audiometer with adherence to the Occupational Safety and Health Administration (OSHA) Hearing Standard, a well-functioning and calibrated spirometer with a properly trained technician, and a vision screener. It may be appropriate to include laboratory, x-ray, and physical therapy or to make provisions for these services by referral.

- The physician providing occupational health care is often viewed as a health consultant to business. Educational activities are an essential component of service delivered by the physician on such issues as the prevention and management of back injuries, substance abuse testing, and the role of lifestyle in promoting health.

- A good working professional relationship with local medical specialists, such as orthopedists, general surgeons, otolaryngologists, pulmonologists, neurologists, and psychiatrists, is advised. Access to professionals such as industrial hygienists, audiologists, or physical therapists can be helpful.

- The goals of an occupational health service include protecting workers from health and safety hazards, protecting the local environment, facilitating safe placement of workers, ensuring adequate medical care and rehabilitation of the occupationally ill or injured, and promoting health.

- A well-run program depends on effective communication between the business facility and the physician. A visit to the business is essential. Awareness of corporate policies and union-sponsored programs can be helpful. University-based teaching centers can serve as a valuable information or referral point.

QUESTIONS

1. Which of the following statements is most correct regarding occupational medicine and the workplace?

A. Occupational disease has only been recognized during the past century.
B. Approximately 90% of businesses in the United States have 100 or fewer employees.
C. Occupational medicine certification is provided by the American Board of Family Practice.
D. According to most sources, there is an excess of specialists in occupational medicine in the United States today.
E. Preplacement testing should be uniform regardless of the job for which the worker is being considered.

*2. In the provision of occupational health services to small businesses, the following items are considered essential **except***

A. An audiometric booth and audiometer
B. A well-functioning and calibrated spirometer
C. A vision screener
D. A properly trained spirometric technician
E. A clinic-based laboratory that conducts toxicologic analysis of biologic and environmental samples

*3. Which of the following is **not** usually a goal of an occupational health service?*

A. Protecting people at work from health and safety hazards
B. Assisting in activities related to health promotion
C. Providing primary care for personal illness
D. Facilitating safe placement of workers according to their physical, mental, and emotional capacities
E. Communicating health information to workers

*4. Which of the following is **not** considered an essential component of an occupational and environmental health program?*

A. Evaluation, inspection, and abatement of workplace hazards
B. Diagnosis and treatment of occupational illnesses
C. Maintenance of occupational medical records
D. Biostatistics and epidemiology assessment
E. Immunization against nonoccupational infectious diseases

*5. In the context of conducting a preplacement evaluation, which of the following is **least correct**?*

A. The purpose of the examination is to recognize medical conditions that may be aggravated by the job duties or that may jeopardize the health and safety of others.
B. The physician conducting the examination should understand the job duties and work environment.
C. OSHA required examinations cannot be performed with preplacement examinations.
D. The arbitrary use of certain tests can be considered discriminatory, legally unsound, and of limited medical utility.
E. Genetic testing is likely to be associated with ethical issues.

2

Legal and Ethical Issues

OBJECTIVES

- Discuss exceptions to the exclusive remedy of workers' compensation
- Explain record-keeping requirements of Occupational Health and Safety Administration (OSHA) and workers' compensation
- Describe OSHA's Hazard Communication Standard
- Discuss the development of workers' compensation law in the United States
- List factors that determine compensability of an injury or illness
- List rules of confidentiality related to medical records of injured workers
- Identify ethical issues involved in the practice of occupational and environmental medicine
- Explain the impact of the Americans with Disabilities Act (ADA) on the workplace and occupational medicine
- Review theories of law under which toxic tort lawsuits can be brought

OUTLINE

I. Workers' compensation law
  A. History and determining when a disorder is occupational
  B. Exceptions to the exclusivity of workers' compensation
    1. The intentional tort exception
    2. The dual-capacity doctrine
  C. Obligations of the occupational physician
II. OSHA's Hazard Communication Standard
  A. Right-to-know laws
III. OSHA and other record-keeping and reporting requirements
  A. OSHA requirements
    1. History
    2. Summary of the new regulations
      a. Work-relatedness
      b. The distinction between injuries and illnesses eliminated
      c. Significant injury or illness
      d. Work at home
      e. First aid
      f. Job restrictions or transfer
      g. Privacy issues
      h. Generation and posting of records
  B. Workers' compensation law requirements

IV. Medical record access
    A. Federal law: OSHA's Exposure Record and Access Standard
        1. Who is covered?
        2. General provisions
        3. The definitions of "toxic substances" and "harmful physical agents"
        4. Medical records
           a. What constitutes a medical record?
           b. Who can review medical records and under what circumstances?
           c. When can access to medical records be refused?
        5. Exposure records
           a. What constitutes an exposure record?
           b. Who can review exposure records and under what circumstances?
           c. Analyses using exposure medical records
    B. State laws
    C. Confidentiality
 V. The ADA
    A. History
    B. Structure of the ADA
    C. Impairments that "substantially limit" major life activities
    D. The ADA's impact on medical examinations
    E. The "direct threat to others" exception
VI. Toxic torts
    A. Background
    B. Theories of law
    C. Analysis

KEY POINTS

- Workers' compensation statutes vary from state to state but represent a series of compromises between employer and employee. Although generally less of a monetary recovery than through suits at common law, payment is made regardless of fault and presumably more quickly. In exchange, employees agree to accept this compensation as their exclusive remedy, based on disability and without other damages. Employees effectively give up their right to sue employers at common law with certain exceptions as outlined later. Disputes are generally decided by administrative bodies rather than by courts.
- At first, during the early development of workers' compensation, only work-related accidents were covered. Illness and disease coverage was later included if the employee's occupation put him or her at a greater risk of getting the disease than the general public or if a work-related accident aggravated or accelerated the underlying disease. Mental stress attributable to the general work environment is not covered, but mental stress causally related to a specific significant employment incident may be compensable. Cumulative trauma disorders (CTDs) are not compensable in jurisdictions that classify them as "ordinary diseases of life." However, some states have found CTDs compensable if the employee had an exposure at work greater than that of the general public and medical evidence attributes the disorder to that motion at work with reasonable medical certainty.
- As to latency of certain diseases, most states have adopted the discovery rule, with the statute of limitations beginning when the claimant becomes aware of the disease and

its potential work-relatedness. Exceptions to the exclusivity of workers' compensation include an injury caused by a deliberate and intentional act of the employer. This might include the employer and physician if the presence of the disease was known and fraudulently concealed from the employee, resulting in an exacerbation. Furthermore, employees might be able to file cases at common law under the dual-capacity doctrine when a relationship other than an employer-employee one is established (e.g., doctor-patient). Good medical and ethical practice, as well as potential for liability, are compelling reasons for being completely candid with the employee regarding a suspected occupational disorder.

- The OSHA Hazard Communication Standard (29 CFR 1910.1200), applicable to all employers covered by the OSHA Act (including importers of chemicals), requires that containers in the workplace be properly labeled, that employees be informed of and trained about the hazards of chemicals to which they are or may be exposed, and that Material Safety Data Sheets (MSDS) detailing the hazards of specific chemicals be made available to employees (see Table 2.1 in the text). In addition, under the Superfund Amendments and Reauthorization Act (SARA), citizens may obtain information regarding hazardous materials in their communities.

- New revisions of the occupational injury and illness recording requirements took effect January 1, 2002. Injuries (except extremely minor ones treated only with first aid) and all deaths and illness that result from a work-related accident or from an exposure in the work environment should be recorded on the OSHA 300 Log and OSHA 301 Incident Report. With new rules, up to four forms are required to post records: the OSHA 300, OSHA 300 A (Annual Summary of Injuries and Illnesses), OSHA 301 (Injury and Illness Incident Report), and the Confidential List of "privacy concern" illnesses or injuries. Privacy concern cases such as sexual assault, mental illness, and human immunodeficiency virus (HIV) cases are entered in a confidential log rather than on the 300 Log.

- Injuries and illnesses resulting in restricted work activity beyond the day of the injury or illness, medical treatment beyond first aid, days away from work, loss of consciousness, or death are recordable. Also recordable are needle stick or sharps injuries and cases involving medical removal because of illness [such as tuberculosis (TB)] under the OSHA standards. A number of exceptions to considering illness or injury to be work-related are noted, such as cases occurring in a parking lot or recreational facility, cases that were the result of a non–work-related condition, self-inflicted wounds, common cold or flu illnesses, and so forth. New regulations list 14 first aid treatments. Employees may have access to logs at their current or previous workplace. Accidents resulting in one or more deaths must be reported to OSHA within 48 hours. It is also imperative that physicians be familiar with the reporting requirements of the workers' compensation laws of the state in which they practice.

- OSHA's Exposure and Medical Record Access Standard "applies to all employee exposure and medical records, and analyses thereof, made or maintained in any manner, including on an in-house or contractual (fee-for-service) basis." Any employer who has employees who are exposed to "toxic substances" or "harmful physical agents" must provide the employee (or his or her authorized representative) access to his or her medical record within 15 days of a request. Written consent (good for up to 1 year) should be obtained. Records regarding employee alcohol, drug abuse, or personal counseling programs are not considered medical records and are not covered by the Medical Record Access Standard, if they are maintained separate from the medical record.

- All medical records must be retained for the duration of the employee's employment plus 30 years. Refusal by a physician for the employer, to permit an employee direct access to his or her medical records, is allowable when the record concerns a <u>terminal illness</u> or a <u>psychiatric condition</u> and <u>viewing it may be detrimental to the employee.</u> However, the records must be shown to the employee's authorized representative. Employers are entitled to counsel about the medical fitness of individuals in relation to work but are not entitled to diagnoses or details of a specific nature. As to work-related disorders, the employer is obliged to know about an employee's condition to provide protection from further exposure and to comply with necessary restrictions on that person's activities. The physician should be aware of the Code of Ethical Conduct of the American College of Occupational and Environmental Medicine (ACOEM).
- Under the ADA, a disabled person is "qualified" if, with "reasonable accommodation," he or she can perform the "essential functions" of the job as well as one who is not disabled. An accommodation is necessarily reasonable if it does not impose on the employer an "undue hardship." Employment-related examinations are allowed only after an offer is made.
- Toxic tort suits are common lawsuits that are brought by workers who claim that exposure to the toxic substance caused them some injury or disorder. Workers can sue their employer's third-party suppliers of materials (e.g., asbestos). In addition to the usual damages for medical expenses, lost earning capacity, and pain and suffering, plaintiffs who claim exposure to toxins may, in some states, seek damages for future risk of illness, fear of future illness, or the cost of medical surveillance.

QUESTIONS

1. Which of the following is correct regarding workers' compensation?

A. Employees give up their right to sue employers at common law and agree to accept a certain sum of money per week for their inability to work as a result of work-related injuries.
B. Employees generally receive a higher monetary recovery than through suits at common law.
C. Only work-related accidents are covered, whereas work-related disease and illness are not.
D. Payment is made according to fault.
E. Courts rather than administrative bodies generally decide disputes.

2. Which of the following is correct regarding the OSHA Hazard Communication Standard?

A. MSDS on chemical hazards must be made available to employees.
B. All containers must be properly labeled.
C. Importers of chemicals are not covered.
D. Employees must be informed of and trained about the hazards of the chemicals to which they are or may be exposed.
E. A, B, and D.

*3. Which of the following statements about compensability for on-the-job injuries and illnesses is **not** correct?*

A. CTDs are not compensable in jurisdictions that classify them as "ordinary diseases of life."

B. Mental stress attributable to the general work environment is covered as is stress causally related to a specific significant employment incident.

C. Exceptions to the exclusivity of workers' compensation include an injury caused by a deliberate and intentional act of the employer.

D. Most states have adopted the discovery rule with the statute of limitations beginning when the claimant becomes aware of the disease and its potential work-relatedness.

E. Employees may file common law cases under the dual-capacity doctrine when a relationship other than employer-employee is established (e.g., doctor-patient).

4. *Regarding OSHA Form 300 (Log of Work-Related Injuries and Illnesses), which of the following is true?*

A. Injuries occurring in a recreational facility at work are recordable.

B. First aid injuries are recordable.

C. A work-related disorder that results in restricted work activity beyond the day of injury should be recorded.

D. Employee access to the OSHA 300 Log is limited to the logs for the establishment where the employee currently works.

E. Injuries and illnesses are not recordable if they are only needle stick exposures.

5. *All of the following are correct **except***

A. Workers can sue their employer's third-party suppliers of materials.

B. Damages for medical expenses and lost earnings capacity may be sought.

C. In some states, damages for future risk of illness and the cost of medical surveillance may be obtained.

D. Damages for pain and suffering are not allowed.

E. In some states, damages for fear of future illness may be obtained.

6. *All of the following statements are correct **except***

A. Employers are entitled to counsel about the medical fitness of individuals in relation to work but are not entitled to diagnoses.

B. Employment-related examinations are allowed before an offer is made.

C. Under the ADA, disabled people are "qualified" if with "reasonable accommodation" they can perform the "essential functions" of the job.

D. An accommodation is reasonable if it does not impose an "undue hardship" on the employer.

E. Employees exposed to "toxic substances" or "harmful physical agents" must be provided access to his or her medical record within 15 days of a request.

3

Role of Regulatory Agencies

OBJECTIVES

- Identify the mandates for various government agencies involved in occupational and environmental health
- List the various types of Occupational Safety and Health Administration (OSHA) standards that impact on the practice of occupational medicine

OUTLINE

KEY POINTS

- OSHA standards, National Institute for Occupational Safety and Health (NIOSH) research activities, and certain EPA regulations should become familiar topics for physicians who provide occupational health care. OSHA standards apply to record-ability of occupational injuries and illnesses, access to employee medical records, occupational noise exposure, medical services and first aid, exposure to blood-borne pathogens, hazard communication, required medical surveillance for specific operations and chemicals, and a number of other areas. However, OSHA does not cover federal, state, or local municipal employers. State OSHA standards are often identical to federal OSHA standards and, in some cases, may be more stringent. Compliance with employee requests for medical records is required within 15 working days.

- Recordability of a condition as an injury as opposed to an illness depends on the duration of exposure. An injury results from an instantaneous exposure. Recordability of occupational injuries is, in part, determined by the requirement for medical treatment as opposed to first aid care (in which simple treatment with over-the-counter medication may be required). First aid care for injuries is not recordable.

- The OSHA standard for occupational noise exposure requires annual examinations for employees exposed to noise of 85 dB or higher on a daily time-weighted average (TWA) basis. Audiograms that show a standard threshold shift (STS) of 10 dB or greater compared with baseline must be evaluated by an audiologist or physician to determine the need for further evaluation. A work-related change in hearing of 10 dB averaged over the frequencies of 2,000, 3,000, and 4,000 Hz is recordable on the OSHA 300 Log provided that such loss exceeds an average of 25 dB from audiometric zero.

- Several OSHA standards require the employee to have a medical examination to determine physical fitness to perform certain jobs or to wear specific personal protective equipment (e.g., respirators). However, not all of these standards specify the content of these medical examinations or their frequency (e.g., respirator standard). There are detailed individual standards for 26 chemicals, each of which includes a section on medical surveillance. Medical surveillance is typically required when airborne exposure levels exceed 50% of the permissible exposure limit for at least 30 days per year. Certain of these standards have provisions for medical removal from work (such as the lead standard for general industry).

- After completion of the medical surveillance examination, the physician must furnish a written opinion regarding risk and fitness for or limitations in use of personal protective equipment.

- NIOSH is a part of the Centers for Disease Control and Prevention (CDC) and protects the health and safety of workers by conducting research on workplace hazards, providing information pertinent to the development of OSHA standards through criteria documents and current intelligence bulletins (CIBs), and conducting HHEs at the request of employees or employers. NIOSH also provides training through Educational Resource Centers (ERCs) for occupational medicine residents and graduate students in occupational nursing, industrial hygiene, and safety.

- The EPA is responsible for implementation of numerous acts of Congress promulgated to protect the environment. Although it is not necessary for most occupational physicians to have detailed knowledge of the specifics of environmental laws and regulations promulgated by bodies like the EPA, it is desirable for them to become more knowledgeable concerning the concepts and process of risk assessment. The Toxic Substance Control Act (TSCA) requires manufacturers or users of a specific chemical to keep a record of any allegation of a heretofore-unknown adverse health effect and to report to the EPA new information that reasonably supports the conclusion that the chemical or mixture presents a substantial risk of injury to health or the environment. The Agency for Toxic Substances and Disease Registry (ATSDR) provides continuing education training for physicians through case studies in environmental medicine.

- Other agencies may impact the practice of the occupational medicine physician such as the Mine Safety and Health Administration (MSHA). The purpose of this agency is similar to that of OSHA except that it only covers workers in the mining industry. The Nuclear Regulatory Commission (NRC) has primary responsibility for regulating hazards from ionizing radiation, including x-rays, gamma rays, and radioactive material that can be taken into the body. Agencies of the Department of Transportation (DOT), such as the Federal Aviation Administration (FAA), Federal Railroad Administration, and the Federal Highway Administration (FHA) set physical qualification standards for their employees and issue regulations dealing with drug and alcohol testing. The Equal Employment Opportunity Commission (EEOC) is charged with enforcing the Americans with Disabilities Act (ADA).

QUESTIONS

*1. Which of the following statements regarding OSHA is **incorrect**?*

A. The act does not cover federal, state, or local municipal employees.
B. The act requires annual examinations for employees exposed to noise of 80 dB or higher on a daily 8-hour TWA basis.
C. The physician must furnish a written opinion that includes any limitations on the use of personal protective equipment after a required medical surveillance examination.
D. The standard for lead in general industry has provisions for medical removal protection based on monitoring of whole blood lead levels.
E. Each of OSHA's chemical specific standards includes a section on medical surveillance.

2. Under OSHA record-keeping requirements

A. Medical records of work-related injuries must be maintained until termination of a person's employment.
B. An injury that requires first aid is recordable.
C. Over-the-counter medication is considered first aid and is, therefore, recordable.
D. Compliance with employee requests for medical records is required within 15 working days.
E. All STSs noted on annual audiometry are recordable.

*3. All of the following chemicals have a specific OSHA standard **except***

A. Asbestos
B. 1,1,2-Trichloroethylene
C. Formaldehyde
D. Vinyl chloride
E. Benzene

4. *All of the following statements regarding OSHA standards are true* **except**

A. Federal standards must be more stringent than state standards.
B. An injury is caused by an instantaneous exposure.
C. The Blood-Borne Pathogen Standard is directed primarily at the health care industry.
D. The Hazardous Waste Operations and Emergency Response Standard requires the employee to have a medical examination to determine physical fitness.
E. The Respiratory Protection Standard does not specify details of the content of the medical examination.

5. *NIOSH*

A. Has responsibility for enforcing OSHA regulations
B. Is part of the Department of Labor
C. Is not allowed to conduct research
D. May conduct HHEs at the request of employers
E. Accredits residency training programs in occupational medicine

6. *Which of the following is true concerning roles or requirements of various agencies?*

A. NIOSH develops health standards for OSHA.
B. OSHA requires that every 12 months a physician determine a worker's ability to wear a respirator.
C. EEOC is charged with enforcing the ADA.
D. ATSDR is responsible for regulating imported chemicals.
E. Under TSCA, physicians are required to report adverse effects of chemicals to the ATSDR.

4

Establishing an Occupational Health Program

OBJECTIVES

- Discuss steps in the development of an occupational health program
- Identify perspectives of the employer, employee, physician/provider, and regulatory agencies
- Define primary, secondary, and tertiary prevention programs and their implementation at a worksite
- Illustrate the benefits of the walkthrough visit and review the components of the evaluation
- Recognize the physician's role in treating and preventing injuries and illnesses in the workplace

OUTLINE

KEY POINTS

- Basic principles of high-quality medical care, effective communication, management, and commitment to prevention are the foundation of a successful occupational health program.
- An understanding of work activities is critical to the development of a quality occupational health program.
- Delivery of occupational medical care has expanded from industrial in-plant clinics to hospital-based clinics, occupational medicine programs, corporate medical departments, and union-supported occupational health programs.
- Developing business relationships among the physicians, employer clients, human resources, and medical and safety departments are vital to the success of occupational health programs. Professional service agreements should address type and price of services, nature of communications, and lines of authority. Occupational health providers must realize that employers often use services of several organizations for reasons such as hours of operation or availability of specialized services.
- Occupational medicine physicians have the unique opportunity to interact freely with individuals of many job titles, expertise, and responsibility. Good verbal and written skills are necessary for both the health care providers and the employer clients. Without effective communication even well-trained competent physicians may founder.
- Designation of specific teams ensures responsibility and accountability by all parties— the employer, physician or health provider, and employee. Physicians who deliver and supervise the clinical services lead the heath program team.
- The range of services includes diagnosis and treatment of injury and illness; exposure surveillance and examinations; drug test review; many specific kinds of physical examinations; interpretation of specialized testing (e.g., hearing, vision, pulmonary function, etc.); and supervision of nurses and midlevel professionals.
- The *employer team* includes the person who is ultimately responsible for the health and safety of workers onsite. It may be a member of senior management who provides leadership and an active interest in safety, or an office manager with little training in the field. In some cases, human resources departments may manage the health programs. Manufacturing companies often have environmental health and safety departments, industrial hygienists, safety engineers, and/or occupational health nurses onsite.
- Occupational medicine is a branch of preventive medicine and holds to the belief that occupational health injuries and illnesses are preventable. Board-certified occupational and environmental medicine (OEM) physicians are trained in areas of public health, toxicology, epidemiology, health promotion of large groups, risk assessment, and health law.
- Public health and occupational professionals identify three types of preventive services: *primary, secondary*, and *tertiary.*
- Primary prevention is an intervention that identifies and addresses a risk for disease or injury in the workplace (e.g., immunization against an infectious disease).
- There is a hierarchy of controls aimed at prevention defined by the National Institute for Occupational Safety and Health (NIOSH). The effectiveness of control decreases as the employer moves down the list. *Substitution* of a toxic substance with a safer one or replacement of a physically hazardous operation by automation may reduce the worker's risk. *Engineering controls* are aimed at improving the design and operation of a process. Proven methods of primary prevention decrease the risk of exposure and, therefore, injury. Having access to Industrial Hygiene (IH) information and Material

Safety Data Sheets (MSDS) allows the physician to make suggestions regarding health implications of certain exposures. *Administrative controls* focus on job descriptions and methods that match the worker to the task.

- The Americans with Disabilities Act (ADA) protects workers from inappropriate job discrimination. Historically, workers were excluded by the preemployment physical examination. Education and regular training are important ways that employers communicate information about health hazards to their employees and are a part of primary prevention. The use of personal protective equipment is low on the hierarchy of primary prevention controls but remains a necessary part of preventive measures at the workplace.
- Secondary prevention refers to early detection of disease and intervention before symptoms appear. The goal is to reverse, halt, or retard the progression of the illness or injury. Key approaches include medical surveillance, the early identification of repetitive motion disorders and high-risk manual-lifting situations, elimination of various physical hazards, and the provision of employee assistance programs. Health risk appraisals and screening examinations are other important examples of secondary prevention.
- Tertiary prevention is exemplified by clinical or case management of the illness or injury to minimize the disability and to reduce the complications and premature deterioration. A goal of tertiary prevention is to enhance timely return to function. Medical ethics, primary loyalties of physicians to patients, and careful consideration of confidentiality all play a role in clinical case management or tertiary prevention of disease.
- Competitive programs include physician onsite walkthrough visits. A preliminary review of the operation and conference with a contact person is helpful. By gathering information in this manner it is possible not only to establish a relationship with the employer representative but also with the employees who will observe your interest in their actual workstations. This may facilitate medical care in the future. General categories to observe for risk include the tasks, environment, equipment, and workers. Several important considerations make the walkthrough more effective. For example, it is helpful to schedule the visit during regular working hours to observe normal operations. It is important to approach workers in a nonthreatening manner. Be sure to wear the same, required, personal protective equipment as all employees in the area. Set a good example. A review of the OSHA 300 injury log will help the physician focus on problem areas or injury types.
- After the site visit, a comprehensive written report will solidify your recommendations and interest in the employer and employees. It offers an opportunity to provide education and training and is a marketing advantage for your program if services are required in the future. Combining quality health promotion programs with an understanding of occupational medicine offers an opportunity to become an employer's exclusive provider.

QUESTIONS

*1. Which of the following statements is **incorrect**?*

A. A major trend in delivery occupational health services is the growth of for-profit or privately held occupational health networks.
B. Employers have reduced their investment in onsite occupational health services because it holds no advantage for employees.

C. Strengths of the private practice model include flexibility and autonomy to the physician, ability to customize services to local employers, and ability to accrue financial benefits.

D. Universities have established internal occupational health programs, primarily to meet the needs of the employees at the university.

E. Union-supported occupational health programs have had an important place in delivering health services to their members since the 1900s.

2. *Which of the following statements is **incorrect**?*

A. Primary prevention is any intervention that addresses a risk factor for an injury or illness.

B. A hierarchy of controls exists for primary prevention that includes substitution, engineering, and administrative controls.

C. Detecting noise-induced hearing loss during annual medical surveillance is an example of secondary prevention.

D. Screening mammography is an example of primary prevention.

E. An example of tertiary prevention is the use of physical therapy in the management of injured workers to minimize the effects of their injury.

3. *Which of the following is the **least** important to the occupational physician conducting a facility walkthrough?*

A. The visit should be scheduled during regular working hours to observe normal work practices.

B. The human resource policy regarding use of a sick leave should be examined.

C. Staff members responsible for health and safety measures should be interviewed.

D. Types of personal protective equipment used should be examined.

E. The physician should bring a preventive health perspective to the evaluation.

4. *What considerations are made before and during an onsite visit to make the walkthrough more effective?*

A. Availability of MSDS
B. A review of the types of injuries that have occurred previously
C. Training procedures regarding hazard communication
D. Speaking directly to workers to get their perspective on safety
E. All of the above

5

Understanding the Americans with Disabilities Act

OBJECTIVES

- Explain the relationship between impairment and disability
- Discuss the basic provisions of the Americans with Disabilities Act (ADA)
- Explain the impact of this law on the practice of occupational medicine
- List the types of examinations allowed by employers under the ADA
- Explain the process involved in determination of fitness-for-duty

OUTLINE

KEY POINTS

- The ADA was built on many provisions of Sections 503 and 504 of the Rehabilitation Act of 1973, which covered government employees and federal contractors. The Civil Rights Act of 1991 strengthened the ADA by allowing punitive and compensatory damages. There are several definitions related to the ADA legislation (see Table 5.1).
- The ADA is intended to bring those with physical and mental disabilities into the mainstream of American society by protecting those individuals with disabilities as defined in the law from improper discrimination. The Equal Employment Opportunity Commission (EEOC) enforces the ADA.
- Title I of the ADA covers employment and applies to all private employers, state and local governments, and education institutions that employ 15 or more persons.

not Federal employers

- The ADA places strong emphasis on evaluation of each individual situation on a case-by-case basis. The relationship between impairment, functional limitation, and disability varies enormously from individual to individual. Disability determination is a non-medical managerial task, whereas health professionals make medical technical judgments about pathology, impairment, and functional limitation within a framework of generally accepted medical principles and practice. The ADA places clear responsibility on management to make appropriate decisions about disability, direct threat, and reasonable accommodation.
- The ADA prohibits preoffer and preemployment medical inquiries, medical examinations, and other medical information gathering (e.g., workers' compensation claims) until after a *bona fide* job offer has been made. Job application forms may ask only about current ability to perform essential job functions. The job offer may be conditioned on satisfactory completion of a postoffer medical examination as long as this is required of all other entering employees in the same job category. Strength testing and agility tests are not considered to be medical procedures and may be required preoffer. Withdrawal of a job offer must be job related (to essential functions) and consistent with business necessity, not based on speculation of future injury, and may occur only if reasonable accommodation is not possible or poses an undue hardship for the employer.
- For current employees, medical surveillance and fitness-for-duty examinations can be required only when mandated by statute or when job related and consistent with business necessity, and then they must be limited to determining ability to perform essential functions on a case-by-case basis.
- Voluntary examinations (e.g., blood pressure, cholesterol screening, health risk appraisal, periodic physician examination, and wellness programs) are permitted.
- The ADA requires that the employer maintain confidential medical records in locked cabinets, separate from personnel files, accessible only to designated persons. If any medical information is to be shared with the employer, the applicant/employee should sign a medical release authorizing dissemination of such medical information. The ADA requires that health professionals share sufficient information with employers to make management decisions about the presence of a disability, direct threat, and reasonable accommodation.
- The medical examiner is not responsible for making employment decisions or determining whether a reasonable accommodation can be made. The physician should advise the employer about two things only: (a) the individual's functional abilities and limitations in relation to functional job requirements and (b) whether the individual can

perform the job without posing a direct threat to the health or safety of himself or herself or others. The ADA does not permit blanket exclusions.

- Testing for illegal drugs is specifically excluded as being a "medical test." The EEOC has recommended informally that employers arrange drug testing, so that any associated medical inquiry is conducted after a conditional job offer. The ADA offers limited protection to recovered/recovering alcoholics and illegal drug users. The critical distinction for illegal drug users is between current and former use. Employers are not required to provide alcohol/drug rehabilitation as a reasonable accommodation.
- The ADA's definition of "any mental or psychologic disorder" is very broad. Nowhere else were symptoms or diagnoses included or excluded with the same degree of specificity (e.g., pyromania, homosexuality, and pedophilia are excluded). Stress and depression may or may not be considered impairments, depending on whether these conditions result from a documented psychologic or mental disorder. Functional job descriptions can include a number of attributes in the psychologic or social realm (e.g., maintain concentration over time).
- Some communicable diseases, such as tuberculosis (TB) and human immunodeficiency virus (HIV) infection, are disabilities for the purposes of the ADA.

QUESTIONS

*1. All of the following statements about the ADA are correct **except***

A. It is a federal law enforced by the EEOC.
B. It places strong emphasis on evaluation of each individual situation on a case-by-case basis.
C. Federal government employers are covered under the act.
D. It is intended to bring those with physical and mental disabilities into the mainstream of American society.
E. Employment provisions apply to all private employers with 15 or more employees.

2. The ADA prohibits discrimination in which of the following employment activities?

A. Hiring and firing
B. Job advertisements
C. Compensation
D. Training and apprenticeship programs
E. All of the above

*3. Before making an offer of employment, the ADA prohibits all of the following **except***

A. Inquiries about the existence, nature, or severity of a disability
B. Inquiries about a past history of drug or alcohol abuse
C. Testing for illegal drugs
D. A medical examination
E. Questions about prior workers' compensation claims

4. Under the ADA, an individual with a disability is a person who

A. Has a physical or mental impairment that substantially limits one or more major life activities

B. Has a record of an impairment that substantially limits one or more major life activities
C. Is regarded as having an impairment that substantially limits one or more major life activities
D. A, B, and C are correct
E. A and B are correct

5. *Physicians conducting work-related physical examinations should advise employers of all of the following* ***except***

A. An individual's functional abilities and limitations in relation to functional job requirements
B. Whether the individual meets the employer's overall health and safety requirements
C. The specific pharmaceutical agents used by the employee that may interfere with his or her ability to do the job
D. Whether a person with a disability can currently perform a specific job with or without an accommodation
E. Whether an individual can perform a job without posing a "direct threat" to the health or safety of himself or herself or others

6. *Under the ADA, all of the following mental and psychologic disorders were specifically excluded as disabilities* ***except***

A. Kleptomania
B. History of heroin addiction
C. Compulsive gambling
D. Pedophilia
E. Pyromania

6

Occupational Health Nursing: Roles and Practice

OBJECTIVES

- Explain the scope of the occupational health nursing practice
- Describe the function of the nurse case manager
- List goals of prevention services
- Describe influences that affect occupational health nursing practice

OUTLINE

KEY POINTS

- The scope of occupational health nursing has expanded significantly in recent decades.
- Economic demands and regulatory mandates are likely to increase primary health care delivery at the worksite, case management, and disability management, but the management, monitoring, and surveillance of work-related illnesses and injuries must remain a priority.
- Occupational health nursing practice is grounded in the principles of public health practice, that is, examining population trends in health, illness, and injury. Individual

care is provided to ill and injured workers; however, the emphasis is on providing programs and services to maintain, improve, and protect the health of the workforce.

- The occupational health nurse is often the only health care professional at the worksite and, as such, has the primary responsibility for the management of worker health and safety with consideration to ethical, cultural, spiritual, and corporate beliefs.
- Seven major roles are identified in the practice of occupational health nursing: clinician/practitioner, administrator, educator, health promotion specialist, case manager, researcher, and consultant.
- The occupational health nurse clinician/practitioner applies the nursing process (i.e., assessment, diagnosis, planning, implementation, and evaluation) in providing nursing care for occupational and nonoccupational health problems and develops health promotion, protection, and prevention programs and strategies based on worker needs and health hazards.
- The occupational health nurse administrator provides direction for the planning, implementation, and evaluation of occupational health services.
- Health education is provided often during a health assessment or visit to the occupational health unit and to groups in informal group meetings.
- As a health promotion specialist, the occupational health nurse designs, implements, and evaluates worksite health promotion programs with the goals of improving the overall health status and productivity of the workforce and reducing health care costs.
- The occupational health nurse case manager establishes a provider network, recommends treatment plans that ensure quality and efficacy while controlling costs, monitors outcomes, and maintains communication among all involved.
- Occupational health nurses may identify and participate in research projects and disseminate the results of such studies.
- A nurse consultant may provide services such as developing policies and procedures, record systems or job descriptions, or performing hazard evaluation and worker job analysis.
- Prevention programs seek to promote, maintain, and restore the physical and psychosocial well-being of the workers to enhance optimal functioning; to protect the worker from hazards that may occur as a result of the work experience; to encourage and participate in a company culture supportive of health; and to collaborate with workers, management, and other disciplines and health care professionals to ensure a safe and healthful work environment.
- There are many factors that affect occupational health nursing programs, including external (economic constraints, sociocultural characteristics of the population, legislation that requires implementation of regulations affecting workplace health and safety, and advances in technology) and internal or work setting influences (the workforce, type of work and related hazards, corporate culture, mission and philosophy, allocation of human and capital resources, interdisciplinary functioning, data/information resources, and the goals of the occupational health unit).

QUESTIONS

*1. Which of the following is **inaccurate** about case management activities?*

A. The case manager establishes a provider network.
B. The case manager orders treatments that control costs.
C. The case manager determines the need for intervention.

D. The case manager develops and conducts an evaluation process for the program.
E. Case management is not limited to occupational injuries.

2. *Which of the following functions is* **least consistent** *with an occupational health services prevention program?*

A. Promotion and maintenance of physical and psychosocial well-being
B. Management of acute injuries
C. Cholesterol screening programs designed for early detection of disease
D. Provision of immunization for influenza
E. Blood pressure screening

7

The Independent Medical Evaluation

OBJECTIVES

- State the purposes and components of the independent medical evaluation (IME)
- Discuss issues concerning injury or illness causality
- Identify the differences between impairment and disability
- Delineate the uses of the functional performance assessment

OUTLINE

I. Challenges in IMEs
   A. Figure 7.1: Example referral letter
   B. Diagnoses
   C. Causal relationship
   D. Prognosis
   E. Maximal medical improvement (MMI)
   F. Permanent impairment
   G. Work capacity
      1. Table 7.1: *Dictionary of Occupational Titles* work demands
   H. Appropriateness of care
II. Conducting an evaluation and preparing a report
   A. Preevaluation
   B. Evaluation
   C. Key components of the evaluation
      1. History
      2. Examination
      3. Pain and disability inventories
      4. Diagnostic studies
   D. Postevaluation
   E. Reports
      1. Table 7.2: Preparation of the IME report

KEY POINTS

- IMEs are examinations performed by a physician who is not involved in the person's care for the purpose of clarifying medical and job issues. Occupational medicine physicians are often the most appropriate specialists to evaluate work-related injuries and to determine whether worksite accommodations may be necessary for certain medical disorders.

- IMEs are performed to provide information for case management and for evidence in hearings and other legal proceedings. IMEs are a component of all workers' compensation statutes, although the specifics vary by state. IMEs also are used in clarifying liability (personal injury) and disability. Insurers, third-party administrators, employers, and attorneys usually request IMEs.
- The physician who performs the IME is not involved in a treating capacity. The physician must be impartial and unbiased in performing the assessment. The physician makes a careful assessment and addresses the issues raised by the referring sources. Physicians with some clinical, consulting, or teaching involvement are considered to be more credible than those who perform only IMEs. The examinee is not necessarily a willing participant.
- Key issues associated with an IME differ from clinical consultations in role and focus. The most common issues are diagnosis, causation, prognosis, MMI, permanent impairment, appropriateness of care, and recommendations.
- Pain, especially chronic pain, may not be associated with significant physical pathology. Pathology may be present without symptoms or dysfunction. Impairment is a measurable decrement in some physiologic function, whereas disability considers not only the physical or mental impairment but also the social, psychological, or vocational factors associated with a person's ability to work. Functional limitations are manifestations of impairment. Chronic pain, the most common problem seen in the performance of IMEs, may not be a symptom of an underlying acute somatic injury but a multidimensional biopsychosocial phenomenon.
- Work-related causation is defined as a problem that "arose out of and during the course of employment." Establishing causation to a reasonable degree of medical probability implies that it is more probable than not (i.e., there is more than a 50% probability) that a certain condition arose out of or in the course of work duties. Possibility implies less than 50% likelihood. Apportionment refers to the extent to which a condition is related to each of multiple factors. Aggravation implies a long-standing effect resulting from an event, which results in a worsening, hastening, or deterioration of the condition. Exacerbation is a temporary increase or flare in symptoms from the condition.
- MMI is a phrase used to indicate when further recovery and restoration of function can no longer be anticipated to a reasonable degree of medical probability. This assessment implies that a condition is permanent and static.
- Impairment is the loss of the use of, or a derangement of, any body part, system, or function. Disability is the limiting loss of the capacity to meet personal, social, or occupational demands or to meet statutory or regulatory requirements. Impairment is considered permanent when it has reached MMI. Impairment is a measurable decrement in health status evaluated by medical means. The medical role usually is limited to evaluating impairment not disability. Subjective complaints such as fatigue or pain, when not accompanied by demonstrable organ dysfunction, clinical signs, or other independent, measurable abnormalities, are generally not ratable. In some workers' compensation jurisdictions, either by law, regulation, or administrative practice, a formula is used, whereby the impairment rating becomes the primary piece of information from which a compensation level is established. This situation is unfortunate because an impairment evaluation can only document a person's health status at a point in time and not the impact on functioning in society or employability.
- Functional performance assessments are more accurate determinations of ability, if the assessment is valid and reliable and relates to particular job tasks. Various methodologies are available. It is customary to express work capacity following parameters in the

Dictionary of Occupational Titles from the Department of Labor. Estimates of lifting and carrying capabilities are usually noted for specific frequencies. Guidelines should be provided for the frequency and duration of tasks such as bending, squatting, and so forth. These capacities are compared with the functional requirements of the job.

- Disability durations that provide information regarding the length of disability typically associated with a diagnosis or disorder may also provide very valuable insight into how much and how long of an impact a problem may have on the functional ability.
- In conducting an evaluation and preparing a report, it is important to review the medical records before the evaluation and to read correspondence from the client, so that the evaluation can be structured to answer specific questions. Pain and functional inventories completed before the evaluation are particularly helpful in identifying behavioral and psychologic components related to an illness or injury. At the beginning of the visit, the physician should explain the nature of the evaluation and that an independent evaluation will be conducted but that no treatment will be performed, there is no patient-physician relationship, and a report will be sent to the requesting client. A signed release to this effect is advised.
- Histories need to include a detailed review of the injury or illness, relevant preexisting conditions, the chronology of events from the time of injury through the present, current status, the person's perceived functional status, a thorough occupational history, and a psychologic history. The meticulous history is followed by a physical examination including a behavioral assessment and a detailed examination of the involved area(s). Available diagnostic studies should be reviewed. Additional studies may be recommended to the referring source; however, they should not be obtained without approval from the referral source to avoid conflicts regarding fiscal responsibilities for the testing. The evaluation should address the specific issues requested by the referring source. Reports should be organized and detailed and present the information obtained during the evaluation.

QUESTIONS

1. Independent medical evaluations or IMEs

A. Are generally performed by the treating physician
B. Are performed to provide information for case management and for evidence in hearings and other legal proceedings
C. Are typically performed by professionals who are not health care providers
D. Should not address questions related to workers' compensation
E. Are requested by insurers and third-party administrators but not usually by employers

2. In performing an IME, it is important to recognize that

A. The examinee usually requests the evaluation and is a willing participant.
B. Chronic pain is always associated with significant physical pathology.
C. Pathology is never present without symptoms or dysfunction.
D. Impairment and disability are equivalent.
E. Functional limitations are usually manifestations of impairment.

3. *Causation is a common question in IMEs. Which of the following is true regarding work-related causation?*

A. It is defined as a problem that "arose out of and during the course of employment."
B. Medical probability and possibility are synonymous terms when drawing causal conclusions.
C. Apportionment refers to the percentage of an individual's body mass affected by a given problem.
D. Exacerbation implies a long-standing effect due to an event that results in a worsening, hastening, or deterioration of the condition.
E. Aggravation is a temporary increase or flare in symptoms from the condition.

4. *All of the following are true concerning MMI **except***

A. It is a phrase used to indicate when further recovery and restoration of function can no longer be anticipated to a reasonable degree of medical probability.
B. It implies that a condition is permanent and static.
C. Residual impairment is the loss of the use of, or a derangement of, any body part, system, or function.
D. Impairment is considered to be permanent at this stage.
E. It is synonymous with total disability.

5. *Regarding functional performance assessments*

A. They are unrelated to particular job tasks.
B. There is only one proper method for their performance.
C. It is customary to express work capacity following parameters in the *Dictionary of Occupational Titles.*
D. Estimates of lifting and carrying capabilities are not standard parts of the analysis.
E. Guidelines related to frequency and duration of tasks performed are not relevant.

6. *All of the following are recommended components of an IME **except***

A. A review of available records
B. Pain and functional inventories
C. Establishment of a doctor-patient relationship
D. A signed release of medical information
E. A comprehensive history

8

The Physician Working with the Business Community

OBJECTIVES

- Discuss opportunities for physicians in the practice of occupational medicine
- Distinguish between types of occupational medicine practice

OUTLINE

I. Overview—into the new millennium
II. The changing occupational health environment
III. The changing physician role
IV. An overview of physician opportunities
   A. Opportunities with hospital-based or hospital-affiliated programs
   B. Freestanding occupational health clinics
   C. Consulting
V. What the astute physician can do now
   A. Gain a basic foundation in occupational medicine
   B. Be prepared to address the occupational medicine continuum
   C. Remain abreast of regulatory measures
   D. Associate interventions in terms of health care cost containment
   E. Be an educator
   F. Be prepared to play multiple roles
VI. Summary—the occupational medicine physician of the future

KEY POINTS

- Opportunities for physicians working with the business community continue to expand.
- Close associations with employers are paramount for physicians and medical centers as the private sector assumes greater influence in directing health care funding and service delivery.
- Several characteristics of the current environment include:

1. Competition for the health care dollar is increasing between health systems, hospitals, and physician groups in most markets.

2. Advanced communication tools (the Internet, audionet conferencing, and telemedicine) are providing health practitioners with heretofore-unimaginable opportunities to communicate directly with the workplace.
3. National concern for terrorist-related fears and activities has spawned a critical new calling for occupational medicine physicians to advise employers on biologic and chemical risks, associated mental health issues, and plans for emergency preparedness.

- Occupational medicine is in the throes of a shift away from injury management toward the provision of health-related consultations.
- Numerous public health regulations [Americans with Disabilities Act, Drug Free Workplace Act, Occupational Safety and Health Administration (OSHA)] affect occupational health practice.
- Perhaps the most profound change in the practice of medicine is the decline of fee-for-service reimbursement in exchange for a variety of managed care arrangements.
- By 2001, an estimated 1,500 or more hospitals of approximately 7,000 in the United States had dedicated programs that provided occupational medical services for employers. Although a small number of programs are still based in emergency departments, freestanding clinics within the hospital, freestanding ambulatory care locations, and networks of clinics are the most common delivery models.
- Freestanding occupational health clinics—with no formal ties to a hospital—grew at a breathless pace during the late 1980s and early 1990s. Although still common, national or regional for-profit occupational health clinic networks have acquired many of the freestanding clinics.
- The shortage of physicians with training in occupational medicine provides yet a third practice option—that of a consultant. The well-trained occupational medicine physician can provide consultative services to provider groups and to employers.
- The consultant occupational health physician should emphasize the following:

1. One-stop shopping—employers are increasingly attracted to programs with a broad range of services that can be provided in one setting, especially by a single physician.
2. A partnership concept—employers envision their future partnership with health care providers as being considerably closer than it is today.
3. Training—employers increasingly recognize the value of training in occupational medicine; the physician should emphasize certification and special training in occupational medicine to potential clients.

- To succeed in occupational medicine, the astute physician should

1. Obtain a basic foundation in occupational medicine
2. Be prepared to address the occupational medicine continuum (i.e., prevention, acute injury treatment, and the return to work process)
3. Remain abreast of regulatory measures
4. Associate interventions in terms of health care cost containment
5. Be an educator
6. Be prepared to play multiple roles

- The emergence of the employer as a key figure in the changing health care delivery system paradigm and as a gatekeeper and financial supporter of the health care system presents an extraordinary opportunity to the physician with training and expertise in occupational medicine.

QUESTIONS

1. All of the following are indicative of the changing occupational medicine environment **except**

A. The private sector is assuming greater influence in directing health care funding and service delivery.
B. The deregulation of the 1980s is being replaced by an emphasis on public health regulation.
C. A shift from managed care arrangements to a fee-for-service system has occurred.
D. Health care cost control leads the agenda for many employers.
E. Many hospitals have programs in occupational health.

2. Which of the following is **least** *representative of the changes in occupational medicine?*

A. Occupational physicians are expected to have clinical expertise and to address broader community health care concerns.
B. Prevention is likely to assume a less important role in the workplace.
C. Occupational physicians frequently work with hospitals.
D. Occupational physicians must work with multiple constituencies.
E. Occupational physicians are expected to be knowledgeable about environmental issues.

3. Which of the following best characterizes hospital-based occupational health?

A. Hospitals have declining interest in occupational medicine services, which are generally unprofitable.
B. Hospitals possess the financial backing, breadth of services, and management support to prosper in competitive markets.
C. Compensation for medical directors of hospital-based programs is usually straight salary.
D. A hospital setting is especially attractive for the physician who prefers autonomy and independence.
E. Hospital-based occupational programs rarely care for the hospital employees.

4. Which of the following is **least likely** *to provide a consultative opportunity for a physician specialist in occupational medicine?*

A. Medical surveillance
B. Worker-management mediation
C. Worker education
D. Health and safety policy and program development
E. Workers' compensation loss control and managed care

5. *Which of the following is **not** a key element in developing a profile that will allow the physician to prosper financially and make a genuine difference when working with the business community?*

A. Remain abreast of regulatory measures
B. Obtain a basic foundation in occupational medicine
C. Associate interventions in terms of health care cost containment
D. Be an educator
E. All of the above

Drug Testing in the Occupational Setting

OBJECTIVES

- Explain the scope of drug testing in the contemporary workplace
- List the types of worksite drug testing
- Discuss problems involved in specimen collection
- Explain the duties of the medical review officer (MRO)
- Discuss controversial issues concerning drug and alcohol tests

OUTLINE

KEY POINTS

- The most essential factor responsible for the extraordinary growth of drug testing has been the availability of simple, inexpensive, immunoassay urine screening tests. Gas chromatography/mass spectrometry (GC/MS) has become the "gold standard" for forensic drug testing.
- Drug testing of public sector employees was shaped by the 1986 Executive Order 12564 and Public Law 100-71, which commissioned the DHHS to develop technical procedures for drug testing.
- In 1990, companies with more than 250 employees were much more likely to have written policies for drug programs. Drugs in the workplace are a concern because 77% of current illicit drug users older than the age of 18 are employed. Illicit drug use is most prevalent among employees age 18 to 25, higher among males than females, and higher in those with less formal education and lower personal income (Table 9.1).
- Illicit drug use among employees is associated with higher rates of absenteeism, accidental injury, involuntary separation, medical care use, and health care costs.
- There are two categories of drug testing: federally regulated versus nonfederally regulated. More than half of all states regulate some aspect of nonfederally regulated workplace drug testing. The DHHS, DOT, Department of Defense (DOD), Department of Energy (DOE), and other agencies govern federally regulated drug testing.
- Federal regulations contain detailed procedures for urine collection, completion of custody and control forms, analysis by laboratories originally certified by the National Institute on Drug Abuse (NIDA) for only five specified illicit drugs [amphetamines, cocaine, marijuana, opiates, and phencyclidine (PCP)—the "NIDA-5"], and mandatory reporting of all results to an MRO for review and interpretation before reporting to the employer.
- Six major drug-testing situations exist: preemployment/preplacement, postaccident/incident, reasonable cause/reasonable suspicion, random, return-to-duty/follow-up, and periodic.
- Unannounced random drug testing provides the highest deterrent against drug use.
- Drug testing can be broken down into three steps: (a) collection of the specimen and completion of custody and control forms; (b) laboratory analysis for screening and confirmation of positive tests; and (c) review, verification, and reporting to the employer of test results.

- Urine specimen collection and custody and control form documentation is a crucial step because so many errors occur here. Most positive drug tests that are invalidated are due to improper urine collection or documentation.
- It is important that in the urine collection process each person is treated with respect and allowed the maximum reasonable privacy while minimizing the opportunity to substitute or adulterate urine specimens.
- There are three ways to conduct urine collection: private collection, monitored, and direct observation. *Private* collection allows the donor to provide a specimen in a carefully prepared separate room with complete privacy. A *monitored* collection is conducted in a restroom or other facility that offers partial privacy. Under *direct observation*, the observer directly observes the urine exiting the urinary meatus during collection.
- Following collection, the collector and the donor should keep the sample in constant view until it is properly sealed and labeled.
- If an employer has requested both a federally mandated drug test and nonregulated testing, separately voided specimens must be collected with separate custody and control forms.
- Federally regulated urine drug tests must be analyzed in laboratories certified by the Substance Abuse and Mental Health Services Administration (SAMHSA). SAMHSA also permits laboratories to perform specimen validity testing to determine whether the specimen is consistent with human urine, whether specific adulterants or foreign substances are added, and whether the specimen was substituted or diluted.
- If the urine specimen has a positive screen, then another aliquot is taken from the specimen for confirmation testing for the identified drug by GC/MS. Administrative cutoff levels for each of the five illicit drugs are specified by the regulation for each form of testing (see Table 9.4).
- When the laboratory identifies a specimen as negative, it is discarded. "Nonnegative" specimens (i.e., positives, adulterated, substituted, or invalid) are frozen and retained at the laboratory for at least 1 full year, and specimen records must be retained for a minimum of 2 years.
- DHHS has issued guidance to laboratories regarding "fatal flaws" that constitute grounds for rejecting a specimen, in which case the MRO will report the test as *canceled* (see Table 9.3). Nonfatal flaws can be corrected by receiving a signed statement of correction from the appropriate individual.
- In federally regulated testing, laboratory results must be reported directly to the MRO. In nonfederally regulated testing, results may be permitted to go directly to the employer, although a growing number of states now require use of an MRO, especially for positive results.
- The most critical MRO function is to interpret and verify each positive, adulterated, substituted, or invalid test result.
- DHHS guidelines describe the MRO as "a licensed physician...who has knowledge of substance abuse disorders and has appropriate medical training to interpret and evaluate an individual's positive test result together with his/her medical history and any other relevant biomedical information." The MRO must understand the urine collection procedures, custody and control form completion, and analytic procedures.
- A substance abuse professional (SAP) as defined by DOT regulations is a licensed physician or psychologist, social worker, certified employee assistance professional, or drug and alcohol ~~addition~~ counselor certified by an acceptable national organization.
addiction

The SAP evaluates employees who have violated DOT drug and alcohol regulations and makes recommendations concerning appropriate education, treatment, follow-up testing, and aftercare.

- In the Omnibus Transportation Employee Testing Act of 1991, Congress extended testing for controlled substances to include testing for misuse of alcohol in preemployment, random, reasonable suspicion, postaccident and posttreatment testing in most transportation sectors. It also provided legislative authority for drug and alcohol testing for mass transit vehicle operators, controllers, and maintenance workers. Although oral swabs for testing saliva may be used for screening, all confirmation tests must use evidential grade breath testing devices approved by the National Highway Traffic Safety Administration (NHTSA). Only in the Federal Railway Administration is blood alcohol testing permitted for postaccident testing.
- In the past, MRO training and credentialing was voluntary. In 2001, the DOT published rules requiring MROs to receive initial qualification training in specified subjects; to receive at least 12 hours of continuing medical education (CME) in pertinent subjects every 3 years; and to pass an examination by an approved national certifying body [American Society for Addiction Medicine (ASAM), the American Association of Medical Review Officers (AAMRO), and Medical Review Officer Certification Council (MROCC)].
- The ADA does not consider testing for controlled substances a medical test. Therefore, drug testing is permitted at any time, including before an offer of employment. Current drug users are not protected under the ADA. Former drug users who are no longer using drugs are protected under the ADA. Testing for alcohol is considered a medical test and may not be performed before the employer makes a job offer.
- The *ACOEM Ethical Guidelines for Drug Screening in the Workplace* lists several features that should be included in any program for the screening of employees and prospective employees for drugs (see Appendix to Chapter 9 in the textbook).

QUESTIONS

1. All of the following statements about illicit drug use in the United States are true **except**

A. Most drug users older than age 18 are employed.
B. Drug use is more common in males than females.
C. Drug use is most prevalent among employees age 18 to 25.
D. Drug users are not likely to be heavy users of alcohol.
E. Drug use is associated with higher rates of accidental injury and absenteeism.

2. Federally regulated drug testing is characterized by all of the following **except**

A. Urine specimens can only be analyzed for cocaine, marijuana, opiates, amphetamines, and PCP.
B. Results of positive urine drug tests can be reported directly to the employer by the laboratory.
C. Only the Nuclear Regulatory Commission can perform onsite drug screening.
D. Split specimens are required for all DOT urine collections.
E. Urine drug tests must be conducted at a laboratory certified by SAMHSA.

3. *Validity testing of urine specimens by laboratories is conducted to determine*

A. Whether the specimen is consistent with human urine
B. Whether specific adulterants or foreign substances were added
C. Whether the specimen was substituted
D. Whether the specimen was diluted
E. All of the above

4. *A donor could have a legitimate medical explanation for all of the following drugs or their metabolites **except***

A. Amphetamines
B. Opiates
C. PCP
D. Cocaine
E. Marijuana

5. *Under the DOT alcohol-testing regulations, prohibited conduct includes*

A. Having a breath alcohol concentration of 0.04 or greater
B. Consuming alcohol while on duty
C. Consuming alcohol within 4 hours [8 hours for flight crews under Federal Aviation Administration (FAA) rules] of performing duty
D. Refusing to take an alcohol test
E. All of the above

6. *In federally regulated drug testing, which of the following errors is **not** considered a "fatal" flaw?*

A. No donor signature and no remark explaining failure to sign
B. Insufficient specimen volume (<30 mL)
C. Specimen identification (ID) number is omitted on specimen bottle
D. Specimen bottle seal is broken or shows evidence of tampering
E. Specimen ID numbers on specimen bottle and custody and control form do not match

Not needed

10

Accreditation of Occupational Health Services

OBJECTIVES

- Explain the rationale for accreditation of occupational health centers
- Review eligibility requirements for accreditation
- List components of the survey process
- Differentiate between the core and adjunct standards required for accreditation
- Identify potential problem areas in achieving accreditation

OUTLINE

I. Accreditation of occupational health services
   A. Overview
   B. Accreditation under Accreditation Association for Ambulatory Health Care (AAAHC)
   C. Survey eligibility
   D. Survey process
II. AAAHC standards
   A. Core standards
   B. Adjunct standards
III. Problem areas in achieving accreditation
   A. Clinical records
   B. Quality management and improvement
   C. Occupational health services
   D. Practical considerations
IV. Rationale for accreditation
V. Other certification requirements

KEY POINTS

- Accreditation is a process used to certify that an organization meets certain criteria. Medical organizations may pursue accreditation to improve operations and quality of care and to gain recognition; accreditation may be desired for financial reasons, ensuring reimbursement through third-party payers. The American College of Occupational and Environmental Medicine (ACOEM) supports the development of standards of practice, the achievement of these standards through self-evaluation, and the participation in accreditation to demonstrate that the standards have been met.

- The development of the AAAHC as a separate organization was prompted by a reorganization of the Joint Commission for the Accreditation of Hospitals [now the Joint Commission for Accreditation of Healthcare Organizations (JCAHO)]. Seeking accreditation in occupational health settings remains a voluntary process. There are 24 individual standards in the AAAHC's handbook; these are divided into two groups: core and adjunct. Core standards apply to all organizations and address issues common to ambulatory health care delivery, such as administration, facilities, and records. Adjunct standards address specific services or activities and only apply if the organization offers the services listed. One of the adjunct standards is occupational and employee health services.
- Eligibility requirements for accreditation surveys include the following:

  1. The organization's primary activity must be provision of health services, and it must have been in operation for at least 6 months.
  2. Either the organization, or its parent organization, must be a formally organized, legal entity.
  3. If required, the organization must be licensed to provide services and must be in compliance with appropriate regulations.
  4. Medical care must be under the direction or supervision of a physician. The health care organization must also share facilities, equipment, and patient care records among its members providing patient care.

- Preparation for an AAAHC survey begins with a self-assessment process including the creation of a committee or team. The process may be lengthy, depending on the status of the organization. A presurvey questionnaire is completed and submitted. The survey consists of an extensive onsite evaluation of policies, procedures, and operations. A primary goal of the surveyors is to determine if the organization is in compliance with the intent of the standards. A second goal is to educate and provide consultation to the organization. Accreditation can be granted for either 1 or 3 years.
- AAAHC has eight core standards: patient rights, governance, administration, quality of care, quality management and improvement, clinical records, professional improvement, and facilities and environment. A separate adjunct standard exists for occupational and employee health services. The opening statement sets the primary goals of occupational and employee health services as ensuring a safe and healthy workplace for employees and patients through the recognition, evaluation, and control of illness and injury in or from the workplace and through meeting the needs of the individuals served.
- The occupational health chapter is divided into two sections. The first deals with employee health in health care settings addressing protection from biologic hazards and chemical hazards, hazard communication compliance, physical hazards such as violence in the workplace and ergonomics, and record keeping. The second section is more comprehensive and applies to occupational health facilities or departments and contains five general standards and eight service-specific standards. These standards focus on several issues such as patient rights; accurate portrayal of occupational health services; appropriate resources needed to evaluate workplace hazards; matching medical status with work demands; inclusion of appropriate elements in medical records;

medical care for individuals with occupational injury or illness; various forms of examination including medical surveillance; laboratory testing programs; consultation, education, and training; and community preparedness and response.
- Other applicable adjunct standards may include immediate and urgent care services; testing (both diagnostic imaging and laboratory services); and other professional and technical services (such as occupational therapy, physical therapy, psychologic services, health education, and audiology).
- Problems in accreditation are usually in one of three areas: clinical records, quality management and improvement, or occupational health services.
- A common problem with clinical records is failing to adequately document the patient encounter. To evaluate care, the medical records must provide sufficient detail so that an outside reviewer can (a) determine the patient's primary complaint, (b) independently confirm the patient's diagnosis based on reported findings, (c) confirm that the treatment was appropriate and necessary, and (d) confirm that the patient's care was appropriate over time. Records must be complete and legible.
- Successful quality management and improvement programs require commitment at all levels of the organization, starting with the governing body. These programs draw on all sources of information for quality improvement initiatives including peer review, audits, patient surveys, suggestions, outcome measurements, and benchmarking. Risk management and practice guidelines are important elements. Practice guidelines are sets of directions or principles used to assist health care practitioners with decisions concerning appropriate medical management.
- The specific goals of the occupational health services standard should be reflected in all other relevant AAAHC standards. Documentation must include preventive activities, knowledge of the workplace, and compliance with all applicable rules and regulations.

QUESTIONS

*1. Which of the following statements concerning the AAAHC is **false**?*

A. It is the largest accreditation body for ambulatory health care facilities.
B. ACOEM formally endorses its accreditation as a means to improve health care quality.
C. It hires experienced administrators to serve as full-time surveyors.
D. Its adjunct standards are specific to occupational health services.
E. Its standards are designed to apply to all occupational health facilities in the United States.

2. Which of the following statements concerning the accreditation process is true?

A. Organizations must be in operation for 2 years before submitting their accreditation application.
B. The surveyor submits his or her observations to AAAHC and is not allowed to discuss findings with the organization.
C. In-plant occupational health departments, supervised and directed by a head nurse, are eligible for accreditation under AAAHC.
D. A typical initial clinic survey involves one surveyor for 4 to 6 hours.
E. The surveyor provides consultative comments to the organization in addition to evaluating the standards.

3. Which of the following is **not** required for accreditation as an occupational health facility?

A. At least one physician board certified in occupational medicine
B. Use of local, state, or national comparison benchmarks
C. A program to identify adverse patient outcomes and "near misses"
D. Preventive counsel in matters regarding occupational health
E. An understanding of the work environment for each of the patients seen in the facility

4. Which of the following is **not** covered under the Quality Management and Improvement Standard?

A. Intervention or quality studies
B. Credentials verification
C. Benchmarking
D. Peer review
E. Risk management

5. Several standards pose greater challenges for occupational health facilities. Which of the following is relatively easy?

A. Clinical records
B. Occupational health standards
C. Quality management and improvement
D. Facilities and environment

11

Health and Productivity

OBJECTIVES

- Describe relationships between worker health and worker productivity
- Understand the occupational physician's role in health promotion and productivity
- Discuss components of worker productivity: absenteeism, presenteeism, quality of work, safety, and health
- Define the Worker's Productivity Index (WPI)
- Discuss how health problems such as allergies, arthritis, asthma, diabetes, mental disorders, influenza, and so forth affect health and worker productivity

OUTLINE

KEY POINTS

- Health has a significant impact on an employee's productivity. In this emerging field, a major challenge has been to develop tools, metrics, and methodology to measure employee performance. Employers and occupational medicine providers realize that promoting and maintaining a healthy workforce facilitates higher levels of productivity. This has both a direct and indirect effect on the financial success of an organization.

- Time off the job is the most commonly accepted measure of worker productivity. Lost workdays resulting from health-related problems are indirect costs to corporations and to society that are largely unmeasured. *Absenteeism* is the label attached to time off the job. Absenteeism and disability costs contribute significantly to an incomplete estimate of the total loss of productivity. This may vary with how absenteeism is defined by the employer [e.g., not only as sick days, but also short- and long-term disability, Family Medical Leave Act (FMLA), unpaid leaves, jury duty, military leave, etc.].

- *Presenteeism* is the amount of work accomplished while on the job or the output per unit of time. It is the decrease in performance that results by remaining at work while impaired by health problems or risk factors. Presenteeism can be measured in terms of costs associated with slowed output, production standards, errors, and additional training time. Health problems have a varying impact on the worker's presenteeism. These measurements depend on distinct job classifications and are developed within a corporation.

- Quality of work is an important contributor to the total value of the output of work. Customer satisfaction can be an outcome measure of quality, including delivery time and number of errors.

- Work-related disability from injuries or illnesses is minimized when safety and health are priorities within an organization. Participating in health promotion programs and job safety training has lowered not only accident rates, but also workers' compensation claims. Xerox Corporation noted that 85% of their workers' compensation costs could be related to excess health risks. Substantial indirect costs of work-related disability are related to recruitment, retention, and turnover of employees.

- In 2000, the Bureau of Labor and Statistics reported that 1.7 million injuries and illnesses in private industry required time away from work. In 1999, the National Safety Council estimated the total annual cost of occupational injuries at $125 billion: $62 billion for wage and productivity losses, $19.9 billion in medical costs, $25.6 billion in administrative expenses, and $16.7 billion in other employer costs.

- Healthy People 2010 has established a goal of reducing work-related injuries to 4.6 per 100 full-time workers. The Occupational Safety and Health Administration (OSHA) lost time recordable injuries/illnesses data are available for most industries and can be expressed as the number of cases per 200,000 hours worked, which is the number of events per 100 employees per year. Identification of workplace hazards, early provision of appropriate medical services, and flexible return-to-work policies are included in effective management of work-related illnesses or injuries. Other important components of total corporate health and productivity programs are safety training programs, regulatory compliance, and case management of workers' compensation benefits. Overall these programs prove beneficial to both the employee and employer.

- The WPI, an objective measure of productivity, was developed to measure the productivity of customer service call center operators. A credit card company employed call operators to answer customer questions. A computer was programmed to record data elements of the calls: waiting time, length of call, time between calls doing paper work, and time logged off. The information was analyzed to determine the performance goals among employees with similar call center tasks. A WPI was calculated using the algorithms derived from the employee's presenteeism together with absenteeism and short-term disability absence.

- Questionnaires are another objective productivity measure used by employers. These are helpful in jobs that involve tasks in which data are not readily available. Such objective measures are important to validate self-reported presenteeism. Several questionnaires are available. It is important to recognize the strengths and weaknesses of some of the more commonly used questionnaires: Endicott Work Productivity Scale (EWPS), Health and Labor Questionnaire (HLQ), MacArthur Health and Performance Questionnaire (MHPQ), Quality of Life SF-36, Stanford/American Health Association Presenteeism Scale (SAHAPS), Work Limitations Questionnaire (WLQ), and Work Productivity and Activity Impairment Questionnaire (WPAI).
- Calculating the cost of replacing workers is critical to understanding the implication of lost productivity. The lost wages method is the number of hours per days absent times the rate of compensation. A better metric is to include both direct and indirect costs or total compensation.
- Health risk appraisals for preventive services raise the employee's awareness about his or her health status. A wealth of information shows that healthy behaviors lower risk factors, lower absenteeism, decrease short-term disability, and increase productivity. Figure 11.2 in the textbook indicates that disease management, screening, preventive services, and risk reduction programs can be effective. Figure 11.3 in the textbook shows the impact of the risk factors on illness days and short-term disability. The same risk factors that are precursors for disease impact hours of lost productivity: smoking, stress, hypertension, high body mass index (BMI), and so forth.
- Chronic conditions account for significant medical disability and lost productivity costs for corporations. There is a dose-response relationship between the number of chronic medical conditions and the probability of any work impairment.
- There is a positive relationship between the health of a country's population and its per capita income. Primary costs of health care are diseases such as heart disease, cancer, diabetes, and stroke. However, the diseases involved in lowering productivity are relatively low cost in health care, such as arthritis, asthma, digestive disorders, headaches, flu, stress, and back pain.
- Mental health conditions including depression are often unrecognized causes of low productivity and lost workdays. Arthritis is the leading cause of disability. Allergies and headaches affect productivity more than absenteeism. Lost workdays resulting from diabetes have declined since 1997 with education, worksite wellness programs, and improved treatment. Vaccination against influenza has decreased the potential impact of absenteeism. Gastrointestinal disorders, in general, are associated with lower productivity but can be improved with treatment for gastroesophageal reflux disease (GERD) and irritable bowel syndrome (IBS).
- The role of the corporate medical director in managing worker productivity has both direct and indirect effects on worker health and overall corporate financial success. Maintaining health and safety; defining modified duty positions; supporting wellness programs; and providing access to timely, quality health care are ways that corporate medical directors have an impact on employee health and productivity.

QUESTIONS

1. Measurement of worker health and productivity include(s) which of the following?

A. Time off the job or lost workdays
B. Decreased productivity in unhealthy workers

C. Quality of work and customer satisfaction
D. Amount of work performed on the job per unit time
E. All of the above

2. *Which of the following does **not** describe costs involved with decreased productivity?*

A. There are both direct and indirect costs.
B. Charges for medical and pharmacy are direct costs.
C. Long- and short-term disability are indirect costs.
D. Cost of wellness programs and health screening appraisals.
E. Absenteeism or time off the job may require replacing the employee with someone less effective.

3. *Which of the following best describes the component of worker productivity known as presenteeism?*

A. White collar employees' work remains at their desks until they return from time off.
B. Presenteeism is the amount of work accomplished while on the job per unit of time.
C. It is the most commonly accepted measure of worker productivity.
D. It is not measured by self-reported or objective factors such as error rate, slowed output, or low quality.
E. Comorbid health conditions do not affect presenteeism.

4. *Which of the following is **least correct** in attracting and retaining employees?*

A. Competitive salary and benefit packages are important.
B. Corporate interest in employee health and well-being encourages retention.
C. Competition by companies for qualified workers during periods of high employment is important.
D. Substantial indirect costs occur when recruiting workers.
E. Investigating causes of turnover rates is not within the scope of retaining qualified workers.

5. *Which one of the following statements is most correct?*

A. Healthy People 2010 has a goal of promoting wellness and is not focused on reducing work-related time off.
B. OSHA recordable data is expressed as cases per 1,000 hours worked, which is the number of events per 100 employees working for 1 month.
C. Transitional return-to-work from a work-related injury can benefit both the worker and the employer.
D. Questionnaires are never used in measuring worker productivity because of the subjective aspects of self-reporting.
E. WPI measures the number of job-specific tasks completed per unit time.

12

Health Promotion

OBJECTIVES

- List benefits of health promotion programs to the employer
- Explain types of programs that may be included
- Identify methods used to determine the effectiveness of such programs

OUTLINE

I. Overview
II. Rationale and justification for worksite health promotion
    A. Health care costs
    B. Absenteeism
    C. Health outcomes
    D. Attitudes toward health and the company
III. A Systematic planning process—getting started and starting over
    A. Establishing the vision, mission, and goals
    B. Data collection
IV. Scope of programs for health promotion
    A. Preventive screenings and examinations
    B. Smoking cessation
    C. Fitness and aerobics
    D. Eating habits/nutrition/cholesterol
    E. Weight management
    F. Blood pressure control
    F. Stress management
    G. Employee assistance
    H. Demand management
    I. Disease management
V. Environmental and organizational interventions
VI. Other programs of interest
VII. Implementation options: what works and what doesn't
    A. The target audience
    B. Program resources
    C. Program logistics
VIII. Evaluating the effectiveness of health promotion
    A. General characteristics
    B. Specific program evaluation considerations
IX. The future—facing the challenges and opportunities

KEY POINTS

- Health promotion is the science and art of helping people change their lifestyle to move to an optimal state of health.
- The scope of health promotion practice today has evolved and strives to change physical, social, and normative environments.
- Health promotion is now central to worksite programming and is recognized as an integral part of occupational health practice.
- The National Health Promotion Survey (see reference in the textbook), conducted by the Office of Disease Prevention and Health Promotion, concluded that 90% of worksites with 50 or more employees offer at least one health promotion activity compared with 81% of worksites in 1992 and 65% in 1985.
- Employers hope that these programs will help to manage health care costs, affect absenteeism, improve productivity, improve employee morale, recruit and retain employees, enhance corporate image, and contribute to the health and well-being of their human resources.
- There is now a compelling body of evidence indicating that there are positive results from health promotion activities, thereby providing substantive rationale to invest in programming.
- Numerous studies have documented lower absenteeism and health care costs for participants of health promotion programs.
- Appropriate health promotion programs depend on the characteristics of the employee population coupled with the goals of both the program and the business.
- At the outset of planning, a clear description of the expectations of the health promotion program is essential.
- There are numerous sources of data that are helpful in the development of health promotion activities and in the measurement of program impact. These include employee assessments, management interviews, health care cost data, and information from health risk assessments. Program participation and employee satisfaction can also be analyzed.
- Some popular programs offered in the business setting include: preventive screenings and examinations, smoking cessation, exercise and aerobics, eating habits/nutrition/cholesterol, weight management, blood pressure control, stress management, employee assistance, demand management, disease management, environmental and organizational interventions, and other programs of interest.
- Biologic screenings and preventive examinations (such as cancer or high blood pressure checks) are central to early detection of disease and, thereby, to prevention efforts. No screening is complete without appropriate follow-up
- Smoking is the single lifestyle behavior that has the greatest impact on health. There are 430,000 tobacco-related deaths each year, with associated medical care costs of $50 billion. It remains the single most important preventable cause of death in our society.
- Sixty percent of U.S. adults are inactive or underactive, making the prevalence for inactivity more than twice that of smoking. The more that this country is faced with a decline in physical activity, the more evidence there is that physical activity has proven health benefits.
- The goal of a fitness and aerobics component is to improve cardiovascular fitness, increase strength, and improve flexibility. The psychosocial benefits and improved morale, attitude, and productivity also cannot be overlooked.

- Approximately one in two U.S. adults is overweight or obese, representing a 25% increase over the past three decades. Increased severity of obesity is specifically associated with high risk for and prevalence of hypertension, type II and gestational diabetes, cardiovascular disease, gallbladder disease, osteoporosis, high birthweight babies, and certain cancers.
- Hypertension treatment and education programs in the workplace have been shown to be more effective in achieving compliance and reduction of health care costs than treatment by any other type of community-based program.
- Effective stress management techniques can improve employees' ability to cope with stress, improve their sense of well-being, and reduce the likelihood of stress-related symptoms.
- Problems from alcohol abuse and various types of psychiatric disorders (e.g., depression) are common. Employee assistance programs have emerged as a viable strategy for early detection, short-term counseling, appropriate referral, and follow-up.
- Demand management attempts to control medical care costs by enhancing the participant's sense of responsibility for his or her own health and health care decisions to reduce unnecessary use, encourage appropriate treatment decisions, eliminate delays in seeking appropriate medical care, and reduce the severity and discomfort of symptoms.
- Disease management interventions are designed to support the needs of employees at the point along the health continuum where they have been diagnosed with and are living with a chronic disease, to prevent progression and complications of the disease, and to help individuals maintain optimal quality of life.
- Worksite health professionals are urged to work with management to incorporate a "culture of health" in the workplace and to investigate workplace practices that have an impact on employee health and well-being.
- Process evaluation measures the participant's perception of the program. A logical indicator of program success is participation numbers and percentages. Impact evaluation measures the extent to which an intervention has had an immediate effect on biometric measures and risk factors. Outcome evaluation determines the effect of interventions on the company or employee population as a whole.
- Current best practices for worksite health promotion programs include those in which: (a) program plans are linked to organizational business strategy; (b) there are effective communication strategies applied; (c) effective (positive) incentives are offered; (d) evaluation is conducted, results shared, and value of results communicated; (e) the environment is health supporting; and (f) there is strong executive support.

QUESTIONS

*1. Which of the following statements regarding worksite health promotion is **not** correct?*

A. They are central to worksite programming and recognized as an integral part of occupational health practice.
B. They can reduce the medical costs for employees.
C. They help control absenteeism.
D. They are mandated by the federal government for companies with 50 or more employees.
E. They are offered currently in 90% of worksites with 50 or more employees.

2. *Which of the following is most correct about a modern comprehensive workplace health promotion program?*

A. An appropriate program depends on the characteristics of the employee population coupled with the goals of both the program and the business.
B. It will narrowly target one or two easily measurable outcomes.
C. There is no compelling evidence to demonstrate positive results from such activities.
D. Wellness programs for executives should have highest priority because a healthy management is likely to encourage a healthy work environment.
E. Company management should treat grassroots efforts to promote wellness with "benign neglect."

3. *Which of the following is **least** important in the design of an effective worksite health promotion program?*

A. Screening for common diseases in the employee population
B. Providing management with a series of lectures that review all major health risks
C. Understanding the social makeup of the employee population, including awareness of the ethnic groups, social class, and cultural backgrounds of the employees
D. Having the employees complete baseline and interval health risk appraisals
E. Interviewing management regarding their concerns about employee health behaviors

4. *Which of the following is **least** likely to be included in a worksite health promotion programs?*

A. Cholesterol screening
B. Smoking cessation programs
C. Treatment for drug abuse
D. Disease management interventions
E. Stress management classes

5. *Which of the following statements is **least consistent** with optimal evaluation of worksite health promotion programs?*

A. Process evaluations should be used to measure a participant's perception.
B. Impact evaluation should be conducted to measure the extent to which an intervention has had an immediate effect on biometric measures and risk factors.
C. Outcome evaluation is necessary to determine the effect of interventions on the company or employee population as a whole.
D. Program evaluation is ideally designed after the health promotion program has been in place for a year.
E. Current best practices for worksite health promotion programs include the use of evaluation, and the results should be shared in the workplace.

13

Principles of Travel Medicine

OBJECTIVES

- Discuss the importance of preventing, recognizing, and treating travel-related illnesses and injuries
- Understand the risks associated with international travel
- List common medical problems associated with travel
- Discuss the importance of vaccine use in travelers and understand the terms *routine, recommended,* and *required* in relation to vaccinations
- Understand the importance of malaria prevention through the use of appropriate medications

OUTLINE

XI. Screening the returning traveler
XII. Specific problems in the returning traveler
    A. Fever
    B. Gastrointestinal problems
    C. Dermatologic problems
    D. Psychologic problems

KEY POINTS

- In 2000, it is estimated that approximately 700 million people traveled internationally.
- International travelers are at risk of injuries and illnesses related to environmental conditions and infectious agents.
- Educating travelers should include discussions about food and water risks in the developing world and motor vehicle safety.
- Acute barotitis media is caused by negative pressure in the middle ear and may be associated with eustachian tube dysfunction, allergy symptoms, or upper respiratory infections.
- DVT and associated pulmonary embolism is a risk factor of travel, especially extended flying. Predisposing factors for DVT include age older than 40 years, pregnancy, blood disorders, altered blood clotting, personal or family history of DVT, recent surgery, and estrogen therapy.
- TD is extremely common. Approximately 40% of travelers to the developing world experience TD.
- Travelers should be advised to carry a medical kit, especially if traveling to the developing world. Travelers should also be advised to use caution if seeking medical care in certain parts of the world.
- Avoiding insect bites while traveling is important. Use of protective clothing and mosquito netting should be considered, as well as the use of insect repellants containing permethrin and DEET.
- Caution in extremes of temperature or altitude should be used. At altitudes above 10,000 feet, there is increased risk of acute mountain sickness (AMS), high-altitude pulmonary edema (HAPE), and high-altitude cerebral edema (HACE). Travelers should avoid overexposure to UV radiation.
- Use of appropriate vaccinations in the international traveler is important. In addition to geographic destination, other factors to consider include age, state of health, use of medications, country of origin, and prior history of vaccination.
- Chemoprophylaxis for malaria should be considered if the traveler enters a country of risk. The choice of medication depends on the region, potential patterns of resistance, and individual needs of the traveler.
- After travel, it is important to evaluate the health of the traveler, especially when fever or gastrointestinal problems occur following travel.

QUESTIONS

*1. In preparation for prolonged travel to a developing country, the physician should routinely recommend all of the following interventions **except**:*

A. The traveler should be advised about food and water sanitation precautions.
B. The traveler should have a tetanus/diphtheria immunization updated every 10 years.

C. The traveler should receive Bacille Calmette-Guérin (BCG) before travel.

D. Unvaccinated adults should receive inactivated polio vaccine (IPV).

2. *Yellow fever disease risk is present in all the following areas **except:***

A. Central America

B. Southeast Asia

C. Sub-Saharan Africa

D. South America

3. *Which malaria species accounts for most malaria-related mortality?*

A. *Plasmodium vivax*

B. *Plasmodium falciparum*

C. *Plasmodium ovale*

D. *Plasmodium malariae*

4. *Travelers to areas with chloroquine-resistant malaria can be given chemoprophylaxis with all the following medications **except:***

A. Doxycycline (Vibramycin)

B. Atovaquone/proguanil (Malarone)

C. Mefloquine (Lariam)

D. Dicloxacillin (Dynapen)

5. *All of the following infections are associated with contaminated food or water **except:***

A. Hepatitis B

B. Typhoid fever

C. Enterotoxigenic *Escherichia coli*

D. Hepatitis A

6. *Which one of the following infections is not transmitted by insects?*

A. Yellow fever

B. Malaria

C. Polio

D. Japanese encephalitis

=14=
Economics of Occupational Medicine

OBJECTIVES

- Explain how occupational health services can support an organization
- List the traditional occupational medical services
- List newer occupational services that may support an organization
- Explain the impact of lifestyle on health and costs
- Describe how occupational health services can be consistent with and support the mission, goals, and objectives of an organization
- Explain how to evaluate the economic benefits of occupational health services and how to communicate these benefits effectively to management

OUTLINE

I. "Traditional" occupational medical services
   A. Preplacement, surveillance, and return-to-work examinations
   B. Medical surveillance
   C. Immunization
   D. Treatment of job-related injuries and illnesses
   E. Rehabilitation and return to work
   F. Consulting activities
   G. Industrial hygiene consultation
II. Newer occupational services
   A. Employee assistance programs (EAPs)
   B. Transitional work
   C. Onsite management of nonoccupational illness and injuries
   D. Chronic disease management
   E. Self-care and wise use of counseling education
   F. Case and disease management
III. Health promotion at the worksite
   A. Impact of lifestyle on health and costs
   B. Effects of health promotion efforts
   C. Screening to promote health
IV. Medical benefits quality and cost management
   A. Benefit design consultation
   B. Utilization management: the gatekeeper concept
   C. Changes in economic incentives

KEY POINTS

- Occupational health programs (OHPs) can play an important role in support of the organizations that they serve by preserving and enhancing the health and productivity of the workforce. The mission, goals, and objectives of the OHP should be congruent with and support the mission, goals, and objectives of the organization. It is important to quantify the benefits provided to the organization, its employees, and their dependents; to match resource needs with benefits provided; and to focus the operations of the OHP. Some occupational physicians have become involved in benefits redesign and in medical management of employee and dependent general health care.

- Adverse health effects from the workplace should be prevented by medical surveillance and control of hazardous exposures. Strategic health management activities can also reduce morbidity, mortality, and disability caused by a number of diseases through informed comanagement by the patient and health professionals. The economic benefits of any of these activities can be evaluated along a number of dimensions, including direct, indirect, and intangible costs.

- Traditional occupational medical services may include preplacement and return-to-work examinations, medical surveillance activities, immunizations, and the treatment of job-related injuries and illnesses. In addition to providing treatment, the occupational medicine physician acts as the medical liaison with the private medical community. Other activities may include rehabilitation services, consulting activities, and industrial hygiene consultation. The key to these activities has been negotiating and assisting with job accommodation for those who have some degree of medical impairment and ensuring quality care for those who have a variety of illnesses, injuries, and medically related impairments.

- The traditional cornerstone of clinical OHPs is the determination of the ability of an applicant or employee to safely perform the essential functions of a job. The Americans with Disabilities Act (ADA) has changed the approach to these examinations to some extent. Under the ADA, a thorough attempt must be made to reasonably accommodate the applicant or employee if the person can perform the *essential*, or key, job functions with accommodation. A number of the actions taken under the impetus of reasonable accommodation actually have made jobs safer for all employees.

- In evaluating the economic effects of medical screening and placement programs, one would balance the cost of the program against decreases in real or projected cost of work-related illness or injuries. All direct and indirect costs, including medical treatment, time lost from work, supervisory time, and other attributable costs, should be included to obtain a proper analysis. Failure to place employees appropriately using essential job function comparison and cost-benefit analysis may result in preventable costs for replacement and retraining, inefficiency, medical treatment, workers' compensation payments, fines under the ADA, actions under the Vocational Rehabilitation Act of 1974 or various state laws, and lost wages.

- A key duty of the occupational health professional is to monitor health-related data on members of the workforce exposed to chemical, radiation, and other physical hazards and to compare the values for exposed and unexposed groups periodically. If an increased prevalence of abnormal laboratory values or symptoms is detected in an exposed group, the exposure should be quantified and controlled through engineering measures, administrative efforts (i.e., rotating employees), or personal protective equipment in that order. The economic value of this type of service depends on the cost of the disease avoided, which can be computed for a population of workers if the probability of illness is known for various levels of exposure. There are many examples of preventable occupationally related complaints or diseases that ultimately have caused great expense including cases of back, upper extremity, and other muscle and tendon pain. Consistent monitoring and changes in job structure are important modes to prevent the occurrence or worsening of these health complaints and disorders.

- Immunization can be instituted to prevent occupational transmission of infectious disease, as in hepatitis B immunization of workers in health care facilities, prisons, and sanitation industries. Immunization of workers against tetanus will prevent many visits to medical facilities for prophylaxis of minor wounds. Diphtheria, influenza, and other routine immunizations will prevent considerable lost work time.

- Treatment of injuries and illnesses onsite can be cost effective for a variety of reasons. Time lost to travel to a health facility and to wait for treatment is avoided. Physicians and nurses who are familiar with the work environment usually have a better understanding of the toxicity of substances used; individual workers' backgrounds, attitudes, and risks; and factors involved in injuries that may complicate the recovery process. When onsite treatment is not feasible, community-based occupational health services can also save time by prompt treatment and effective management of work-related injuries. Knowledge of the job is critical for appropriate placement of workers returning to work following an illness or injury. There are physical, mental, and economic advantages from early return to work.

- Beyond the clinically based activities of placement, treatment, medical management, and rehabilitation, occupational health professionals often serve as internal consultants to an organization in areas of industrial hygiene, job modification, employee assistance, and other special problems. Occupational health practitioners have the opportunity to prevent illnesses and injuries caused by chemical and physical hazards at the worksite in several ways. They can advise managers about the presence, nature, and magnitude of hazards. They can also evaluate the adequacy of barriers and procedures intended to protect employees from exposure, both by inspection and by epidemiologic surveillance of the workforce. The occupational physician should work closely with the industrial hygienist if one is available. Intangible effects of control measures include avoidance of liability for delayed or negligently caused health problems, and enhanced public image.

- Newer occupational medical services include EAPs, transitional work, onsite management of non-work-related health problems, assistance with the management of chronic disease, self-care instruction and counseling, and case management services. In addition, worksite health promotion programs are increasingly common.

- A small group of employees at most worksites use significantly more medical services than other employees and are absent a great deal because of somatization of psychologic conflicts. Resolution of these somatization disorders by providing cognitive services has resulted in benefit-cost ratios of up to 10:1. EAPs also provide savings by early intervention in mental health problems, which can prevent hospitalization and long-term illness.

- Injury and reinjury in taxing jobs can be prevented by gradually increasing workload or time at the job. This is termed *transitional work*. The value obtained from reconditioning workers appears to significantly outweigh the cost of professional time and lost production. It is clear that onsite transitional duty is much less expensive and more supportive of reintegration than extensive simulated work conditioning and work hardening performed by clinics off-site.

- Many employers, especially those who are self-insured, have noted the advantages of providing comprehensive health care for both occupational and nonoccupational illnesses and injuries at the worksite. Advantages include earlier treatment with reduced morbidity, better health supervision, ready access to practitioners who understand the work environment, and lower unit cost. Management or comanagement of certain conditions such as hypercholesterolemia, diabetes, asthma, coronary artery disease, and hypertension may be more effective at the worksite, primarily because of ease of access to medical care, close follow-up, and coordination with managing physicians.
- Education of patients in self-care for minor illnesses and injuries has reduced health care costs. Educating employees in the best way to use the medical care system has resulted in increases in the quality of care and substantial decreases in inappropriate utilization.
- Case management of both chronic diseases and catastrophic and complex cases can have a significant effect on total costs. Close management of seriously ill, injured, or chronically ill employees or those undergoing treatment is valuable to avoid unnecessary procedures, ensure appropriate therapy, and aid in proper discharge planning and early return to work. Costs for lifestyle-related problems have been estimated at 10 to 15 times as much as for work-related illness and injuries.
- There is evidence from both epidemiologic studies and clinical trials to show that morbidity and mortality are reduced if risk factors are decreased. Studies on the net cost effectiveness of health promotion programs demonstrate a significant positive benefit-to-cost ratio. Although much of the risk screening done today is nonproductive, early detection of hypertension, hypercholesterolemia, and cervical and breast cancer has a significant benefit-to-cost ratio. In asymptomatic individuals, other tests, such as chest and back films, multichannel chemistries, and resting and stress electrocardiograms, are of minimal value and may result in unnecessary costs involved in ruling out false positives.
- Astute occupational medicine physicians can be of great value to a company's benefits organization by recommending appropriate medical services to be covered (including preventive services) and reimbursement schemes that discourage the use of medically unnecessary services. Occupational medicine physicians can assist benefits managers in selecting among various approaches to utilization management, such as use of a gatekeeper to authorize hospitalizations and certain procedures, redesign of benefits plans to discourage inappropriate utilization, and capitated payment systems to health care providers.

QUESTIONS

1. The determination of the ability of an individual to safely perform the essential functions of a job

A. Does not require consideration of work accommodation

B. Has indirectly made jobs safer for all employees by providing for reasonable accommodation under the ADA

C. Carries no liability risk

D. Does not reduce preventable costs
E. All of the above

2. *Failure to place employees appropriately using essential job function comparison and cost-benefit analysis may result in preventable costs for*

A. Replacement and retraining
B. Workers' compensation payments
C. Fines
D. Lost wages
E. All of the above

3. *If workplace medical surveillance efforts reveal an increased prevalence of abnormal laboratory values or symptoms among an exposed work population*

A. The exposure should be quantified and controlled through engineering measures, administrative efforts (i.e., rotating employees), or personal protective equipment in that order.
B. The exposure should be quantified and controlled through personal protective equipment, administrative efforts (i.e., rotating employees), or engineering measures in that order.
C. The affected workers should be terminated.
D. Medical surveillance efforts should cease, so that worsening problems would not be apparent in the event of an Occupational Safety and Health Administration (OSHA) inspection.
E. None of the above.

4. *Immunizations offered in the work setting*

A. Should be avoided because there are no occupationally related infectious diseases
B. Should be considered for health care workers who may sustain exposure to hepatitis B
C. May reduce lost workdays (e.g., influenza)
D. Could reduce costs associated with minor injury (e.g., tetanus)
E. B, C, and D

5. *Treatment of injuries and illnesses onsite can be cost effective because*

A. Doctors are not permitted to bill for these services.
B. It increases the time spent away from the work setting.
C. The employer is then permitted to authorize further evaluation and treatment.
D. Physicians familiar with the work environment usually have a better understanding of the toxicity of substances used and factors that may complicate the recovery process.
E. All of the above.

6. *Regarding the cost benefit of OHPs, all of the following statements are true **except***

A. EAPs can prevent hospitalization of employees with mental health problems by directing them to outpatient treatment that emphasizes early rehabilitation.

B. Placing an employee in a transitional work program that gradually increases the workload may prevent reinjury by allowing acclimation over time.

C. Education of patients and workers in self-care for minor illnesses and injuries has reduced health care costs.

D. Educating employees in the best way to use the medical care system has resulted in increases in the quality of care and substantial decreases in inappropriate utilization.

E. Employees who are off work for an extended period related to a work injury are more likely to return fully recovered.

7. *Which of the following risk screening approaches is **not** likely to demonstrate a favorable benefit-to-cost ratio?*

A. Early detection of hypertension
B. Identification of hypercholesterolemia
C. Annual electrocardiograms
D. Breast cancer screening
E. Cervical cancer screening

=15= *Not needed*

Educational Opportunities

OBJECTIVES

- Describe the role of occupational medicine in the provision of medical care
- Outline components of occupational medicine residency training programs
- List available training programs that can help primary care physicians improve their knowledge about occupational and environmental medicine (OEM)
- Describe other resources in OEM

OUTLINE

I. OEM and the physician-in-training
II. Need for physicians in OEM
    A. What is an OEM physician
III. Specialization and residency training programs
    A. Board certification and accredited training in occupational medicine
    B. Two pathways to specialty certification in OEM
    C. Traditional residency training programs for OEM
    D. Nontraditional academic year training
    E. Nontraditional practicum year training
IV. Continuing medical education (CME) and related educational resources
    A. Professional societies
    B. Education and research centers
    C. Schools of public health
    D. Federal and state agencies
    E. Journals and computer databases
    F. Books and other reference materials
V. Conclusions
VI. References

KEY POINTS

- Each week, thousands of workers ask physicians for advice about fitness for job duties or work-relatedness of symptoms.
- In the United States, OEM remains a field in which most practitioners do not have formal training because most medical schools have little curricula or faculty with expertise in OEM.

- The Institute of Medicine (IOM) has estimated a shortage of 3,100 to 5,500 physicians with special competence in OEM, and has recommended that all primary care physicians be able to identify possible occupationally or environmentally induced conditions and make appropriate referrals for follow-up.
- OEM is a specialty that focuses on prevention of illness and injury. The OEM physician deals primarily with a healthy workforce and often focuses on medical surveillance of workers to identify potentially hazardous exposures at a stage when disease can be prevented.
- A reference set of competencies for OEM has been defined and published by the American College of Occupational and Environmental Medicine (ACOEM) (*http://www. acoem.org/oem/oem.asp*).
- The American Board of Preventive Medicine (ABPM) administers board certification in occupational medicine. Pathways for eligibility to sit for the certifying examination include completion of an accredited residency in occupational medicine followed by a period of relevant practice experience or an alternative pathway that requires, in addition to specific medical training, successful completion of graduate-level courses in biostatistics, epidemiology, health services administration, and environmental health. Requirements for board certification are periodically revised.
- The Residency Review Committee (RRC) of the Accreditation Council for Graduate Medical Education (ACGME) provides oversight and accreditation for occupational medicine residency training programs.
- Distance learning techniques currently allow academic and didactic material to be learned off-campus. In addition, innovative practicum year training experiences have been developed to help physicians with a midcareer shift into OEM.
- Several CME programs are available from a variety of sources. The National Institute for Occupational Safety and Health (NIOSH) has established Educational Resource Centers (ERCs) to provide multidisciplinary educational resources in occupational health. They have also created a comprehensive curriculum for use by primary care residency training programs to teach the fundamentals of OEM to nonspecialists.
- ACOEM sponsors seminars and courses related to the specialty. These programs are offered each spring and fall in conjunction with national meetings.

QUESTIONS

1. The IOM has recommended that "all primary care physicians be able to identify possible occupationally or environmentally induced conditions and make appropriate referrals for follow-up." Which of the following would be helpful to meet this goal?

A. Integration of occupational medicine into the medical school curricula
B. Availability of faculty with expertise in OEM
C. Regular inclusion of an occupational history by physicians-in-training
D. Review of federal regulations concerning blood-borne pathogens
E. All of the above

2. ACGME requires some element of occupational medical training in which of the following residencies?

A. Orthopedic surgery
B. Family practice

C. Dermatology
D. Obstetrics
E. None of the above

3. Which of the following statements regarding the specialty of OEM is most correct?

A. It is a specialty that focuses on treatment of disease and minor injury.
B. A major aspect of practice in this specialty is observing employees at the worksite.
C. Company management determines much of injury treatment.
D. The majority of an occupational physician's patient population is injured.
E. The possession of excellent clinical skills is all that a physician needs to deliver competent services.

4. Which of the following statements regarding residency training of OEM physicians is most correct?

A. There is a slight excess of residency-trained occupational medicine physicians in the United States.
B. ACGME provides oversight and accreditation for in-hospital residency programs but does not provide accreditation for OEM residency programs.
C. In the United States, approximately 75 to 100 OEM residents graduate each year.
D. OEM residency training consists entirely of classroom didactic study of such subjects as epidemiology, biostatistics, and health services administration.
E. OEM residency programs consist of 3 years of clinical work, which is divided approximately evenly among large corporation medical departments, hospital occupational health departments, state health departments, and free-standing occupational health clinics.

5. Which of the following statements is most correct?

A. NIOSH-funded ERCs only provide training programs designed for safety professionals and industrial hygienists.
B. Schools of public health offer courses in biostatistics and epidemiology, but these offer little insight into OEM issues.
C. Postgraduate courses offered by the ACOEM are available only to members.
D. ACOEM's basic curriculum provides nonoccupational medicine specialists with a useful overview of occupational medicine topics.
E. Occupational medicine is too small a specialty to provide much active participation in state medical societies.

====16====

Computers and Informatics in Occupational Medicine Practice

OBJECTIVES

- Explain how computers and informatics benefit the practice of occupational medicine
- Describe components of an occupational health information system (OHIS) and an integrated health data management system (IHDMS)
- Summarize the uses of the Internet within the practice of occupational medicine
- Describe guidelines for evaluation and selection of computer software
- Explain regulatory requirements and compliance issues using informatics

OUTLINE

I. Introduction and types of informatics systems
II. Benefits of computerization and applications
   A. Advantages of automation
      1. Improved efficiency, accuracy, and productivity
      2. Enhanced quality, decision making, and documentation
      3. Regulatory compliance and litigation assistance
      4. Provisions for supplemental services
III. OHISs
   A. Evolution of OHISs
      1. First generation—mainframe systems
      2. Second generation—minicomputer systems
      3. Third generation—microcomputer systems
      4. Fourth generation—Internet-connected or Web-based
   B. Using the Internet and databases to deliver highly customized occupational health (OH) services
   C. Managed care and the growth of practice guidelines
   D. IHDMS
   E. Establishing an OHIS/IHDMS—practical guidelines
   F. Components of an OHIS/IHDMS
IV. Currently available software
V. Practical guidelines for evaluating, selecting, and/or developing software
   A. Evaluating and selecting software
   B. Working with a software vendor
VI. Future directions for OH information management technology

    A. Legal climate and regulation
      1. Food and Drug Administration (FDA) regulation of medical software
      2. Reasonable accommodation under Americans with Disabilities Act (ADA)
      3. The Health Insurance Portability and Accountability Act of 1996 (HIPAA)
    B. Computer hardware
    C. Software
    D. Networks and servers
    E. Information access
    F. Connectivity
    G. Summary

KEY POINTS

- Informatics (i.e., the use of computers, automated data, the Internet, telecommunications, etc.) is common in today's occupational medicine practice.
- There are three types of informatics: (a) office automation; (b) health applications, including OHIS and IHDMS; and (c) information databases through compact disks (CDs) or the Internet.
- Informatics is quickly becoming an essential management tool in all aspects of OH. Informatics can significantly improve an organization's ability to achieve its goals through (a) improved efficiency, accuracy, and productivity; (b) enhanced quality, decision making, and documentation; (c) regulatory compliance and litigation assistance; and (d) the ability to inexpensively create supplemental and new services, such as Web sites customized to meet highly specific client and employee needs.
- OHIS have paralleled the evolution of computer systems. This evolution has progressed from room-filling first-generation mainframe programs; second-generation minicomputer systems; third-generation desktop computers (that interface to modems, scanners, and medical testing equipment) to today's Internet or Web-based systems.
- The Internet can be used to deliver client- or patient-specific customized services by fostering a 24 hours per day, 7 days per week (24/7) one-on-one relationship with the client or patient. Examples include the homebound injured worker's access to resources that speed recovery and return to work.
- Contemporary case management systems contribute to quality improvement and cost-containment initiatives. These case management systems can feature disability duration guidelines, medical protocols, and sophisticated scheduling and follow-up programs.
- Implementation of IHDMS can prevent unnecessary duplication of effort, foster coordination among units, assist in regulatory compliance, and provide a clearer picture of a company's health expenditures and priorities.
- Some components of an OHIS may include
  1. Automation of office work
  2. Maintenance of updated personnel information
  3. Benefits information
  4. Work history and job tracking
  5. Functional job requirements
  6. Work restrictions
  7. Appointment scheduling
  8. Regulatory requirements
  9. Medical record keeping and retrieval
 10. Health history

11. Medical examination results
12. Medical problems, treatments and disease coding
13. Injury monitoring and management
14. Case management and disability management
15. Ergonomics and health promotion
16. Drug and alcohol testing
17. Employee assistance programs (EAPs)
18. Medical surveillance
19. Exposure monitoring
20. Chemical inventory
21. Toxicology data
22. Safety and training
23. Financial and administrative information
24. Analytic and reporting
25. Epidemiologic and statistical analysis
26. Linkages to other systems and databases

- OHISs are now linked to regulatory requirements such as Occupational Safety and Health Administration (OSHA), ADA, and HIPAA.
- Regulatory requirements from HIPAA virtually require informatics to track the flow of confidential information within an organization, allow patients access to their own records, and maintain rigorous controls regarding data and medical records security.
- OHISs of the future will be based on networked personal computers that are linked to many internal databases, as well as Web-based databases of medical management and treatment guidelines.
- Connectivity to internal databases, peripheral medical equipment, and Web-based resources are mandated by the American National Standards Institute (ANSI) standard for Health Level Seven (HL7) that provides standards for information exchange.

QUESTIONS

*1. Benefits of an automated clinic management system for occupational medicine include all **except** which one of the following?*

A. Increased efficiency, productivity, and accuracy
B. Enhanced quality of care and decision making
C. Reduced office personnel costs
D. Regulatory compliance and litigation assistance
E. Provision of additional supplemental services

2. The practice of occupational medicine makes extensive use of Internet and Web-based databases. Which application would be improper in the clinical setting?

A. Providing the patient/client with highly individualized services with up-to-date databases
B. Offering the opportunity for one-on-one communication between the health care provider and the client on a 24/7 basis
C. Providing a secure means of communication between the patient and the doctor
D. Providing the "at home" patient with self-help and support information to help speed recovery and return to work

3. *The application of informatics to legal and regulatory functions of OH services can fully justify the cost and time commitments to select, install, train, and use these multicomponent systems. Before using them, which of the following must be ensured?*

A. Compliance with OSHA testing requirements
B. Compliance with HIPAA requirements
C. Compliance with FDA regulations
D. Compliance with ADA regulations

4. *There are many components of IHDMSs and OHISs to choose from. Which function from the following list is likely to be the most important component?*

A. Regulatory reporting assistance
B. Clinical decision-making and practice guidelines
C. Integration of OH data management, OH information, and office automation
D. Telecommunications via the Internet to Web-based information databases

International Occupational Medicine

OBJECTIVES

- Distinguish between traditional practice of occupational medicine (OM) and international practice
- Recognize differences between exposure in the international environment compared with those in developed nations
- Identify unique exposure risks for waste handlers
- List global issues in international OM

OUTLINE

I. Introduction
II. Health risks related to occupation
   A. Occupational risks of waste handlers
   B. Susceptibility
   C. Occupational hygiene/industrial hygiene in the international setting
III. Global occupational issues
IV. International health programs
V. Expatriate health

KEY POINTS

- Instead of being responsible only for injuries or illnesses resulting from workplace risks, as in the United States, international practice may include health care of employees and families for all medical problems. The international occupational physician must understand the national health system of the host country and provide appropriate support for national workers, managers, and expatriates.
- Health risks present in an international setting may be similar to the risks experienced in developed countries, but exposures may be quantitatively greater. Chemicals, minerals, and other substances (e.g., asbestos, pesticides, leaded gasoline, lignite coal, chlorinated hydrocarbons) that have significant economic value despite health risks are a major global issue.
- Biologic risks are of more serious concern. Although bacterial and viral diseases (malaria; hepatitis A, B, and C; and others) have been the traditional focus, the global impact of emerging infectious diseases such as prions and mad cow disease has been significant.
- Physical hazards (heat, humidity, cold, radiation, altitude, noise) are also global risks.

- Waste collection in developing countries is primitive. It requires lifting and unprotected waste handling. Exposure to infectious agents is constant. Workers have significant increases in diarrhea, respiratory diseases, and blood-borne diseases. Burning of wastes also increases particle exposures.
- Susceptibility of workers may be increased because of the use of child labor or migrant workers, warfare, and poverty.
- Occupational hygiene services may be unavailable because of a lack of equipment or laboratories. In the absence of quantitative exposure levels, hazard recognition is important.
- Standardization of medical surveillance, exposure limits, measurement systems, audit programs, policies, and procedures and regulations are major international challenges.
- In many countries, the OM program provides nonoccupational health care for expatriates, short-term assignees and visitors, managers, workers and their families, and, in some cases, extended families.
- Emergency transportation and evacuation plans must be outlined for victims of injury or illness in developing countries.
- Local procurement or importation of pharmaceuticals may be difficult. International transportation of prescription drugs by mail is generally illegal, and hand carrying of medications for workers and family members by other workers is often necessary. Some drugs that are legal in the United States may be illegal in other countries.

QUESTIONS

*1. Which of the following statements is **least** correct about international OM?*

A. International practice may include health care of employees and families for all medical problems.
B. Health risks present in an international setting may be similar to the risks experienced in developed countries, but exposures may be quantitatively greater.
C. Biologic risks are of little concern for the international worker.
D. LASER may not be regulated in developing nations.
E. Consideration of local government and culture is critical.

2. Which of the following factors contribute to enhanced disease risk in developing nations?

A. Child labor
B. Migrant workers
C. Impoverished workers
D. Populations in a war zone
E. All of the above

*3. Which of the following statements about international OM is **incorrect**?*

A. Occupational hygiene services are generally available.
B. There may be little standardization of medical surveillance, exposure limits, measurement systems, audit programs, policies, and procedures and regulations.
C. It is important to develop emergency transportation and evacuation plans for employees in developing countries.

D. The OM program may need to provide nonoccupational health care for expatriates, short-term assignees, visitors, managers, and workers and their families.
E. Preassignment health screening is critical for employees and for family members if they accompany the employee.

4. *With regard to prescription drug use in the international community, which of the following statements is **least correct**?*

A. Procurement of pharmaceuticals locally may be difficult.
B. International transportation of prescription medication by mail may be illegal.
C. It is rarely necessary for other workers to hand carry medications for workers and family members.
D. Some drugs that are legal in the United States may be illegal in other countries.
E. It is important to provide ample supplies of required medication before foreign assignment.

18

Workers' Compensation

OBJECTIVES

- Describe the evolution of modern workers' compensation in the United States
- Explain the structure and function of the workers' compensation system and the types of benefits available
- Describe trends in the rate of occupational illness and injury and in the costs associated with workers' compensation in the United States
- Describe incentives and disincentives relating to workers' compensation
- Outline the administrative roles for occupational health professionals and others in workers' compensation
- Describe clinical best practices in caring for ill or injured workers
- Describe best practices in managing impairment and functional recovery

OUTLINE

   I. Introduction
  II. The modern workers' compensation system
    A. Overview
    B. Evolution of workers' compensation laws
    C. Goals and objectives of workers' compensation
    D. Types of workers' compensation systems
    E. Coverage
    F. Benefits
    G. Adequacy of coverage and benefits
 III. Financial aspects
    A. Costs
    B. Insurance markets
    C. Financial condition of the workers' compensation insurance industry
    D. Incentives and disincentives
       1. Immediate versus delayed investment and rating
       2. Risk spreading and payment lags
       3. Perverse incentives within organizations
       4. Provider and patient incentives
       5. Legal factors
  IV. Epidemiology of death, illness, and injury
    A. Mortality
    B. Morbidity

KEY POINTS

- Before the development of workers' compensation in the United States, injured workers had to prove that their injuries were due to employer negligence, which resulted in a slow, costly, and uncertain legal process. As a defense, the employer could claim that the employee contributed to the injury, that he or she had assumed risk by taking the job, or that negligent acts of fellow workers were responsible for the injury.
- Injured workers did not receive timely compensation. As a result, a series of "no fault" workers' compensation laws were passed on a state-by-state basis. Workers' compensation laws represented a compromise or "lesser peril" for both employers and employees. These laws were supposed to ensure rapid payment to injured workers for lost wages and medical costs regardless of fault. In exchange, employers' liability for occupational injuries, illness, and death was limited if they participated in a compensation system. Under this system, employers generally were exempt from damage suits, unless gross negligence could be proved. Occupational disease laws were not passed until later for fear of liability because of the long latencies of disease. Compensation laws are elective or compulsory. Under an elective law, the employer may accept or reject the compensation act.

- The goals of workers' compensation systems are typically to prevent work-related illness and injury; to make injured workers whole physically, mentally, and/or economically; and to return workers to productive work in their original or, if necessary, some alternative capacity.
- All industrial and most service employment is covered by workers' compensation statutes; however, very small businesses, business owners, farm labor, domestic service, and casual employees are usually exempted from the laws.
- Railroad and merchant marine workers are generally not covered by state workers' compensation acts, but may seek damage under the Federal Employee Liability Act (FELA) or the Jones Act, respectively.
- Workers' compensation provides benefits for wage replacement, medical and legal expenses, and permanent impairment. The two traditional criteria for eligibility for workers' compensation benefits are termed *AOE/COE*—arising out of employment (AOE) and in the course of employment (COE). Most states limit compensation to two thirds of previous wages and cover all medical costs. For a variety of reasons, some employers have elected to offer benefits equivalent to or coordinated with their short-term disability programs, which typically fully replace wages. Because these payments are tax exempt, they actually exceed the value of the average weekly wage.
- Impairment is defined as a loss of or damage to a body part or function due to illness or injury, whereas disability is defined as the inability to perform a specific task based on the functional requirements of the job, education, social factors, and other issues in addition to the medical impairment. In fact, one can be impaired but not disabled. Generally, physicians determine impairment and personnel administrators or supervisors determine disability.
- When claims are contested, there are three fundamental provisions of all workers' compensation programs. First, the insurer or self-insured company is entitled to contest permanent disability claims and, in most cases, all claims. Second, state compensation boards or court systems adjudicate all contested claims. Third, the burden of proof is on the worker in any contested case.
- Several incentives and disincentives affect workers' compensation. One reason why workers' compensation costs have not led to an increased investment in loss control technology or prevention is that it is generally less expensive to buy insurance now than to install costly engineering controls. In many companies or nonprofit organizations, losses are not allocated back to the department in which they were incurred. This policy is an intracompany version of risk spreading that provides a disincentive to improvement and safety records. Furthermore, many managers have productivity incentives. Therefore, they prefer not to return employees to work on limited duty. This disincentive clearly prevents rapid return to work, which is associated with shorter recovery times and reduced payments. With reductions in group-health benefits, there has been a tendency to ascribe injuries to the worksite because workers' compensation will pay 100% of the medical bills and provide wage replacement. Because workers' compensation pays 100% of charges, there has been an apparent increase in cost shifting.
- Accidental work deaths per 100,000 population have dropped more than 83% from 1912 to 1999. Forty-three percent of work-related fatalities in the United States in 1999 were due to transportation incidents. The occupations with the highest relative risk are in construction.
- Ninety-three percent of the nonfatal occupational illness and injury cases were reported as injuries. Truck drivers had the highest rate in 1999. Grouped by mechanism, repeti-

tive motion cases had the longest median absence. According to Occupational Safety and Health Administration (OSHA) statistics, the back was the body part most commonly affected by disabling work incidents.

• Reasons for underreporting work injuries include fear of reprisal, a belief that pain is a normal consequence of aging or work, lack of management responsiveness to previous complaints, and a desire not to be moved to another job. Corporate safety objectives may have an indirect effect on reporting because managers attempt to reduce injury rates to meet goals.

• It is important for all participants in the workers' compensation system to understand each other's roles and responsibilities to have this conflict-prone system function more smoothly. Employers, employees, payers, regulators, and health care providers all have important roles to play.

• The physician or other health professional can play a pivotal role as diagnostician, medical expert on causation and evidence-based medicine, and care and disability manager. To do so, one must obtain a detailed health and work history, perform a careful and complete yet focused physical examination, and use analytic skills to make and explain the most effective recommendations at each stage of the care of the ill or injured worker.

• At a minimum, providers caring for workers with health concerns should provide excellent care and foster functional recovery. Doing so requires a broader and arguably more neutral approach than nonoccupational health care. In addition to diagnosing the problem and providing treatment, providers should take a complete occupational history to determine causation, understand the hazards that caused the problem to prevent further adverse effects, facilitate functional recovery using modified work and other proven effective methods, and dispassionately evaluate impairment at maximal medical improvement.

QUESTIONS

1. State and provincial workers' compensation systems are generally intended to

A. Reasonably "cure and relieve" adverse health effects of work
B. Mitigate the economic consequences of ill health caused by work
C. Provide benefits regardless of fault for work-related illnesses or injuries
D. Limit employers' liability for work-related illnesses or injuries
E. All of the above

2. Currently accepted employer defenses in workers' compensation cases include

A. The employee contributed to the injury.
B. The employee had assumed risk by taking the job.
C. Negligent acts of fellow workers were responsible for the injury.
D. The employee was not acting in the course of employment when injured.
E. The employee owns stock in the company and is, therefore, unable to pursue workers' compensation.

3. Disincentives for returning to work following an occupational health complaint include which of the following?

A. Dislike of the work climate or personnel

B. Wage replacement equal to preinjury wages net of taxes
C. Litigation in progress
D. Perceptions that the job causes pain
E. All of the above

4. *Barriers to return to work on modified duty might include all of the following **except***

A. Productivity incentives
B. Central funding of the costs of workers' compensation
C. Cost sharing of employee's pay between salary and workers' compensation
D. Insistence on being able to do all job tasks
E. Job dissatisfaction

5. *Which of these causes of occupational morbidity is **least** common?*

A. Low back pain
B. Hand and wrist discomfort
C. Head injuries
D. Neck pain
E. Internal derangement of the knee

6. *Reasons for underreporting of work-related illnesses or injuries include*

A. Fear of reprisal
B. Lack of management responsiveness to previous complaints
C. Ongoing treatment through a health maintenance organization (HMO) group health plan
D. All of the above
E. All except C

7. *Which of the following causes of occupational mortality is **least** common?*

A. Transportation accidents
B. Overdoses
C. Falls
D. Assaults and violent acts
E. Constructions accidents

8. *Which of the following is **not** considered to be a best practice in occupational disability management?*

A. Maximizing impairment ratings to ensure the greatest worker benefit
B. Having an occupational physician take a complete occupational history and perform a focused physical examination to determine causation
C. Facilitating functional recovery using modified work
D. Coordination of return to work among the payer, provider, employee, and employer
E. Reassessing treatment when the patient's functional recovery has ceased to improve

=19=

Not needed.

Health Care Management

OBJECTIVES

- Understand issues for employers that address the rising cost of health care
- Illustrate the shift from cost containment models to purchasing based on informed consumer choice, outcomes and quality, cost-sharing arrangements, and disease management
- Discuss occupational medicine (OM) and its focus on health issues impacting employers, employees, and the workplace
- Define employer-based health benefits programs, managed care systems, preferred provider organizations (PPOs), health maintenance organizations (HMOs), capitation, point of service, insurance plan designs, and utilization reviews
- Describe efforts of employers, occupational physicians, and insurance carriers to improve quality of care, employee satisfaction, health promotion, prevention, and productivity

OUTLINE

   I. Overview
  II. Employer-based health benefits programs
     A. Rising health care costs and the federal government
     B. Cost shifting
     C. Evolution from managed care
     D. Insurance plan design
 III. Managing the delivery of health care
     A. Utilization review
     B. Quality and employee satisfaction
 IV. Opportunities for occupational physicians
  V. Health and productivity
 VI. Prevention and health promotion
VII. Summary

KEY POINTS

- There has been a shift from pure cost containment to more innovative purchasing methodologies based on informed consumer choice, disease management, outcomes and quality, and cost-sharing arrangements between employers and employees.
- Employers and the federal government are the two largest purchasers of health insurance in the United States.

- Integrating health benefits with disability management and workers' compensation has not resulted in significant cost reductions or the medical management goals of employers who have used cost shifting.
- Investments in employee health and safety can improve productivity, focus on quality of care and outcomes, reduce absenteeism, and reduce total health care expenditures.
- Employee-based health benefits provide most U.S. citizens with health insurance. The Health Care Financing Administration (HCFA) estimates that businesses spent approximately $250 billion on health care in 1992. Health care spending in the United States is expected to double over the next decade to $2.6 trillion, with businesses bearing a significant portion of the tab.
- Linking medical insurance to employment was a product of the statutory wage freezes of World War II, as labor and management turned to health benefits as an alternative to increased compensation to employees. The Great Depression, in part, brought about the founding of Blue Cross and Blue Shield, as concerns about insolvency led hospitals and doctors to form third-party organizations to finance their operations. Health benefits have been tax exempt since their inception, creating a financial incentive for companies.
- A recent study of 2,800 employers estimated that the average cost per employee for health care benefits rose 11.2% to $4,924 in 2001, the largest increase in 9 years. Some estimate that the cost per employee will exceed the average wage by 2030. The Mercer survey predicts that 40% of large employers will require employees to pay higher deductibles and copayments.
- Insurance brokers and consultants believe that corporate health costs will continue to grow until employers focus their attention on creating value, increasing the cost sharing with the consumers of health benefits (employees and their dependents), and moving toward a defined contribution approach.
- The government entered the health care market with the establishment of Medicare and Medicaid in 1965. The Center for Medicare and Medicaid Services (CMS), formerly known as HCFA, is the single largest purchaser of health care in the world, with $476 billion paid for health care services in 2001 on behalf of 70 million disabled, elderly, and poor beneficiaries.
- In 1977, HCFA was created to manage Medicare and Medicaid. Currently, the Social Security Administration is responsible for managing Medicare. State governments operate Medicaid with federal oversight.
- Since 1996, HCFA has been responsible for implementing 700 provisions of five major laws: the Reconciliation Act of 1996, the Health Insurance Portability and Accountability Act of 1999, the Balanced Budget Act of 1997, the Balanced Budget Refinement Act of 1999, and the Benefits Improvement and Protection Act of 2000. Regulating private health insurance and establishing electronic-data standards for the health care industry are some of the provisions contained in these laws.
- The Balanced Budget Act reduced Medicare payments to virtually every clinical laboratory, hospital, skilled nursing facility, and home health agency, with an estimated total reduction of $112 billion for the period from 1998 through 2002.
- *Cost shifting* is a term that refers to providers' shifting of the burden of payment for care to private employers. It is estimated that almost 30% of the increases in employer-based premiums of the last decade have been due to this cost shifting. Small and mid-sized businesses are assuming a larger portion, up to two to three times the portion of the larger companies, as the total size of the health care budget is growing.
- *Managed care* is a system of medical care designed to control some aspects of that care (standardization of performance and contractual relationship between providers and

buyers), which are usually not part of indemnity plans. Although employers have been a prime force in reshaping the delivery of health care (e.g., managed care), reshaping health care delivery has not delivered long-term price control, patient satisfaction, or improved outcomes.

- *PPOs* apply to discount pricing, prepayment for care, and utilization management. The agreement is typically a contract between providers and a financing entity such as a self-funded employer, an insurance company, a government program, or an independent entity. There is also a separate contract between each *employee* and the *financing organization*. Except for the contract of prepaid care, PPOs do not fix the total price of services; price and volume management features can occur separately or together and apply to physicians, hospitals, and/or other providers.
- *HMOs* were developed under a system of capitation, a payment mechanism that pays a provider a sum of money for ongoing care. The sum is set in advance of the actual period of service, and it represents a prediction of the amount of money that will be required to provide that care. In a staff model HMO, the physicians are generally employed by the entity to accept the risk entailed by prepayment and to configure care so that the costs fall within that prepaid amount.
- Physician network or *independent practice association (IPA)* contracts, based on capitation, may involve only a small fraction of a physician's patients. Managed care may include rules about referrals, requirements for precertification, and selective contracting for ancillary services such as imaging, physical therapy, or consultation of specialists.
- Employee cost-sharing devices (such as copayments and deductibles) are the most common insurance plan designs that spread the cost between the employer and employee. *Deductibles* are fixed amounts paid by the employee before expenses are covered by insurance. Once the deductible is satisfied, the employee's price for the service reduces to a percentage of the cost of the care, in the form of a copayment (usually 20%). A hybrid approach, in the form of flexible benefits or "cafeteria plans," can be implemented; the hybrid approach gives the employee a budget to purchase various types of insurance. *Stop losses* refer to limits of responsibility after which copayments no longer apply. Certain incentives for employees to use generic drugs or shop for less expensive physician services include rolling over unused money into the next year.
- *Utilization review* is the process in which services are reviewed by third parties to determine if they are medically appropriate and necessary. Payment is tied to this review. Popular forms of utilization review are preadmission and preprocedure certification. Other forms include case management, second surgical opinions, and "carving out" specific high cost areas such as mental health and pharmacy services.
- Corporations and the federal government share concerns that health plans and providers may compete by skimping on services to reduce prices. The National Committee for Quality Assurance (NCQA) is a not-for-profit organization that is the leading accreditor of managed care plans. An employer's willingness to pay for quality depends on preserving productivity and controlling medical costs. These are good reasons to implement worksite programs and to design health benefits that encourage prevention of diseases.
- *Quality of care* has been addressed by a number of approaches: evidenced-based medicine, total quality management, accreditation, professional development, and patient empowerment. All of these are viewed as powerful tools for the achievement of effective and efficient care. Physician report cards or profiles from systematic data collection are tools for external accountability. *Total quality management* and *continuous*

quality improvement emphasize efforts to improve teamwork, provide stable infrastructure, and build a culture of quality.

- The *Leapfrog Group,* a coalition of 60 corporate members providing health benefits for more than 20 million Americans, spends more than $40 billion per year on health care. They have focused on promoting change in the hospital setting to increase efficiency, improve quality, and subsequently reduce waste and cost.
- OM physician input is critical, but few are integrally involved in health care purchasing decisions. Only a small percentage of the 12,000 members of the American College of Physician Executives, doctors involved in health care management, are also occupational physicians.
- The American College of Occupational and Environmental Medicine (ACOEM) has developed programs and courses of medical management topics. Failure to take a lead role may be due to perceived potential ethical dilemmas of being between medicine and management.
- OM physicians are an integral part of implementing programs for health and productivity. Onsite health risk appraisals and screenings have been shown to reduce time away from work.
- The Health Enhancement Research Organization (HERO), a national not-for-profit coalition of employers interested in health-related productivity and health promotion, was launched in 1996 by a group of proactive employers. Corporate medical directors, human resource personnel, Fortune 500 benefit executives, smaller companies, private physicians, and government research agencies have united to promote research objectives and expertise in health and productivity.
- Employee Assistance Programs (EAPs) have favorable cost-to-benefit ratios and serve as initial points of contact for employees with personal or mental health challenges. Mental health benefits have been rapidly increasing.

QUESTIONS

*1. Which of the following statements is **least correct** concerning the OM physician's role in health care costs?*

A. The physician should focus on a pure cost containment model to avoid complicated cost-sharing arrangements between employers and employees.
B. The physician should be involved with employers, employees, and health insurance carriers in addressing corporate health care expenditures.
C. The physician should become knowledgeable about health insurance benefits.
D. The OM physician should become involved in onsite wellness programs, health risk appraisals, and recommendation of health care benefit services.
E. The physician should be aware of ethical dilemmas that occur between physician and employer as a result of a worker's eligibility for disability and future employability.

*2. Which of the following is **least correct** about health care management?*

A. Investments in employee health and safety may improve productivity and reduce absenteeism.
B. Creating value, increasing the cost sharing with consumers of health care benefits, and educating employees about costs will help reduce health care expenses.
C. Employers can involve employees in accepting a portion of the costs by copayments, deductibles, and monthly contributions for flexible benefits.

D. Using forms of utilization review to monitor the delivery of medical benefits is unethical.

E. Employer's willingness to pay more for quality care depends on the connection between overall health and productivity.

3. *Which of the following is correct concerning health insurance in the United States?*

A. Medical insurance was partially a product of statutory wage freezes of the World War II era.

B. Blue Cross was founded in 1929 partially because of the Great Depression.

C. HCFA is the federal agency that is the single largest purchaser of health care in the world.

D. In 1965, Congress created Medicare for the elderly and Medicaid for the poor.

E. All of the above are true.

4. *Which of the following is **incorrect**?*

A. HCFA was created in 1977 to manage Medicare and Medicaid.

B. HCFA is responsible for provisions of major laws including the Balanced Budget Act of 1997.

C. The Balanced Budget Act failed to reduce Medicare payments between 1998 and 2000.

D. Small and midsized businesses have faced a second cost shift and higher burden of the total health care costs because large employers have been able to leverage their size to get discounts from providers.

E. PPOs refer to discount pricing, prepayment for care, and utilization management.

5. *Which of the following statements about capitation is **incorrect**?*

A. It refers to payment of a specific sum of money to a provider for the ongoing care of a person or group of people for a particular period of time.

B. The sum is set in advance of the actual period of service and represents an agreed-on estimate of the amount of money that will be required to provide that care.

C. Organizations that arrange care under a system of capitation attempt not only to buy care, but also to manage care.

D. Capitated contracts have no associated risk because the payment amount is set in advance of service.

E. Technically, a contract based on capitation can include or exclude almost any medical service.

Answers to Chapters 1–19

CHAPTER 1 ANSWERS

1. The answer is B. (Ref: pp. 1–2)

The history of occupational medicine can be traced back to antiquity. Observations related to increased rates of illnesses and mortality among miners date back to Roman times; however, explanations for this phenomenon were often attributed to the fact that workers were slaves and, thus, of a more feeble constitution. It was not until the late seventeenth century, when an Italian physician published *Disease and Occupations,* that physicians were formally urged to pay attention to the role of one's work in the development of certain illnesses.

Although occupational medicine has been a distinct discipline within the American Board of Preventive Medicine since 1954, a considerable shortage of well-trained and certified specialists in this field exists. In large part, this shortage is due to a deficiency of postgraduate training positions. The situation is now changing.

A relatively unknown fact is that more than 90% of businesses in the United States and in the world have 100 or fewer employees. It is rarely economically feasible for these enterprises to provide anything other than meager health care and, in some cases, at best first aid.

2. The answer is E. (Ref: p. 6)

Ancillary services refer to laboratory and related procedures conducted as part of clinical evaluations. The type and level of ancillary services depend on the practice setting and the local medical community. In the provision of occupational health services to small businesses, however, the following items are considered essential: an audiometric booth and audiometer, a well-functioning and calibrated spirometer, and a vision screener. Optional services include laboratory, x-ray, and physical therapy; however, the appropriateness of including these services will vary. In some cases, it may be suitable to employ referral services.

3. The answer is C. (Ref: p. 9)

The goals of an occupational health service include the following:

1. To protect people at work from health and safety hazards
2. To protect the local environment
3. To facilitate safe placement of workers according to their physical, mental, and emotional capacities
4. To ensure adequate medical care and rehabilitation of the occupationally ill and injured
5. To assist in measures related to personal maintenance

4. The answer is E. (Ref: Tables 1.1 and 1.2; pp. 2–3)

5. The answer is C. (Ref: pp. 3–4)

The purpose of a preplacement evaluation is to ensure that the person examined does not have any medical condition that may be aggravated by the job duties or that may affect the health and safety of others. Incumbent on physicians conducting preplacement examinations is a thorough understanding of the job duties and the *work environment.*

TABLE 1.1. *Occupational and environmental health programs: essential components*

- Health evaluation of employees
- Preplacement
- Medical surveillance
- After illness or injury
- Diagnosis and treatment of occupational and environmental injuries or illnesses, including rehabilitation
- Emergency treatment of nonoccupational injury or illness
- Education of employees about potential occupational hazards
- Implementation of programs for personal protective equipment
- Evaluation, inspection, and abatement of workplace hazards
- Toxicologic assessments, including advice on chemical substances that have not had adequate toxicologic screening
- Biostatistics and epidemiology assessments
- Maintenance of occupational medical records
- Immunization against possible occupational infections
- Medical interpretation and participation in governmental health and safety regulations
- Periodic evaluation of the occupational or environmental health program
- Disaster preparedness: planning for the workplace and community; local emergency planning committees
- Assistance in rehabilitation of alcohol- and drug-dependent employees or those with emotional disorders

Adapted from Scope of occupational and environmental health programs and practices, report of the Occupational Medical Practice Committee of the American College of Occupational and Environmental Medicine. *J Occup Med* 1992;34:436, with permission.

Preplacement evaluations can also be of value in complying with certain Occupational Safety and Health Administration (OSHA) standards and in serving as a baseline for health improvement programs. For example, the OSHA standard for occupational exposure to asbestos requires that workers undergo a chest x-ray film and pulmonary function studies before job assignment. In some cases, when workers are exposed to substances regulated by OSHA standards, such evaluations are legally mandated.

Arbitrary use of certain tests can also be considered discriminatory, legally unsound, and of limited medical utility. Random use of low back films to "predict" future back disorders falls under this category.

TABLE 1.2. *Elective components of occupational and environmental health programs*

- Palliative treatment of nonoccupational disorders
- Management of nonoccupational conditions prescribed and monitored by personal physicians
- Assistance and control of illness-related job absenteeism
- Assistance and evaluation of personal health care
- Immunization against nonoccupational infectious diseases
- Health education and counseling
- Termination and retirement administration
- Participation in planning and assessing the quality of employee health benefits
- Participation in research efforts (27)

Adapted from Scope of occupational and environmental health programs and practices, report of the Occupational Medical Practice Committee of the American College of Occupational and Environmental Medicine. *J Occup Med* 1992;34:436, with permission.

CHAPTER 2 ANSWERS

1. The answer is A. (Ref: p. 14)

Until the early years of the twentieth century, if employees were injured in their place of employment, the only remedy against the employer was a suit at common law. In the early twentieth century, employers and employees in the various states changed this system. The new system was known as workers' compensation. The workers' compensation statutes vary a bit from state to state (each state has its own workers' compensation law), but each is composed of several compromises:

1. Employees gave up their right to sue employers at common law and agreed to accept a certain sum of money per week for their inability to work as a result of work-related injuries. They agreed to accept this compensation as their exclusive remedy against the employer.
2. Employers agreed to give injured employees a certain sum of money per week, if they were unable to work as a result of work-related injuries. Thus, payment would be made, regardless of fault. Monetary recovery may be less than through suits at common law.
3. Payment would be automatic unless disputes arose. The disputes over issues of work-relatedness, amounts of entitlement, timeliness of claim, and so forth would (generally) be decided by administrative bodies rather than by courts.
4. Payments would only be made for disability (i.e., inability to work).[1] No damages would be allowed as a punishment of the employer (punitive damages).

At first, most of the state workers' compensation systems covered only work-related accidents. Illness and disease coverage were added later.

2. The answer is E. (Ref: p. 18)

In recent years, many states and the Occupational Safety and Health Administration (OSHA) have enacted rules mandating that employees be provided with information about the chemical exposures they are receiving in the workplace and how those exposures may affect their health. OSHA's rule is known as the Hazard Communication Standard (HCS). The HCS originally covered only entities in the manufacturing sector and importers of chemicals.

Because of the potential for conflicting regulations, OSHA expanded the coverage of the HCS to all employers covered by the OSHA Act.

Generally, the HCS requires that

1. Containers in the workplace that contain hazardous chemicals[2] must be labeled with the chemical's identity, appropriate hazard warnings, and the identity of the manufacturer.

---

[1]Most state laws did contain scheduled awards, in which a certain percentage of impairment resulted in a certain payment of compensation, even though the employee continued to work. Thus, loss of a finger or partial loss of vision or hearing might result in payment of a number of weeks of compensation, even though it did not affect ability to work.

[2]Hazardous chemicals are defined in the HCS as being those chemicals that present one of several physical hazards (e.g., flammability, reactivity, or explosiveness) or a health hazard. Health hazards include carcinogens, mutagens, teratogens, and toxins to any of the body's organ systems [29 CFR 1910.1200(c), (d)]. A determination as to what constitutes a hazard must be made by the manufacturer or importer, but downstream users may also make that determination [29 CFR 1910.1200(d)(1), (2)].

TABLE 2.1. *Information provided on Material Safety Data Sheets (MSDS)*

1. The label identity of the chemical
2. The chemical and common names including synonyms
3. If the substance is a mixture that has been tested as a whole to determine its hazards, the chemical and common names of the ingredients that contribute to the known hazards.
4. If the substance is a mixture that has not been tested as a whole, the chemical and common names of all ingredients that have been determined to be health hazards and that constitute 1% or more of the mixture (or 0.1% or more, if the hazard is a carcinogen)
5. The chemical and common names of all ingredients that have been determined to present a physical hazard
6. The physical and chemical characteristics of the chemical
7. The physical hazards of the chemical
8. The health hazards of the chemical, including signs and symptoms of exposure, and any medical conditions that can be aggravated by exposure to the chemical
9. The primary routes of exposure
10. The Occupational Safety and Health Administration (OSHA) permissible exposure limit, the American Conference of Governmental Industrial Hygienists (ACGIH) threshold limit value, or any other recommended exposure limit
11. Whether the substance is listed on the National Toxicology Program's "Annual List of Carcinogens" or has been found to be a potential carcinogen by the International Agency for Research on Cancer or OSHA
12. Known precautions for safe handling and use
13. Applicable control measures
14. The date of preparation of the latest MSDS or its latest change
15. The name, address, and telephone number of the manufacturer, importer, employer, or other responsible party preparing or distributing the MSDS, who can provide additional information on the hazardous chemical and appropriate emergency procedures

2. Employees must be trained about the hazards of chemicals to which they are or may be exposed.
3. Material Safety Data Sheets (MSDS), which set out in considerable detail the hazards of specific chemicals, must be made available to employees who may be exposed to those chemicals (Table 2.1).

3. The answer is B. (Ref: p. 16)

Mental stress attributable to the general work environment is NOT covered by workers' compensation, although stress related to a specific significant employment incident (such as witnessing a shooting at work) might be compensable.

4. The answer is C. (Ref: pp. 23–24)

The OSHA 300 Log is used to record all injuries (except extremely minor ones treated only with first aid) and all deaths and illness that result from a work-related accident or from an exposure in the work environment. Many specific requirements apply. Injuries and illnesses resulting in restricted work activity beyond the day of the injury or illness, loss of consciousness, medical treatment beyond first aid, or days away from work are recordable. Also recordable are needle stick or sharps injuries and cases involving medical removal due to illness (e.g., tuberculosis) under the OSHA standards. New regulations list 14 first aid treatments that are not recordable. "Privacy concern cases" such as sexual assault and mental illness and human immunodeficiency virus (HIV) cases are entered in a confidential log. With new rules, up to four forms are required to post records: the OSHA 300, OSHA 300 A, OSHA 301 and the Confidential List of "privacy concern" illnesses or injuries.

Employee access to the OSHA 300 Log is limited to the logs for the establishment where the employee worked or formerly worked.

All employers must report to OSHA, within 48 hours, accidents that result in one or more deaths or in the hospitalization of five or more employees.

5. The answer is D. (Ref: pp. 27–28)

Damages for medical expenses, lost earning capacity, and pain and suffering are allowed in toxic tort lawsuits. In some states, damages may be obtained for future risk of illness, fear of future illness, and the cost of medical surveillance. The toxic tort is a possible concern for the practitioner of occupational medicine. Toxic tort suits are suits at common law, brought by those who claim that exposure to the toxic substance caused them some injury or disorder. Workers can sue third-party suppliers of materials (e.g., asbestos) to their employers. Consumers of products (e.g., pharmaceuticals such as diethylstilbestrol) or those exposed to allegedly toxic waste in the environment (e.g., a Superfund site) can also bring a civil suit. Therefore, workers' compensation is NOT the exclusive remedy in toxic tort cases.

6. The answer is B. (Ref: pp. 26–27)

Under the Americans with Disabilities Act (ADA), all employment-related examinations are allowed only after an offer is made.

Under the ADA, a disability is (a) a physical or mental impairment that substantially limits one or more of the major life activities of an individual, (b) a record of such impairment, or (c) a situation in which an individual is regarded as having such impairment. The thrust of the ADA (relevant to employers) is that employees or job applicants with such disabilities may not be discriminated against in any aspect of the employment relationship if that employee or applicant is qualified for the job. A disabled person is qualified if, with reasonable accommodation, he or she can perform the essential functions of the job as well as one who is not disabled.

With regard to preplacement or periodic examinations, physicians should be aware of the Code of Ethical Conduct of the American College of Occupational and Environmental Medicine (ACOEM), originally adopted in 1976 and updated in 1994: "Employers are entitled to counsel about the medical fitness of individuals in relation to work, but are not entitled to diagnoses or details of a specific nature."

The OSHA Exposure and Medical Record Access Standard requires employers who expose employees to toxic substances or harmful physical agents to provide employees (or their authorized representative) with access to their medical records within 15 days of a request.

CHAPTER 3 ANSWERS

1. The answer is B. (Ref: pp. 30–33)

The Occupational Safety and Health Administration (OSHA) Act does not cover federal, state, or local municipal employees. However, executive branches of the federal government are expected to have equivalent regulations, and most state-run programs cover state and local municipal employees.

This OSHA standard requires annual examinations for employees exposed to noise of 85 dBA or higher on a daily 8-hour time-weighted average (TWA) basis.

In general, the OSHA standards require the physician to furnish the employer a written opinion on whether the employee has any medical conditions that would place the employee at increased risk of impairment from the work or use of protective equipment. The physician must provide in writing any limitations on the employee's assigned work. The employee should be informed of any conditions that require further examination or treatment and be referred to private physicians, as necessary.

There are detailed individual standards for 26 chemicals. Each of these standards includes a section on medical surveillance. In all standards, medical examinations are required if certain conditions are met.

Some of the more recent standards also include provisions for medical removal protection and multiple physician review (e.g., lead and methylene dianiline). In some cases, the criteria for medical removal may be straightforward. In lead exposure, for example, temporary removal from exposure is required if the average of the last three blood tests for lead is greater than 50 g/100 g whole blood and the last test is more than 40 g/100 g whole blood.

2. The answer is D. (Ref: pp. 20–21, 31)

An injury that requires only first aid care as opposed to medical treatment is not recordable. In contrast, all illnesses are recordable regardless of how trivial they may be. Employers greatly appreciate injuries being given first aid rather than medical treatment whenever this level of care is sufficient. OSHA also has definitions of what is first aid and what is medical treatment. For example, use of over-the-counter medication is first aid; use of prescription medication is medical treatment. Likewise, use of a Band-Aid is first aid, whereas use of a Steri-Strip is considered medical treatment. For minor injuries, the selection of treatment can determine OSHA recordability.

Records must be maintained for the duration of a person's employment plus 30 years. This time period is much longer than that typically required for non-work-related inactive patient files. OSHA also requires that medical records be released to designated representatives, including the employee, on presentation of signed consent. Compliance with such requests is required within 15 working days.

Audiograms that show a standard threshold shift (STS), which is defined as an age-adjusted decrease of 10 dB or greater in either ear averaged for the frequencies of 2,000, 3,000, and 4,000 Hz, must be evaluated by an audiologist or physician to determine the need for further evaluation.

Based on current OSHA field directives, a work-related change in hearing of 10 dB averaged over the frequencies of 2,000, 3,000, and 4,000 Hz must be recorded on the OSHA Form 300 as a disorder resulting from repeated trauma.

3. The answer is B. (Ref: See Table 3.3, p. 32)

4. The answer is A. (Ref: pp. 30–34)

Some states have taken advantage of an option in the OSHA Act to establish and administer their own state OSHA plan. Standards promulgated by these states are usually identical to the federal OSHA standards but in some cases may be more stringent.

Injuries and illnesses are recorded on an OSHA Form 300 by the employer. The threshold of recordability is different depending on whether the case is an injury or illness. OSHA defines these terms differently than they have been traditionally defined in medicine. OSHA's definition of an injury is something that is caused by an instantaneous exposure, for example, in the snap of the fingers. An illness is anything caused by a longer exposure even if it is as short as a couple of seconds.

Several OSHA standards, including Hazardous Waste Operations and Emergency Response, Respiratory Protection, and some Chemical Specific Standards, require the employee to have a medical examination to determine physical fitness to perform certain jobs or to wear specific personal protective equipment (e.g., respirators). None of these standards specifies details of the medical examination, which are left to the discretion of the examining physician. Employers may specify requirements.

OSHA's standard on blood-borne pathogens is directed primarily at the health care industry, but also affects blood processing and research activities using human blood or other body fluids, as well as any employer who has designated first-aid responders.

5. The answer is D. (Ref: pp. 34–35)

The National Institute for Occupational Safety and Health (NIOSH) is the research agency created by the OSHA Act. In 1973, NIOSH became part of the Centers for Disease Control and Prevention (CDC). The institute is mandated to protect the health and safety of workers by conducting research on workplace hazards.

NIOSH plays an important role in providing information pertinent to the development of OSHA standards. Before making specific recommendations, NIOSH performs research and conducts a literature review of human and animal literature and other test systems.

At either employee or employer request, NIOSH may conduct a Health Hazard Evaluation (HHE), which includes an industrial hygiene study and appropriate medical evaluation of an occupational health problem.

The majority of the training and educational services provided by NIOSH are conducted at 15 Education Resource Centers (ERCs), which were established in 1977 because of the shortage of occupational health professionals. A variety of programs are offered, including occupational medicine residencies and graduate school training in occupational nursing, industrial hygiene, and safety.

6. The answer is C. (Ref: pp. 34–38)

NIOSH develops health standards for Mine Safety and Health Administration (MSHA), but only advises OSHA concerning health standards.

Regulations issued by the Nuclear Regulatory Commission (NRC) require that every 12 months a physician must determine a worker's ability to wear a respirator. This is in contrast to OSHA's standard, in which an annual review was suggested but longer time intervals are acceptable.

The Equal Employment Opportunity Commission (EEOC) is charged with enforcing the Americans with Disabilities Act (ADA).

The Toxic Substance Control Act (TSCA) Section 8c requires manufacturers or users of a specific chemical to keep a record of any allegation of a heretofore-unknown adverse health effect.

TSCA requires manufacturers, producers, and users of chemicals to report to the Environmental Protection Agency (EPA) new information that reasonably supports the conclusion that the chemical or mixture presents a substantial risk of injury to health or the environment.

The Agency for Toxic Substances and Disease Registry (ATSDR) is primarily concerned with the potential adverse health effects associated with environmental exposure to toxic substances. ATSDR's mission is to support activities designed to protect the public from the adverse health consequences of toxic chemical exposure. Part of its mission is to conduct research about the health effects of toxic materials.

ATSDR is mandated to establish a disease and exposure registry to provide an information base of health effects of toxic substances. It also provides continuing education training for physicians through case studies in environmental medicine.

CHAPTER 4 ANSWERS

1. The answer is B. (Ref: p. 42)

Employer-based programs are also more likely to provide an extended range of health services, including health promotion, disease management, and absentee monitoring. However, employers who have reduced their onsite services have pointed out that establishing and managing health services is outside the scope of their core business. Continued investment in onsite services may prove difficult for corporate managers with emphasis on the "bottom line" and difficulty calculating the cost effectiveness. Each of the other choices is discussed in the text, and choice E is possibly an unexpected response. Since the 1900s, unions have paid less attention to health and safety, focusing their energies on job security, salary, and benefits. Nevertheless, union-supported occupational health programs have an important place in selected locations. Some unions hire occupational and environmental medicine (OEM) physicians on a consultative basis to ensure that government standards are met and that scientific research is appropriately interpreted or to aid in lobbying for a stronger regulatory protection in the workplace.

2. The answer is D. (Ref: pp. 46–48)

Primary prevention addresses risk factor(s) for illness or injury. Primary prevention includes a hierarchy of controls to prevent illness or injury. (See Table 4.1. Substitution, enclosure, engineering controls, personal protective equipment, and administrative controls.) Secondary prevention represents detection at an earlier, treatable stage. Screening tests such as screening mammography are secondary prevention.

3. The answer is B. (Ref: pp. 49–54)

Each of the components mentioned except the sick leave policy is a consideration that an OEM physician can use to better establish an occupational health program to meet specific needs of the employer. Sick leave policy, other than modified duty availability, is usually a human resource issue and is not a part of the occupational health service.

4. The answer is E. (Ref: pp. 49–54)

Occupational health services depend on all of the items listed. Working with employers and employees in establishing a program involves interaction and knowledge about the potential hazards and methods of preventing injury and illness.

TABLE 4.1. *Hierarchy of controls*

Substitution
Enclosure
Engineering controls
Personal protective equipment
Administrative controls

CHAPTER 5 ANSWERS

1. The answer is C. (Ref: pp. 57–58)

The Equal Employment Opportunity Commission (EEOC) is the federal agency responsible for enforcement of the Americans with Disabilities Act (ADA). Title I of the ADA covers employment, Title II covers access to public services, Title III covers public accommodations and services operated by private entities, and Title IV covers telecommunications.

Federal government employers are covered by the Rehabilitation Act of 1973, which incorporates the requirements of the ADA. Complaints of discrimination by federal employers are processed by different procedures.

The purpose of the ADA was to allow those with physical and mental disabilities to participate in mainstream American society, including employment. Private employers with 15 or more employees are required to comply with the employment provisions of the ADA.

2. The answer is E. (Ref: p. 57)

The ADA prohibits discrimination in any aspect of employment, including all of those listed. Other employment activities covered include job assignment or employee classification; transfer, promotion, layoff, and recall; recruitment; testing; use of company facilities; fringe benefits; pay, retirement, and disability leave; or other terms and conditions of employment.

3. The answer is C. (Ref: pp. 59, 70)

Before an offer of employment, there are strict limitations on the types of inquiries that employers can make. Inquiries regarding disabilities and medical conditions are prohibited until a job offer has been made. A job offer may be conditioned on results of a medical examination, but only if the examination is required for all entering employees in the same job category.

Under the ADA, drug tests are not considered to be medical tests. Therefore, preemployment drug tests are allowed. Alcohol testing is considered a medical test and should be conducted after a job offer is made.

4. The answer is D. (Ref: pp. 58–59)

An individual with a disability as defined by the ADA is a person who has, has a record of, or is regarded as having a physical or mental impairment that substantially limits one or more major life activities. Examples of major life activities include walking, breathing, seeing, hearing, speaking, learning, and working.

5. The answer is C. (Ref: p. 62)

The ADA requires that the employer maintain confidential medical records in locked cabinets, separate from personnel files, and accessible only to designated persons. Specific pharmaceutical information should be considered confidential.

Medical examiners should not put themselves in the position of making employment decisions or determining whether a reasonable accommodation can be made. They do have the responsibility to advise employers about a person's functional abilities and limitations with regard to functional job requirements and whether or not the person meets the employer's overall health and safety requirements.

6. The answer is B. (Ref: pp.70–71)

A history of drug or alcohol abuse or dependence is not excluded; however, current abuse is not protected. Mental and psychologic disorders are the only categories in which the ADA specifically included or excluded certain symptoms or diagnoses. Certain disorders, such as kleptomania, pyromania, and pedophilia, were specifically excluded. Other mental and psychological disorders may or may not be considered disabilities or impairments as defined by the ADA. To be considered a "disability," an impairment must "substantially limit" one or more major life activities of the individual and must be evaluated in light of any mitigating measures such as medication and therapy.

CHAPTER 6 ANSWERS

1. The answer is B. (Ref: p. 79)

Specific functions of the occupational health nurse case manager generally include the following:

- Determines the need for case management intervention
- Establishes criteria to identify workers who would benefit from case management services
- Identifies goals, objectives, and actions as part of a comprehensive case management plan in collaboration with the worker and other health care providers
- Develops and conducts an evaluation process for the case management program
- Monitors, documents, and evaluates the quality of individual worker outcomes and makes adjustments as necessary

2. The answer is B. (Ref: p. 81; Table 6.1)

Within a framework of prevention, the primary goals of occupational health nursing practice are to:

- Promote, maintain, and restore the physical and psychosocial well-being of the workers to enhance optimal functioning
- Protect the worker from hazards that may occur as a result of the work experience
- Encourage and participate in a company culture supportive of health
- Collaborate with workers, management, and other disciplines and health care professionals to ensure a safe and healthful work environment

TABLE 6.1. *Examples of occupational health nursing practice activities within a prevention framework*

Primary	Secondary	Tertiary
Immunizations	Health assessment and surveillance	Work hardening
Wellness programs	Preplacement/periodic examinations	Rehabilitation
Nutrition education	Screening programs (e.g., high blood pressure, mammography)	Disability management
Exercise/fitness programs		

CHAPTER 7 ANSWERS

1. The answer is B. (Ref: p. 86)

Independent medical evaluations (IMEs) are performed to provide information for case management and for evidence in hearings and other legal proceedings. IMEs are a component of all workers' compensation statutes, although the specifics vary by state. IMEs also are used in clarifying liability (personal injury) and disability. Insurers, third-party administrators, employers, and attorneys usually request IMEs. States may impose limitations on the number of examinations an injured person may have and may specify qualifications for evaluating physicians. IMEs may also have different roles, dependent on the context of the evaluation. For example, in some states, examinations performed by an agreed-on examiner or requested directly by the court or commission may be given particular credence.

The physician who performs the IME is not involved in a treating capacity. No direct clinical management is provided, and the party requesting the examination pays the fee. The information obtained is presented to the client in a written report. The physician must be impartial and unbiased in performing the assessment. Ethics and moral character must be without question.

Assessments are often requested because of a lack of medical information or conflict on specific matters, especially regarding the cause of the condition and a person's ability to work. The physician makes a careful assessment and addresses the issues raised by the referring sources. The assessment process must be precise and detailed to ensure that conclusions are valid, reliable, defensible, and useful. Many assessments undergo legal scrutiny, and the physician must be able to support the conclusions in deposition or testimony.

2. The answer is E. (Ref: p. 88)

Pain, pathology, impairment, residual functional capacity, and disability are separate concepts. *Pain*, especially chronic pain, may not be associated with significant physical pathology. *Pathology* may be present without symptoms or dysfunction. *Impairment* is a measurable decrement in some physiologic function, whereas *disability* considers not only the physical or mental impairment but also the social, psychologic, or vocational factors associated with a person's ability to work. Functional limitations are manifestations of impairment.

Chronic pain, the most common problem seen in the performance of IMEs, may not be a symptom of an underlying acute somatic injury but a multidimensional biopsychosocial phenomenon.

3. The answer is A. (Ref: p. 88)

Causation is a critical issue in work-related and liability cases. A work-related problem is defined as one that "arose out of and during the course of employment."

The physician must establish *causation* to a reasonable degree of medical *probability*, which implies that it is more probable than not (i.e., there is more than a 50% probability) that a certain condition arose out of or in the course of work duties. *Possibility* implies less than 50% likelihood. Stating that a problem is work related implies that, based on the available information, to a reasonable degree of medical certainty, work activities caused the problem. States may vary in the definition of causation, particularly for cumulative trauma disorders and preexisting conditions.

Causation can be ultimate or proximate. Ultimate causation refers to the initial factor that leads to the effect. Proximate cause is the factor that immediately or closely precedes the effect.

A medical condition may be the result of one or multiple factors. *Apportionment* refers to the extent to which a condition is related to each of the multiple factors. For example, a worker may have sustained an injury with one employer, then returned to work and sustained a similar injury with another employer. In reviewing the case, it may be necessary to apportion current dysfunction between the two parties. It also may be necessary to apportion responsibility between work- and non-work-related conditions. Assigning apportionment depends largely on clinical judgment because the science supporting apportionment is in its infancy.

Unique causation occurs when a condition is due to a specific cause, for example, asbestosis. Multifactorial causation, in which there are several possible causes, is more common; the apportionment that goes with it is also assigned to multiple factors.

Work activities may influence underlying problems. An *aggravation* implies a long-standing effect due to an event, resulting in a worsening, hastening, or deterioration of the condition. An *exacerbation* is a temporary increase in symptoms from the condition. Thus, an aggravation has an ongoing substantial impact on the physical condition, whereas an exacerbation results in a *flare* of symptoms, without a significant change in the underlying pathology.

4. The answer is E. (Ref: p. 90)

Maximal medical improvement (MMI) is a phrase used to indicate when further recovery and restoration of function can no longer be anticipated to a reasonable degree of medical probability. This assessment implies that a condition is permanent and static. Considerations include whether the current or proposed treatment will result in functional improvement, if surgery has occurred recently, and whether enough time has passed for the process to be stable.

Often, a physician is asked to conduct an *impairment evaluation* as part of the assessment. To physicians who are not independent medical evaluators, an impairment evaluation and an independent assessment are synonymous, but they are not. The basic philosophies have been detailed in the American Medical Association's *Guides to the Evaluation of Permanent Impairment* (the *Guides*), which is the most widely used and accepted reference for evaluating permanent impairment. The *Guides* distinguishes between an *impairment* evaluation and a *disability* evaluation. According to the *Guides, impairment* is "the loss of, the loss of use of, or a derangement of any body part, system or function" and *disability* is "the limiting loss of the capacity to meet personal, social or occupational demands, or to meet statutory or regulatory requirements." Impairment is considered permanent when it has reached MMI, meaning that it is well-stabilized and unlikely to change substantially in the next year with or without medical treatment.

Impairment is a measurable decrement in health status evaluated by medical means; disability is the gap between what a person can do and what he or she needs to do, partly because of a diminished health status. Disability is assessed by the consideration of non-medical issues, such as the person's educational and vocational skills; experience; age; and, in workers' compensation cases, potential for future loss of wages. Assessing education, vocation, and potential for future loss of wages is not a skill most physicians possess, and thus, the medical role usually is limited to evaluating impairment not disability.

5. The answer is C. (Ref: p. 91)

Functional performance assessments are more accurate determinations of ability, if the assessment is valid and reliable and relates to particular job tasks. Caution should be exercised because various methodologies are available. A structured protocol is essential. It is customary to express work capacity following parameters in the *Dictionary of Occupational Titles*, Department of Labor, which are based primarily on lifting requirements. (see Table 7.1 in the textbook).

The examining physician should estimate capacities as carefully as possible, including the number of hours of work per day, based on endurance and tolerance for sitting, standing, and walking. Estimates of lifting and carrying capabilities are noted for specific frequencies. Guidelines should be provided for the *frequency* and *duration* of tasks such as bending, crouching, squatting, pushing/pulling, climbing stairs, climbing ladders, reaching above shoulder level, lifting above shoulder level, balancing, and working on uneven ground or at heights.

These capacities are compared with the functional requirements of the job, obtained from job descriptions, videotapes, or direct observations. Specific assessments of work capacity based only on a clinical evaluation may be difficult. As a result, a functional performance assessment may be particularly helpful when incorporated into the IME.

6. The answer is C. (Ref: pp. 92–94)

The IME process should address the issues posed by the referral source. The assessment consists of three phases: preevaluation, evaluation, and postevaluation.

It is important to review the medical records before the evaluation and to read correspondence from the client, so that the evaluation can be structured to answer specific questions. The examinee may be asked to complete a questionnaire before the evaluation, to facilitate the interview. Pain and functional inventories are particularly helpful in identifying behavioral and psychologic components related to an illness or injury.

At the beginning of the visit, the physician should explain the nature of the evaluation and that an independent evaluation will be conducted but that no treatment will be provided. There is no patient-physician relationship, and a report will be sent to the requesting client. The person should sign a release.

The meticulous history is followed by a physical examination including a behavioral assessment and a detailed examination of the involved area(s).

The evaluation should address the specifically issues requested by the referring source.

CHAPTER 8 ANSWERS

1. The answer is C. (Ref: pp. 97–98)

Perhaps the most profound change in the practice of medicine is the decline of fee-for-service reimbursement in favor of a variety of managed care arrangements.

Close associations with employers are becoming a paramount positioning strategy for both physicians and medical centers as the private sector assumes greater influence in health care funding and medical service delivery.

Health care delivery is moving toward managed competition, with greater emphasis on employer responsibility.

Several significant changes have occurred in the regulatory environment that affects occupational medical practice. The deregulatory fervor of the 1980s has been overshadowed by public health regulation, especially enforcement activities. Recent initiatives include the Americans with Disabilities Act, the Drug-Free Workplace Act, and the Occupational Safety and Health Administration (OSHA) Blood-Borne Pathogens Standard.

Health care cost control is a major motivator for employers to establish partnerships with providers, especially physicians, the essential ingredients for addressing the complex occupational and environmental health issues facing business today.

2. The answer is B. (Ref: p. 98)

Prevention is likely to assume a more pronounced role, both in reducing workplace risk factors and in using the workplace as a forum for health education.

By 2001, an estimated 1,500 or more hospitals of approximately 7,000 in the United States had dedicated programs that provided occupational medical services for employers. Although a small number of programs are still based in emergency departments, freestanding clinics within the hospital, freestanding ambulatory care locations, and networks of clinics are the most common delivery models.

The practice of medicine in the United States appears poised for a significant change in which physicians are evaluated on both their ability to address broad community health care concerns and their clinical skills.

Occupational medicine necessitates the ability to work as part of a team; deal with multiple constituencies (e.g., employers, workers, insurance carriers); and show leadership.

3. The answer is B. (Ref: p. 99)

By 2001, an estimated 1,500 or more hospitals of approximately 7,000 in the United States had dedicated programs that provided occupational medical services for employers. Although a small number of programs are still based in emergency departments, freestanding clinics within the hospital, freestanding ambulatory care locations, and networks of clinics are the most common delivery models.

Hospitals possess a breadth of services to offer a comprehensive approach in one setting and typically have the financial resources to withstand a development period that may last 12 to 18 months. They can also profit from existing personnel in management, finance, and marketing to offer immediate support for a program.

The physician/medical director is a critical part of the hospital-affiliated program team. Given the chronic undersupply of trained occupational medicine physicians, compensation and negotiation leverage is favorable for the physician. Compensation for medical directors is becoming more creative and ranges from direct salary, to salary plus incentive, to salary plus fee-for-service. A hospital setting is especially attractive for the physician who thrives in a team atmosphere and is interested in environmental and clinical challenges.

4. The answer is B. (Ref: p. 99)

Labor relations are generally not within the purview of occupational medicine practice.

Opportunities to work directly with employers are considerable, including more than one employer on a part-time basis. The more compelling opportunity, however, may be to develop a relatively narrow niche of expertise and provide replicable services to large numbers of organizations. Examples of services include advice related to medical surveillance, training, health policy, program development, and regulatory compliance. Cost-containment activities such as workers' compensation loss control and managed care are increasingly discussed with occupational medicine consultants.

5. The answer is E. (Ref: p. 100)

Employers are increasingly recognizing the value of training in occupational medicine, and, in some cases, they put a premium on it. The physician should emphasize certification and special training in occupational medicine to potential clients.

To succeed in occupational medicine, the astute physician should:

- Obtain a basic foundation in occupational medicine
- Be prepared to address the occupational medicine continuum (i.e., prevention, acute injury treatment, and the return-to-work process)
- Remain abreast of regulatory measures
- Associate interventions in terms of health care cost containment
- Be an educator
- Be prepared to play multiple roles

CHAPTER 9 ANSWERS

1. The answer is D. (Ref: p. 103)

Seven percent of employees are heavy drinkers. There is a 30% overlap between employees who are heavy drinkers and those who use illicit drugs. All of the other statements regarding illicit drug use are true.

2. The answer is B. (Ref: pp. 105, 119)

In federally regulated drug testing, all laboratory-confirmed positive test results must be reported to a medical review officer (MRO) for review and interpretation. Following verification of the result as positive by the MRO, the result is reported to the employer. All of the other statements are correct.

3. The answer is E. (Ref: p. 109)

Using specific guidelines, laboratories are permitted to perform specimen validity testing by Substance Abuse and Mental Health Services Administration (SAMHSA). Validity testing determines whether the specimen is consistent with human urine, whether specific adulterants or foreign substances were added, and whether substitution or dilution of the specimen has occurred.

4. The answer is C. (Ref: pp. 114, 115)

Only phencyclidine (PCP) has no legitimate medical explanation because a donor could have no valid medical reason for its use. Interpretation and verification of legitimate medical explanations for positive tests often requires clinical judgment and is the most critical function of the MRO.

5. The answer is E. (Ref: pp. 116–117)

All of the statements regarding Department of Transportation (DOT) alcohol testing regulations are correct. In addition, consuming alcohol after an accident before a test has been conducted or within 8 hours (whichever comes first) is also prohibited conduct for individuals in qualified safety-sensitive functions.

6. The answer is A. (Ref: Table 9.3, p. 110)

Under the DOT drug testing rules, fatal flaws require that the laboratory reject the specimen for testing. Permanently fatal flaws cannot be corrected and require that the MRO report the test as canceled to the employer. Nonfatal flaws can be corrected by receiving a signed statement of correction from the appropriate individual.

CHAPTER 10 ANSWERS

1. The answer is C. (Ref: pp. 128–129)

Accreditation Association for Ambulatory Health Care (AAAHC) does not hire surveyors nor do they rely on administrators. They use practicing occupational health care professionals who volunteer their time and are trained by AAAHC. Use of these individuals ensures true peer review for occupational health settings.

2. The answer is E. (Ref: pp. 125–127)

Consultative comments are an important component of the onsite survey. The remainder of the answers is false. Organizations can immediately apply for accreditation under the early option accreditation plan. Surveyors review all pertinent observations with the organization before the end of the survey. All medical facilities accredited by AAAHC must provide health services under the supervision or direction of a physician or dentist. The duration and number of surveyors vary from organization to organization, but all require more than one surveyor for 4 to 6 hours.

3. The answer is A. (Ref: p. 129)

The organization must determine which types of health professions are needed to provide high-quality care. The standards do not specifically require a board-certified occupational health physician, occupational nurse, or industrial hygienist. The remaining statements are true.

4. The answer is B. (Ref: pp 130–131)

The quality management standard focuses on programs that assess and improve health care and clinical outcomes. Verification of credentials is an important component of an organization's governance and administration, but it, in and of itself, does not improve quality. The remaining elements in the list do. They are included in the Quality Management and Improvement Standard.

5. The answer is D. (Ref: p. 128)

The remainders listed are generally the most difficult standards for an organization undergoing accreditation. The facilities standard is involved but well defined and relatively easy for most health care organizations.

CHAPTER 11 ANSWERS

1. The answer is E. (Ref: p. 141)

New measurement and data management techniques are available that include assessing the direct costs of medical treatment and indirect costs of long- and short-term disability; absenteeism; and presenteeism, which is the amount of work performed on the job per unit time. Employees who work while feeling ill or in pain show a decrease in productivity.

2. The answer is D. (Ref: pp. 142–143)

Corporate time and expense spent supporting wellness programs and safety and health screening appraisals has been shown to substantially reduce lost workdays and improve worker productivity.

3. The answer is B. (Ref: p. 142)

Presenteeism is a productivity metric that depends on distinct job classifications. It is the amount of work performed on the job per unit time. Absenteeism, or time off the job, is the most commonly accepted measure of worker productivity. Either self-administered questionnaires or job productivity data may be used as tools to measure presenteeism. It is true that salaried or "white collar" or "knowledge" workers return to work after time off and find that their work remains on their desk. Thus, measuring productivity by time off the job does not capture the true loss of productivity; however, this is not the definition of presenteeism.

4. The answer is E. (Ref: p. 143)

All of these are important in attracting and retaining qualified workers. Investigating the cause(s) of high turnover rates would allow appropriate changes to be made and lower the cost of retraining or rehiring workers. It would follow that turnover rates may be due to poor design, unrealistic completion times, and/or uncomfortable working conditions.

5. The answer is C. (Ref: pp. 142–143)

One of the primary goals of the Healthy People 2010 study is to reduce work-related time off. Occupational Safety and Health Administration (OSHA) recordable data is expressed as cases per 200,000 hours worked, which is the number of events per 100 employees working for 1 year. As mentioned previously, questionnaires are used to gather data about presenteeism, and self-reporting is acceptable. The Worker's Productivity Index (WPI) uses algorithms derived from presenteeism together with absenteeism and short-term disability absence. Answer choice E is the definition of presenteeism.

CHAPTER 12 ANSWERS

1. The answer is D. (Ref: pp. 153–154)

There is no federal mandate requiring health promotion programs. As a result of more than 2 decades of program proliferation, health promotion is now central to worksite programming and is recognized as an integral part of occupational health practice. A 1999 Health Promotion Survey by the Office of Disease Prevention and Health Promotion concluded that 90% of worksites with 50 or more employees offer at least one health promotion activity.

There has been a desire on the part of employers to manage health care costs, impact absenteeism, improve productivity, improve employee morale, recruit and retain employees, enhance corporate image, and contribute to the health and well-being of their human resources. As such, the stated mission of worksite health promotion is to support these interests of senior management. The good news is that there is growing empirical evidence that worksite health promotion is contributing to the achievement of management goals.

2. The answer is A. (Ref: p. 157)

The possibilities for program scope, the options for delivery, and potential for targeting not only risks and diseases but also select subsets of the employee population are extremely varied. Appropriate choices depend on the characteristics of the employee population coupled with the goals of both the program and the business.

3. The answer is B. (Ref: pp. 157–158)

Some of the popular programs offered in the business setting today include preventive screenings and examinations; smoking cessation; exercise and aerobics; eating habits, nutrition, and cholesterol; weight management; blood pressure control; stress management; employee assistance; demand management; disease management; environmental and organizational interventions; and other programs of interest.

At the outset of planning, a clear description of the expectations of the health promotion program is most essential.

Employee assessments, taking the form of surveys and focus groups, are a good place to begin. The goal is to understand the wants and needs of the population, as well as the ethnic, cultural, social, and organizational characteristics.

Management interviews gather another perspective, that of the leadership and supervision in the company. It is critical that the needs of the business are understood and that the issues of managers are taken into consideration.

Health care cost data, illness and injury absence data, and demographic data should be used to determine the prominent disease categories that are driving costs and for which groups of employees.

Finally, data from health risk appraisals (HRAs) can be used to develop and aggregate a view of population, information that is essential to program planning.

4. The answer is C. (Ref: pp. 158–165)

Some of the more popular programs offered in the business setting are smoking cessation; exercise and aerobics; nutrition, cholesterol, and weight management; blood pressure control; stress management; employee assistance programs; and preventive examinations.

Treatment of disease can only be coordinated with the patient's physician.

5. The answer is D. (Ref: pp. 170–171)

The evaluation component should be developed at the beginning of the program when the interests of all stakeholders are considered.

Evaluations can be focused on measures of process, impact, and outcomes. Process evaluation measures the participant's perception of the program. A logical indicator of program success is participation numbers and percentages. Impact evaluation measures the extent to which an intervention has had an immediate effect on biometric measures and risk factors. Outcome evaluation determines the effect of interventions on the company or employee population as a whole.

Current best practices for worksite health promotion programs include those in which (a) program plans are linked to organizational business strategy; (b) there are effective communication strategies applied; (c) effective (positive) incentives are offered; (d) evaluation is conducted, results shared, and value of results communicated; (e) the environment is health supporting; and (f) there is strong executive support.

CHAPTER 13 ANSWERS

1. The answer is C. (Ref: pp. 178–179)

Food and water are sources of significant risk to the traveler in developing countries. Travelers should be cautioned about the importance of safety practices with foods, beverages, and general hygiene.

Both tetanus and diphtheria are found in many countries of the world. Following primary immunization in childhood, a booster is recommended every 10 years. If primary (Td) immunization is required, it should be given as a series of three doses (the first two separated by 1 to 2 months, and a third dose 6 to 12 months later).

Bacille Calmette-Guérin (BCG) is a live-attenuated vaccine made from *Mycobacterium bovis.* It is not routinely given before travel and has not been used in the United States because of concerns over efficacy, problems with purified protein derivative (PPD) interpretation after use, and relatively low prevalence of tuberculosis (TB) in the United States.

Adults who received the primary series of polio vaccine in childhood should receive one booster dose of the injectable inactivated polio vaccine (IPV) before travel. This is especially important if travel will include polio endemic areas such as sub-Saharan Africa, the Middle East, the Indian subcontinent, and the island of Hispaniola (Haiti and the Dominican Republic). Persons who have not had prior polio vaccination should receive three doses (the first two separated by 1 to 2 months, and a third dose 6 to 12 months after the second).

2. The answer is B. (Ref: p. 186)

Yellow fever is a mosquito-borne viral infection. The disease is endemic in South America, Central America, and sub-Saharan Africa. Yellow fever is not found in Southeast Asia.

3. The answer is B. (Ref: pp. 186–187)

Plasmodium falciparum malaria accounts for the majority of mortality attributed to malaria disease. *P. falciparum* results in a high parasitemia rate among those infected and is associated with serious complications such a renal failure, pulmonary edema, and cerebral dysfunction.

4. The answer is D. (Ref: pp. 186–187)

Travelers to areas with chloroquine-resistant malaria should be given chemoprophylaxis to prevent malaria disease. All of the regimens listed except dicloxacillin can be used for malaria prophylaxis in chloroquine-resistant areas. Dicloxacillin does not have antimalarial action.

5. The answer is A. (Ref: pp. 188–189)

Enterotoxigenic *Escherichia coli,* typhoid fever, and hepatitis A are all associated with exposure to contaminated food or water. Hepatitis B is contracted by exposure to infected blood or body fluids. Hepatitis B can be transmitted sexually and after exposure to non-sterile needles or instruments.

6. The answer is C. (Ref: pp. 184–185, 188)

Polio is a viral illness spread via the fecal-oral and oral-oral routes. Children are the most common reservoirs. Yellow fever, Japanese encephalitis, and malaria are all spread through mosquito bites.

CHAPTER 14 ANSWERS

1. The answer is B. (Ref: p. 194)

The traditional cornerstone of clinical occupational health programs is the determination of the ability of an applicant or employee to safely perform the essential functions of a job. The Americans with Disabilities Act (ADA) has changed the approach to these examinations to some extent. Under the ADA, a thorough attempt must be made to reasonably accommodate the applicant or employee if the person can perform the *essential,* or key, job functions with accommodation. A number of the actions taken under the impetus of reasonable accommodation actually have made jobs safer for all employees.

In evaluating the economic effects of medical screening and placement programs, therefore, one would balance the cost of the program against decreases in real or projected cost of work-related illness or injuries. All direct and indirect costs, including medical treatment, time lost from work, supervisory time, and other attributable costs, should be included to obtain a proper analysis. Failure to place employees appropriately using essential job function comparison and cost-benefit analysis may result in preventable costs for replacement and retraining, inefficiency, medical treatment, workers' compensation payments, fines under the ADA, actions under the Vocational Rehabilitation Act of 1974 or various state laws, and lost wages.

2. The answer is E. (Ref: p. 195)

See answer 1.

3. The answer is A. (Ref: pp. 195–196)

A key duty of the occupational health professional is to monitor health-related data on members of the workforce exposed to chemical, radiation, and other physical hazards and to compare the values for exposed and unexposed groups periodically. If an increased prevalence of abnormal laboratory values or symptoms is detected in an exposed group, the exposure should be quantified and controlled through engineering measures, administrative efforts (i.e., rotating employees), or personal protective equipment in that order. The economic value of this type of service depends on the cost of the disease avoided, which can be computed for a population of workers if the probability of illness is known for various levels of exposure. There are many examples of preventable occupationally related complaints or diseases that ultimately have caused great expense including cases of back, upper extremity, and other muscle and tendon pain. Consistent monitoring and changes in job structure are important modes to prevent the occurrence or worsening of these health complaints and disorders.

4. The answer is E. (Ref: pp. 196–199)

Immunization can be instituted to prevent occupational transmission of infectious disease, as in hepatitis B immunization of workers in health care facilities, prisons, and sanitation industries. Immunization of workers against tetanus will prevent many visits to medical facilities for prophylaxis of minor wounds. Diphtheria, influenza, and other routine immunizations will prevent considerable lost work time.

5. The answer is D. (Ref: pp. 199–200)

Treatment of injuries and illnesses onsite can be cost effective for a variety of reasons. Time lost to travel to a health facility and wait for treatment is avoided. Physicians and nurses who are familiar with the work environment usually have a better understanding of the toxicity of substances used; individual workers' backgrounds, attitudes, and risks; and factors involved in injuries that may complicate the recovery process. Where onsite treatment is not feasible, community-based occupational health services can also save time by prompt treatment and effective management of work-related injuries. Knowledge of the job is critical for appropriate placement of workers returning to work following an illness or injury. There are physical, mental, and economic advantages to early return to work.

6. The answer is E. (Ref: pp. 201–203)

Knowledge of the job is critical for appropriate placement of workers returning to work following an illness or injury. The occupational physician can prescribe modified duties in light of availability of proper assignment and medical limitations.

There are physical, mental, and economic advantages to early return to work. First, return to work benefits the injured worker, who becomes a part of the work milieu again. Improvements in self-worth that result can aid in the recovery process. Second, many musculoskeletal problems such as regional low back pain become worse with inactivity. Inactivity is one of the risks for significant delays in functional recovery. Furthermore, the rate of return-to-work declines substantially after several months' absence and is very low after 6 months to a year. Many of these employees could work in some capacity if graduated accommodation were made.

A small group of employees at most worksites use significantly more medical services than other employees and are absent a great deal because of somatization of psychologic conflicts. Resolution of these somatization disorders by providing cognitive services has resulted in benefit-to-cost ratios of up to 10:1. Employee assistance programs also provide savings by early intervention in mental health problems, which can prevent hospitalization and long-term illness.

Injury and reinjury in taxing jobs can be prevented by gradually increasing workload or time at the job. This is termed "transitional work." The value obtained from reconditioning workers appears to significantly outweigh the cost of professional time and lost production. It is clear that onsite transitional duty is much less expensive and more supportive of reintegration than extensive simulated work conditioning and work hardening performed by clinics off-site.

Education of patients in self-care for minor illnesses and injuries has reduced health care costs. Educating employees in the best way to use the medical care system has resulted in increases in the quality of care and substantial decreases in inappropriate utilization.

7. The answer is C. (Ref: pp. 203–204)

There is evidence from both epidemiologic studies and clinical trials to show that morbidity and mortality are reduced if risk factors are decreased. Studies on the net cost effectiveness of health promotion programs demonstrate a significant positive benefit-to-cost ratio. Although much of the risk screening done today is nonproductive, early detection of hypertension, hypercholesterolemia, and cervical and breast cancer has a significant benefit-to-cost ratio. In asymptomatic individuals, other tests, such as chest and back x-ray films, multichannel chemistries, and resting and stress electrocardiograms, are of minimal value and may result in unnecessary costs involved in ruling out false positives.

CHAPTER 15 ANSWERS

1. The answer is E. (Ref: p. 209)

Unfortunately, most medical school curricula do not adequately expose students to the field at an early stage in their medical education. A survey of medical schools in 1996 found that, of 116 of 126 schools responding, 24% had no curricula content in environmental medicine (EM). Those who did include EM gave an average of 7 hours of instruction. Only 68% of schools reported having faculty with occupational and environmental medicine (OEM) expertise.

2. The answer is B. (Ref: p. 210)

The Accreditation Council for Graduate Medical Education (ACGME) now requires some element of occupational medicine training in accredited family medicine training programs.

3. The answer is B. (Ref: p. 210)

The most fundamental distinction is that OEM is a specialty that focuses on the *prevention* of illness and injury. Thus, one goal of OEM practitioners is to deliver consultative and clinical services designed to prevent illness and injury. Often a sentinel illness or injury will provide the lead for identifying a problem workplace. What sets the OEM practitioner apart is the desire and expertise to go to the workplace and help formulate measures that will prevent recurrence of the condition among other workers. In instances in which illness is identified, the physician must have enough knowledge about the workplace and specific job activities of the person to render a judgment regarding the relative contribution of the workplace. To competently deliver OEM services, one must be more than just a good clinician.

The practitioner must think in terms of *populations of workers* and have an understanding of epidemiology and biostatistics to interpret trends in illness or presence of certain sentinel abnormalities in disease or laboratory surveillance measures.

4. The answer is C. (Ref: pp. 211–212)

In 2000, 38 residency training programs in occupational medicine were accredited by the ACGME in the United States. Occupational medicine residencies vary widely in size, but nationwide approximately 75 to 100 physicians graduate each year. Occupational medicine residency training includes three distinct components. The first year consists of an ACGME-accredited clinical internship (PG1). The second year of the residency consists of a broad curriculum of study, generally leading to a master of public health (MPH) or equivalent degree. Required courses work includes biostatistics, epidemiology, health services organization and administration, environmental and occupational health, and social and behavioral influences on health. The third year of the typical residency program consists of a series of rotations provided at a variety of occupational medicine settings to gain practical experience. Termed the "practicum," this phase of training usually includes supervised training at industrial sites, occupational medicine clinics, labor organizations, and government agencies such a the Occupational Safety and Health Administration (OSHA), National Institute for Occupational Safety and Health (NIOSH), and Agency for Toxic Substances and Disease Registry (ATSDR).

5. The answer is D. (Ref: p. 214)

The American College of Occupational and Environmental Medicine (ACOEM) sponsors seminars and courses related to the specialty. In addition to postgraduate seminars and courses offered at the national meetings in the spring and fall of each year, the college periodically sponsors 1- or 2-day courses of particular interest to practitioners. Examples include medical review offer (MRO) courses and seminars on the Americans with Disabilities Act (ADA). The ACOEM also offers the basic curriculum, a structured series of three 2-day segments designed to provide the nonoccupational medicine specialist with useful information and an introduction to OEM.

Education and Research Centers (ERCs) were established by NIOSH to provide multidisciplinary educational resources in occupational health. Each center was required to maintain at least three of the four educational components of occupational health as determined by NIOSH: occupational medicine, occupational health nursing, safety, and industrial hygiene.

CHAPTER 16 ANSWERS

1. The answer is C. (Ref: pp. 218–219)

Computers are quickly becoming essential management tools with valued applications in all aspects of occupational health (OH). The use of a successful occupational health information system (OHIS) can significantly improve an organization's ability to achieve its goals through (a) improved efficiency, accuracy, and productivity; (b) enhanced quality, decision making, and documentation; (c) regulatory compliance and litigation assistance; and (d) the ability to inexpensively create supplemental and new services, such as Web sites customized to meet highly specific client and employee needs.

2. The answer is C (Ref: pp. 220–222)

The Internet represents a technology that can both reduce the complexity and enhance the value of OHIS. The Internet provides both low- and high-speed connections among most computers in the world. Internet access software programs (browsers) provide an easy-to-use tool for linking computers and data to a desktop personal computer (PC). Privacy is a major issue.

Harnessing computer and Internet technologies makes it easier to shift clients away from price sensitivity by gaining a competitive advantage based on delivering highly individualized services developed with the help of these continually updated knowledge bases.

Applying one-to-one principals when providing employee health services are likely to be more technology intensive given the pure numbers involved. One exciting approach can provide the homebound injured worker with a highly customized 24 hour, 7 days a week Web portal providing easily accessible resources to help speed recovery and return to work.

3. The answer is B (Ref: pp. 232–233)

The Health Insurance Portability and Accountability Act of 1996 (HIPAA) contains five principles:

1. Consumer control. The standards provide consumers with important new rights, including the right to see a copy of their medical records, the right to request a correction to their medical records, and the right to obtain documentation of disclosures of their health information.
2. Accountability. The statute includes new civil and criminal penalties for violations of a patient's right to privacy.
3. Public responsibility. Privacy protections must be balanced with the public right to support such national priorities as protecting public health, conducting medical research, improving the quality of care, and fighting health care fraud and abuse.
4. Boundaries. With few exceptions, an individual's health care information should be used for health purposes only, including treatment and payment.
5. Security. Organizations that are entrusted with health information must protect it against deliberate or inadvertent misuse or disclosure. The standards require each covered organization to establish clear procedures to protect patients' privacy, designate an official to monitor that system, and notify their patients about their privacy protection practices. In addition, those who get information and misuse it would be subject to the penalties outlined in the proposal. These comprehensive national med-

ical record privacy standards are complex and subject to continuing legislative review.

4. The answer is C (Ref: pp. 223–225)

One of the most important components of an OHIS system—indeed, perhaps the most important component—is support of the office staff in the pursuit of everyday tasks. Word processing, spreadsheets, contact and time managers, project timelines, electronic mail, and Web access are all important parts of general office automation support. Without integration of these functions, the OHIS may not be used.

CHAPTER 17 ANSWERS

1. The answer is C. (Ref: pp. 238–239)

Biologic risks are of more serious concern in international occupational practice. Although bacterial and viral diseases (malaria; Hepatitis A, B, and C; and others) have been the traditional focus, the global impact of emerging infectious diseases such as prions and mad cow disease has been significant.

2. The answer is E. (Ref: p. 239)

Susceptibility of workers may be increased due to use of child labor or migrant workers, warfare, and poverty.

3. The answer is A. (Ref: p. 239)

Occupational hygiene services may be unavailable due to a lack of equipment or laboratories. In the absence of quantitative exposure levels, hazard recognition is important.

Standardization of medical surveillance, exposure limits, measurement systems, audit programs, policies, and procedures and regulations are major international challenges. In many countries, the occupational medicine program provides nonoccupational health care for expatriates, short-term assignees and visitors, managers, workers and their families, and, in some cases, extended families. Emergency transportation and evacuation plans must be outlined for victims of injury or illness in developing countries.

4. The answer is C. (Ref: p. 241)

Procurement of pharmaceuticals locally, or importation of pharmaceuticals may be difficult. International transportation of prescription drugs by mail is generally illegal, and hand-carrying of medications for workers and family members by other workers is often necessary. Some drugs that are legal in the United States may be illegal in other countries.

CHAPTER 18 ANSWERS

1. The answer is E. (Ref: p. 240)

The goals of workers' compensation systems are typically to prevent work-related illness and injury; to make injured workers whole physically, mentally, and/or economically; and to return workers to productive work in their original, or, if necessary, some alternative capacity.

In the days before workers' compensation, injured workers did not receive timely compensation. As a result, a series of "no fault" workers' compensation laws were passed on a state-by-state basis. Workers' compensation laws represented a compromise or "lesser peril" for both employers and employees. These laws were supposed to ensure rapid payment to injured workers for lost wages and medical costs regardless of fault. In exchange, employers' liability for occupational injuries, illness, and death was limited if they participated in a compensation system. Under this system, employers generally were exempt from damage suits, unless gross negligence could be proved.

2. The answer is D. (Ref: p. 243)

The two traditional criteria for eligibility for workers' compensation benefits are termed "AOE/COE"—arising out of employment (AOE) and in the course of employment (COE).

In the days before workers' compensation, there were a number of accepted common law defenses when an employee sued an employer. The employer could claim that the employee contributed to the injury, that he or she had assumed risk by taking the job, or that negligent acts of fellow workers were responsible for the injury.

Workers' compensation laws were intended to modify common law defenses and limit employers' liability. Neither of these initiatives led to equitable and timely compensation for injured workers. As a result, a series of "no fault" workers' compensation laws were passed on a state-by-state basis.

3. The answer is E. (Ref: p. 247)

With reductions in group-health benefits, there has been a tendency to ascribe injuries to the worksite because workers' compensation will pay 100% of the medical bills and provide wage replacement. There is also an economic incentive to undertake workers' compensation claims as benefits payments increase. Dissatisfaction with one's job, monotonous and repetitive tasks, and the feeling of fatigue at the end of the workday are associated with greater absenteeism and disability leave. Attorney involvement was the strongest predictor of disability in one extensive study.

4. The answer is C. (Ref: pp. 247–248)

In many companies or nonprofit organizations, losses are not allocated back to the department in which they were incurred. This policy is an intracompany version of risk spreading that provides a disincentive to improvement and safety records. Furthermore, many managers have productivity incentives. Therefore, they prefer not to return employees to work on limited duty. This disincentive clearly prevents rapid return to work, which is associated with shorter recovery times and reduced payments. The availability of light work or modified duties is key to reducing accident severity rates. Several studies show that absenteeism and disability with low back pain are significantly reduced when light duty is available.

5. The answer is C. (Ref: pp. 253–254)

In an analysis of 12 states' workers' compensation data for 1998 by International Classification of Diseases (ICD)-9 code, soft tissue complaints accounted for many of the top 10 diagnostic groups for all workers' compensation cases. The top 10 in Texas, for example, included low back soft tissue complaints (17%), shoulder soft tissue complaints (7%), neck soft tissue complaints (6%), hand and wrist superficial trauma (4%), knee internal derangements (3.8%), hand and wrist soft tissue complaints (3.4%), multiple body parts soft tissue complaints (3.2%), low back nerve compression (2.4%), ankle and foot soft tissue complaints (2.4%), and hand and wrist nerve compression (2.4%).

According to Occupational Safety and Health Administration (OSHA) statistics, the back was the body part most commonly affected by disabling work incidents accounting for about one fourth or 424,300 cases of the 1.7 million total. Finger injuries were next (149,500 cases), then knees (128,000) and shoulder injuries (93,800). The most common types of disabling injuries and illnesses were sprains and strains (739,700); bruises and contusions (156,000); cuts and lacerations (132,400); and fractures (113,700). A total of 27,900 cases of carpal tunnel syndrome requiring days away from work (DAW) were reported in 1999, ranking sixth overall. There were 16,600 tendonitis cases with DAW reported as well.

6. The answer is E. (Ref: p. 254)

A number of authors have documented significant underreporting of work-related disorders for other reasons. Reasons for underreporting include fear of reprisal, a belief that pain is a normal consequence of aging or work, lack of management responsiveness to previous complaints, and a desire not to be moved to another job. Corporate safety objectives may have an indirect effect on reporting because managers attempt to reduce injury rates to meet goals.

7. The answer is B. (Ref: p. 254)

There were 6,023 work-related fatalities in the United States in 1999, down from 6,055 in 1998 despite an increase in employment. Forty-three percent were due to transportation incidents, 17% to objects and equipment, 15% to assaults and violent acts, 12% to falls, and 9% to harmful substances or environments. Motor vehicle accidents accounted for more than one half of the transport fatalities. The number of homicides at work has declined almost 40% from 1994 to 1999. Homicide dropped from second to third among leading causes. Accidental work deaths per 100,000 population have dropped more than 83% from 1912 to 1999.

8. The answer is A. (Ref: p. 262)

It is important for all participants in the workers' compensation system to understand each other's roles and responsibilities to have this conflict-prone system function more smoothly. Employers, employees, payers, regulators, and health care providers all have important roles to play.

At a minimum, providers caring for workers with health concerns should provide excellent care and foster functional recovery. Doing so requires a broader and arguably more neutral approach than nonoccupational health care. In addition to diagnosing the problem and providing treatment, providers should take a complete occupational history to determine causation, understand the hazards that caused the problem to prevent further adverse effects, facilitate functional recovery using modified work and other proven effective methods, and dispassionately evaluate impairment at maximal medical improvement (MMI). Excellent management of workers' compensation provides a challenge to the administrative and clinical skills of the occupational physician. The effort, however, can benefit both the injured worker with more effective medical care and the employer by increasing availability for work and decreasing unnecessary costs.

When the injured worker has recovered to the extent possible, the attending physician is typically asked to certify that MMI has been reached. This is usually the point at which further medical care would not have substantial benefit. It does not mean that the worker might not require palliative care or care for an exacerbation of a problem in the future. The physician may also be asked to forecast the future medical needs of the patient. This opinion should be as quantitative as possible.

At MMI, the attending physician may also be asked to rate any residual impairment. This is a somewhat specialized skill that many physicians are not comfortable with.

CHAPTER 19 ANSWERS

1. The answer is A. (Ref: p. 267)

Rather than focusing on a pure cost-containment model, occupational physicians should shift to more innovative purchasing methodologies based on informed consumer choice, disease management, outcomes, and quality, and cost-sharing arrangements between employers and employees. This provides the physician with an opportunity to expand the roles of both the corporate medical director and the physician consultant.

Studies have shown that there are financial incentives for companies to offer onsite wellness programs, and it is critical for occupational physicians to become involved. There is a perception that ethical values may potentially be violated because of a professional relationship with the employer and that this may somehow affect medical decisions concerning an employee's financial status, future employment, or disability.

2. The answer is D. (Ref: pp. 270–271)

Utilization review is a process in which services are reviewed by third parties to determine if they are medically appropriate and/or necessary. Payment for services depends on this review. In one survey, 10% of the cases contributed to more than 50% of the total costs. To monitor aspects of the delivery of benefits, employers use utilization review. All other statements are true.

3. The answer is E (Ref: pp. 268–269)

Linking medical insurance to employment was a product of the statutory wage freezes of World War II, as labor and management turned to health benefits as an alternative to increased compensation to employees. The Great Depression, in part, brought about founding of Blue Cross and Blue Shield, as concerns about insolvency led hospitals and doctors to form third-party organizations to finance their operations. Health benefits have been tax exempt since their inception, creating a financial incentive for companies.

The government entered the health care market with the establishment of Medicare and Medicaid in 1965. The Center for Medicare and Medicaid Services (CMS), formerly known as Health Care Financing Administration (HCFA), is the single largest purchaser of health care in the world, with $476 billion paid for health care services in 2001 on behalf of 70 million disabled, elderly, and poor beneficiaries.

4. The answer is C (Ref: p. 269)

The most controversial of the five major laws in which HCFA made provisions was the Balanced Budget Act of 1997. The other four laws are the Reconciliation Act of 1996, Health Insurance Portability and Accountability Act of 1999, the Balanced Budget Refinement Act of 1999, and the Benefits Improvement and Protection Act of 2000. Some of the provisions in these laws called for the agency to regulate private health insurance and to establish electronic-data standards for the entire health care industry. The Balanced Budget Act of 1997 reduced Medicare payments to clinical labs, hospitals, skilled nursing facilities, and home health agencies in the United States, with an estimated reduction of $112 billion for the period from 1998 through 2002.

5. The answer is D (Ref: p. 270)

Capitated contracts create some degree of risk. The payment amount is set in advance of the service; it may turn out afterwards to have been the wrong amount. Someone has to make up the difference if the capitated fee is too low, and someone stands to gain if it is too high. Nothing about capitation specifies who assumes the risk.

20

Suspecting Occupational Disease: The Clinician's Role

OBJECTIVES

- Explain the importance of work-related causes in the differential diagnosis
- Discuss the extent of occupational illness in the United States
- Explain obstacles to physicians in the recognition of work-related and environmental health problems
- Illustrate an organized approach to history taking and diagnosis of occupational or environmental illness
- Identify examples of environmental causes of medical problems
- Identify examples of common dangerous household products
- Identify examples of hazards in hobbies
- List examples of occupational sentinel health events

OUTLINE

I. Introduction
II. Occupational/environmental (O/E) health survey of all patients
III. Defining and describing the sources of exposure
    A. Workplace
    B. Home surroundings
    C. Quantifying exposures
    D. Further follow-up and consultations
IV. Resources
    A. Figure 20.1: Systematic approach to history taking and diagnosis of occupational or environmental illness
    B. Table 20.1: Examples of environmental causes of medical problems
    C. Table 20.2: Examples of common dangerous household products
    D. Table 20.3: Examples of hazards in hobbies
    E. Appendix to Chapter 20: Occupationally related unnecessary disease, disability, and untimely death (sentinel health events—occupational)

KEY POINTS

- Persons suffering from work-related illness enter clinicians' offices every day. However, consideration of work-related causes rarely enters the practitioner's differential diagnosis. As a result, clinicians may miss the chance to make diagnoses that might influence the course of a disease in some and that might prevent disease in others (by stopping exposure).

- It is difficult to estimate the full extent of occupational illness in the United States because of the lack of accurate information. The Bureau of Labor Statistics (BLS) in the Department of Labor reports statistics based on surveys of private companies with greater than 11 employees, excluding the self-employed, farmers, and government employees. BLS reported 5.7 million nonfatal injuries and illnesses or 6.1 per 100 full-time workers in 2000. Of the 362,500 new illness cases reported, 67% were disorders related to repeated trauma, such as carpal tunnel syndrome and noise-induced hearing loss.
- Clinicians have an important role to play in identifying potential workplace risks and possible work-related health problems in their patients. One obstacle to physicians' recognition of job-related health problems is insufficient education. A survey in 1983 showed that 50% of medical schools taught courses in occupational health, but the average curriculum time was only 4 hours. The Institute of Medicine has recommended methods to foster the role and education of the primary care physician in environmental and occupational medicine, and there are now many resources available. Another impediment to the recognition of work-related illness is a lack of uniqueness in the clinical manifestations of many occupational illnesses. A long latency (the period from initial exposure to presentation of disease) is another factor that leads to underrecognition of some occupational diseases.
- To detect cases of occupational disease, an O/E history, even if brief, should be taken on *every* patient. With this in mind, the first step in the O/E history is a brief survey of all patients that could include (a) a list of current and longest held jobs and a current job description; (b) attention to the chief complaint (or diagnosis) for clues suggesting a temporal relationship to activities at work or at home; (c) a review-of-systems type question about exposures to fumes, dusts, chemicals, loud noise, radiation, or musculoskeletal stresses; and (d) observance of the presence of other triggers that prompt further inquiry, such as a sentinel health event diagnosis, disease in an unlikely person, symptoms with unknown cause, and/or the patient with concerns about exposures.
- In the case of allergic reactions, it may take months of exposure before sensitization and clinical allergy develops. Symptoms related to current exposures may initially improve on nonworkdays or vacations, but prolonged exposure can lead to the persistence of symptoms beyond the workday. Exposure to substances in the workplace or environment can also aggravate underlying medical conditions. Other triggers such as the presence of a sentinel health event (occupational) may prompt the need for further inquiry. This is a disease, disability, or untimely death that is occupationally related and whose occurrence may provide the impetus for evaluations (such as epidemiologic studies or industrial hygiene evaluations) and interventions to prevent future cases.
- Responses elicited in the O/E history survey questions may raise the practitioner's suspicions that the patient's condition is related to an environmental or work exposure, thus prompting further questioning and gathering of information about work and home exposures. This may require a detailed evaluation of the work history not only regarding jobs held, places of employment, and description of operations performed but also including (a) inquiry about illnesses in other workers on relevant jobs; (b) content, type, and manner of handling substances; (c) personal protective equipment used; and (d) potential modes of entry (ingestion, inhalation, or skin absorption). To obtain this information, the practitioner can ask the worker or manufacturer for the Material Safety Data Sheet (MSDS) that usually lists the product's ingredients, physical proper-

ties, and some environmental protection information. It is frequently very useful to obtain and review any industrial hygiene or air quality evaluations that may have already been performed.

- The routine survey questions may suggest that the symptoms relate to hazardous materials or conditions in the home. Possible sources of such hazards include internal sources, such as use of household chemicals and pesticides; the performance of certain hobbies; the presence of biologic contamination, faulty heating systems, or water and food contamination; and the transport of toxic dust or chemicals into the home on work clothes.

- Once potential sources have been identified, the next question is whether or not exposure has actually occurred and if so to what degree. Documenting and quantifying exposures can involve performing biologic monitoring tests on the affected person, as well as an evaluation of the work or environmental site. Within the office setting, the patient can be tested for evidence of exposure in body fluids (biologic monitoring) or for adverse health effects on target organs. The practitioner must know what agent to look for, the desirable test medium (urine, blood, hair, or tissue), appropriate timing, and influences on test results. With exposure data in hand, the clinician can go on to determine if the symptoms and medical findings in the particular patient are consistent with the health effects and time course of toxicity associated with a particular hazardous exposure.

QUESTIONS

*1. All of the following factors contribute to the underrecognition of work-related health conditions by medical practitioners **except***

A. The rare nature of occupational illness and injury in the United States
B. Lack of physician education
C. Long latency of certain occupational diseases
D. Lack of uniqueness in the clinical manifestations of many occupational illnesses
E. Inadequate occupational history

*2. Which of the following is **least** important when taking a brief survey of the patient's O/E history?*

A. A list of current and longest held jobs and a current job description
B. Attention to the chief complaint (or diagnosis) for clues suggesting a temporal relationship to activities at work or at home
C. The pay level awarded in all prior jobs
D. A review-of-systems question about exposures to fumes, dusts, chemicals, loud noise, radiation, or musculoskeletal stresses
E. Potential sentinel health events

3. Triggers in the O/E history brief survey that may prompt further inquiry include

A. A sentinel health event diagnosis
B. Disease in an unlikely person
C. Symptoms with unknown cause
D. Patient with concerns about exposures
E. All of the above

4. *Which of the following statements about occupational illness is correct?*

A. Allergic sensitization to occupational chemicals is always clinically apparent after the first exposure.
B. Symptoms rarely improve when away from the work setting.
C. Exposure to O/E substances can also aggravate underlying medical conditions.
D. All of the above are true.
E. None of the above are true.

5. *A sentinel health event—occupational is*

A. A work-related condition that occurred historically but is now all but extinct
B. An occupational illness that is always infectious
C. An occupational condition that lasts only for a short time
D. A work-related problem that never occurs after the age of 18 years
E. A disease, disability, or untimely death that is occupationally related and whose occurrence may provide the impetus for evaluations and interventions to prevent future cases

6. *A detailed evaluation of the work history may be indicated on the basis of a brief O/E survey. Necessary elements of such a history may include all of the following **except***

A. A list of jobs held, places of employment, and description of operations performed
B. A directory of the names and addresses of coworkers
C. Review of available MSDS
D. Personal protective equipment used
E. Review of available industrial hygiene data

7. *Possible sources of hazards in the home environment include*

A. Household chemicals and pesticides
B. Hobbies
C. A faulty heating system
D. A and B only
E. All of the above

8. *Documenting and quantifying exposures can involve performing biologic monitoring tests of the affected person. Which of the following is (are) true regarding biologic monitoring?*

A. It is a measure of the adverse health effect on an organ.
B. Tissue levels of a chemical or metabolite are always long lasting and can be measured months after exposure.
C. Levels of a chemical or metabolite are dependent entirely on environmental levels and health effects always correlate closely.
D. None of the above are true.
E. All of the above are true.

═══21═══
Occupational Pulmonary Disease

OBJECTIVES

- List four major categories of occupational lung disorders
- Cite differences between latency in acute and chronic occupational lung disease
- Explain the range of tests used for the evaluation of occupational lung disease
- State the contributions of the B-reader
- Explain complications that may develop from toxic exposure to the respiratory tract

OUTLINE

KEY POINTS

- An occupational lung disorder is an acute or chronic lung condition that arises, at least partly, from the inhalation of an airborne agent in the workplace. Occupational lung disorders include diseases caused solely by workplace exposures and conditions such as asthma that may predate workplace exposures but are exacerbated by them.
- If malignancy is excluded, occupational lung disorders fall into four major categories: pneumoconioses or "dust-related" disease, irritant reactions, asthmatic responses, and hypersensitivity reactions.
- The diagnosis of occupational lung disease can only be made if a physician is in the habit of asking a patient about his or her work. Acute lung disorders, such as irritant or hypersensitivity reactions, are more likely to be related to workplace exposures at the time symptoms first appear. Some diseases that cause chronic progressive disability (such as advanced silicosis, asbestosis, or coal worker's pneumoconiosis) generally have a period of at least 10 years of exposure to the relevant dust; even with 10 years of exposure, it may be 20 or more years from first exposure before evidence of a pneumoconiosis appears.
- Information that other workers in the same area or doing similar jobs were affected similarly is supportive of a work-related cause.
- A chest x-ray and spirometry are essential to the assessment of occupational lung disease. When any of the pneumoconioses, asbestos-related pleural disease, or berylliosis is suspected, the chest x-ray films should be read according to the classification that has been developed by the International Labor Office (ILO) of the World Health Organization based on the nature, size, and extent of opacities. Only certain radiologists and physicians are certified to read films according to this classification. These physicians are termed B-readers.
- Lung function tests can be used to assign respiratory impairment in terms of abnormal spirometry. By convention, ventilatory abnormalities are described either as being *restrictive* [an abnormally decreased forced vital capacity (FVC)] or *obstructive* with well-preserved forced expiratory volume in 1 second (FEV_1) to FVC ratio. Bronchial provocation tests are particularly useful when assessing patients with possible occupational asthma. Nonspecific airway challenge tests determine whether an individual's airways are unusually "reactive" to a nonspecific bronchoconstrictor stimulus, such as methacholine. Specific airways provocation tests involve exposure of the subject to the agent(s) thought to cause asthma.
- Other studies that may be helpful include fiberoptic bronchoscopy and brushings, transbronchial biopsy, and bronchoalveolar lavage.
- Immune-mediated occupational lung disorders include asthma and "extrinsic allergic alveolitis." Specific immunoglobulin E (IgE) has been demonstrated for several causes of occupational asthma, and antibodies may be detected by the radioallergosorbent test (RAST). Immune testing seems to have the greatest predictive value in chronic beryllium disease in which the lymphocyte transformation test is used.

- Silicosis is the most common pneumoconiosis worldwide. People who work in mines or who are involved in blasting and drilling operations are at risk of exposure to silica. Other high-risk groups include sandblasters and foundry workers.
- A definite increase in the risk of pulmonary tuberculosis is attributed to silica exposure. A variant of silicosis occurs in patients who have rheumatoid arthritis or circulating rheumatoid factor; these patients can develop necrobiotic nodules several centimeters in diameter that frequently cavitate and become infected (Caplan's syndrome).
- Asbestosis is a form of lung fibrosis of the "usual interstitial type" that results from the inhalation of asbestos fibers. The term *asbestosis* refers only to this type of parenchymal lung disease and excludes pleural thickening or fibrosis that may accompany the parenchymal lesions. Asbestos bodies (or ferruginous bodies) are composed of an asbestos fiber that has been subjected to attack by alveolar macrophages with the resulting deposition of proteinaceous materials and iron on the surface of the fiber.
- Many gases, fumes, and aerosols are directly toxic to the respiratory tract by causing acute inflammation of the respiratory mucosa and lung parenchyma. The principal sites in the respiratory tract where different agents have the greatest effect are determined by their water solubility and particle size. Highly soluble agents dissolve readily in the upper respiratory tract and airways; less-soluble agents exert their main effects in the peripheral, small airways and in the lung parenchyma. Particles larger than 10 μm in diameter tend to settle in the upper respiratory tract; those 3 to 10 μm settle mainly in the airways; those smaller than 3 μm deposit mainly in the lung parenchyma and small airways.
- Exposures to high air concentrations of water-soluble agents cause extensive inflammatory changes throughout the respiratory tract. In severe cases, this amounts to a chemical burn of the respiratory mucosa and is a medical emergency. Two principal problems that may result are laryngeal edema and severe lung edema, which may require assisted ventilation and oxygen. The serious sequel of toxic irritants is not always apparent at the time of exposure but may develop 24 to 48 hours later. Long-term complications of toxic edema may include lung fibrosis and occasionally bronchiolitis obliterans.
- Reactive airways dysfunction syndrome (RADS) may follow acute exposures to lung irritants. Individuals may develop asthma or experience the return of asthma after many years.
- Occupational asthma may be diagnosed by (a) demonstrating that an individual has asthma (using lung spirometry or, if baseline lung function is normal, by showing that the individual has nonspecific airway hyperactivity) and (b) demonstrating a causal link between workplace exposure and alterations in lung function. Bronchial challenge in the laboratory or at the worksite with the agent(s) of interest may be useful. Specific bronchial provocation tests are best performed by experienced personnel in a laboratory where the nature of the exposure can be controlled and where urgent treatment can be administered promptly for an acute severe reaction. Once a diagnosis of occupational asthma is established, prompt job transfer to an area of no exposure is necessary.
- Farmer's lung is a type of hypersensitivity pneumonitis that resembles recurrent pneumonia. It is most commonly due to the bacteria *Micropolyspora faeni* and various fungi, such as thermophilic actinomyces species. Current theory attributes pathogenesis of hypersensitivity pneumonitis (extrinsic allergic alveolitis) to T lymphocytes (suppressor cells) and epithelioid granulomas, reflecting a type IV immune response. Diagnosis is made by taking a careful history of exposure because chest x-ray films and blood test results may vary.

• Prevention of occupational respiratory disease is accomplished by engineering controls, use of personal protective equipment such as respirators, and administrative controls. Administrative controls are usually the least effective method to prevent pulmonary disease from airborne hazards.

QUESTIONS

*1. Occupational lung disease includes all of the following categories **except***

A. Hypersensitivity reactions
B. Asthmatic responses
C. Pneumoconioses
D. Paraneoplastic syndromes
E. Irritant reactions

2. Which of the following is (are) true regarding the effect of water solubility and particle size on absorption of gases, fumes, and aerosols?

A. Highly water-soluble agents dissolve readily in the upper respiratory tract.
B. Particles of 3 to 10 µm settle mainly in the airways.
C. Particles smaller than 3 µm deposit mainly in the small airways and lung parenchyma.
D. Less-soluble agents exert their effects in the upper respiratory tract.
E. A, B, and C above.

*3. Which statement is **incorrect** regarding hypersensitivity pneumonitis?*

A. It commonly results from bacteria *M. faeni* and various fungi.
B. It has findings that suggest recurrent pneumonia.
C. It is an immune disease mediated by IgE.
D. It is thought that T lymphocytes are important in its pathogenesis.
E. Chest x-ray film and serum findings are nonspecific.

*4. Pneumoconioses are dust inhalation diseases that are characterized by chest x-ray abnormalities and clinical respiratory impairment. Which one of the following is **false** about pneumoconioses?*

A. Asbestosis is a form of interstitial lung fibrosis.
B. Ferruginous bodies are composed of an asbestos fiber that has been attacked by alveolar macrophages with resulting deposition of iron and proteins.
C. Caplan's syndrome is found in patients with silicosis and circulating rheumatoid factor; patients may develop necrobiotic nodules several centimeters in diameter.
D. Pulmonary tuberculosis is infrequently seen in patients with silicosis.
E. The term *asbestosis* excludes pleural thickening.

5. The ILO system for classification of chest x-ray films is characterized by which of the following?

A. Chest x-ray films are analyzed for the nature, size, and extent of opacities.
B. B-readers are experts certified to read films according to this classification.
C. Only radiologists may be B-readers.

D. Pneumoconioses x-ray films should be read according to this classification.
E. A, B, and D above.

6. *Which of the following is correct regarding occupational asthma?*

A. Bronchial provocation tests such as methacholine are useful in assessing patients.
B. Onset of symptoms may be abrupt and in the workplace.
C. Once the diagnosis of occupational asthma is established, prompt job transfer to an area of no exposure is advised.
D. Onset may be delayed for several hours after exposure.
E. All of the above.

22

Musculoskeletal Disorders

OBJECTIVES

- List the importance of acute back injuries from workplace exposure
- Enumerate the essentials of the evaluation of low back pain
- List therapeutic steps after low back injury
- Distinguish between acute and chronic low back pain
- State important issues in the prevention of back injuries
- Describe soft tissue injuries of the neck, shoulder, and knee
- List various types of cumulative trauma disorders that involve the upper extremity

OUTLINE

I. Rates of occupational injuries
II. Back disorders
   A. Acute back injuries
   B. The diagnosis of low back pain
      1. History
      2. Physical examination
      3. Diagnostic imaging
      4. Acute management of low back pain
      5. Medical follow-up of low back injury
   C. Chronic back disorders
      1. History
      2. Laboratory testing
      3. Electromyography/nerve conduction velocity (EMG/NCV)
      4. Treatment
      5. Rehabilitation and return-to-work status
   D. Prevention of back injuries
      1. Proper selection and placement
      2. Maintenance of a healthy back
III. Shoulder disorders
IV. Knee injuries
V. Cumulative trauma disorders
   A. Carpal tunnel syndrome
      1. History
      2. Physical examination
      3. EMG/NCV
      4. Treatment

KEY POINTS

- Occupational back pain is the most common musculoskeletal complaint in the workplace. Risk factors for low back pain include heavy repetitive lifting, pushing, and pulling as well as exposure to industrial and vehicular vibration. In addition, other psychosocial risk factors include previous back injury claims, job dissatisfaction, poor ratings from supervisors, repetitive boring tasks, younger age, shorter duration of employment, smoking, and a history of nonback injury claims.
- Most low back pain problems are diagnosed and treated by primary care physicians.
- Low back pain may be due to a variety of causes including (a) musculoligamentous injuries; (b) vertebral fractures; (c) degenerative changes; (d) spinal stenosis; (e) anatomic anomalies, such as spondylolisthesis; (f) herniated intervertebral discs; (g) systemic diseases such as cancer, spinal infections, and ankylosing spondylitis; and (h) visceral diseases unrelated to the spine.
- The cornerstones of treatment for low back pain arising from a work-related episode are rest and symptomatic relief of discomfort. Bed rest should not be advised for more than 2 days.
- Frequent follow-up examinations, especially in the early phase of an injury, are advisable.
- Chronic back pain refers to back pain that has been present for over 6 weeks and that has not responded to conservative measures.
- An effective program for prevention of back injuries depends on proper selection and placement of employees, appropriate job design, maintenance of health through edu-

cation, and physical fitness. Back belts and education on lifting techniques have not been shown to be effective in preventing back injuries.

- Routine lumbosacral spine x-ray films have failed to be effective in the identification of individuals predisposed to back injury.
- A variety of disorders of the shoulder occur in occupational settings and include impingement syndrome, biceps tendonitis, rotator cuff tears, and shoulder dislocation.
- Knee injuries are common in the occupational setting and include meniscal tears, collateral ligament sprains, and anterior and posterior cruciate ligament tears.
- Cumulative trauma disorders (also known as repetitive motion injuries) are thought to be due to repetitive performance of a task and primarily affect the upper extremities.
- Carpal tunnel syndrome is due to the compression of the median nerve as it traverses the carpal tunnel in the wrist.
- The National Institute for Occupational Safety and Health (NIOSH) criteria for diagnosis of work-related carpal tunnel syndrome (CTS) include (a) symptoms suggestive of carpal tunnel syndrome; (b) objective findings, which can include either a positive Tinel's or Phalen's sign, decreased sensation in the distribution of the median nerve, or abnormal electrodiagnostic findings of the median nerve across the carpal tunnel; and (c) evidence of work-relatedness.
- The hand-arm vibration syndrome, formerly known as vibration white finger, is thought to be due to arterial spasm (similar to Raynaud's phenomenon) and muscle fatigue as a result of the vibration of a tool.
- Epicondylitis involving either the medial or lateral epicondyle of the elbow may be due to excessive stress on the muscle groups around the elbow and forearm.
- Neck injuries involving muscular strain and spasm are common in the occupational setting.

QUESTIONS

1. Which of the following is **not** a significant risk factor for disabling occupational back pain?

A. Vehicular vibration
B. Poor ratings from supervisors
C. Cigarette smoking
D. Job dissatisfaction
E. Longer duration of employment

2. NIOSH criteria for diagnosis of work-related carpal tunnel syndrome include all of the following **except**

A. A positive Tinel's or Phalen's sign
B. Decreased sensation in the distribution of the median nerve
C. Evidence of work-relatedness, such as forceful repetitive tool use
D. Numbness and burning in the fifth digit
E. Abnormal electrodiagnostic findings of the median nerve

3. Plain x-ray films of the lumbosacral spine are indicated in the evaluation of all of the following conditions **except**

A. Identification of individuals predisposed to back injury
B. Back pain after a severe fall
C. Weight loss and back pain
D. Back pain in a patient previously treated for cancer
E. None of the above

4. *An effective program for prevention of back injuries depends on which of the following factors?*

A. Physical fitness
B. Appropriate job design
C. Proper selection and placement of employees
D. Back belts and education on lifting techniques
E. A, B, and C

=23=

Occupational Cancers

OBJECTIVES

- Explain theories of carcinogenesis
- Recall methods used in the identification of carcinogens
- Review clinical settings that relate to questions about carcinogen exposure

OUTLINE

KEY POINTS

- Carcinogens can be chemicals, physical agents (such as ionizing radiation), or biologic agents (such as viruses or aflatoxin).

- Although current knowledge of carcinogenesis remains incomplete, experimental work with animal models suggests that there are two stages: initiation and promotion.
- Initiation is an event in which an irreversible change occurs in the cell's genetic material known as the alteration of deoxyribonucleic acid (DNA).
- Promotion consists of interactions that would not by themselves cause cancer to occur but would push forward the step after initiation, leading to cancer. Transformed cells proliferate, developing a nodule, then a malignant tumor, and finally a metastasis.
- Studies of ribonucleic acid (RNA) viruses reveal that some viruses code for genetic sequences, which can cause malignant transformation when inserted into host genomes. These are called oncogenes. Suppressor genes such as the *p53 gene* may mutate. When suppressor genes become inactivated, the likelihood of neoplastic transformation is increased.
- Some carcinogens can damage DNA directly, but most require metabolic activation by enzymes. The enzymes responsible for metabolic activation are primarily those of the cytochrome P450 system. The level of aryl hydrocarbon hydroxylase, one common P450 enzyme that is active in metabolizing polycyclic aromatic hydrocarbons, can vary several thousand times among humans.
- Latency refers to the period of time between onset of exposure to a carcinogen and the clinical detection of cancer. The latency period for hematologic malignancies is 2 to 5 years, but the latency period for solid tumors is 10 to 50 years.
- *Threshold* is a safe level of exposure to a carcinogen, below which carcinogenesis does not occur. Whether thresholds exist is controversial.
- Synergistic or multiple factor interactions may increase the risk of cancer. Asbestos and cigarette smoking together result in more than a 50-fold increased risk of lung cancer, a synergistic effect.
- Carcinogens may be identified by epidemiologic studies, animal studies, *in vitro* test systems, and structure-activity relationships analysis. Epidemiologic studies are potentially the most definitive source of information on human carcinogenicity because they are based on human exposure data.
- The International Agency for Research on Cancer (IARC) classifies chemical carcinogens into three categories: group 1 includes chemicals and processes established as human carcinogens, group 2 includes those that are "probably" (group 2A) or "possibly" (group 2B) carcinogenic to humans, group 3 includes agents that are not classified, and group 4 includes agents that are probably not carcinogenic.
- In the event of exposure to a carcinogen, a physician should take steps to end such exposure by replacement of the carcinogen, enclosure of the process, or by the use of personal protective equipment.
- Carcinogens or their metabolites have been directly measured in biologic media, such as blood and urine, for many years. Perhaps the most direct approach to exposure measurement is to assess the "biologically effective dose" of a carcinogen at its ultimate target, DNA, by measuring DNA adducts. As a proxy, RNA adducts and protein adducts may also be studied.
- Markers of risk may emerge from advances in molecular biology. Three general categories are (a) markers of unusually high or low ability to metabolize carcinogens, (b) markers of low ability to repair damaged DNA, and (c) markers of other cancer-prone states.
- Markers of effect are increasingly available. These signal that a carcinogen has reached a target tissue and caused changes in genetic material that might predict the development of cancer. Cytogenetic abnormalities, such as sister chromatid exchanges and

micronuclei, have been measured since the 1970s and have been found to be elevated in many working populations, including those exposed to benzene, epichlorhydrin, styrene, vinyl chloride, asbestos, and ethylene oxide. Such tests, however, are not yet adequately standardized.

- New techniques of rapidly assessing DNA through polymer chain reactions or other tests are not ready for routine application yet but may offer options in the future.
- The Occupational Safety and Health Administration (OSHA) requires monitoring of workplace populations who are exposed to certain carcinogens such as asbestos and benzene. Medical records must be maintained for 30 years following cessation of employment with a particular employer.
- The issue of cancer causation in an individual patient is difficult to address. Information from IARC, National Institute for Occupational Safety and Health (NIOSH), and other databases identify known carcinogens. Exposed workers should be counseled about avoiding further exposure to carcinogens. In a legal setting, the usual question is whether it is more likely than not that an individual's specific cancer was caused by exposure to a specific carcinogen. How multiple causes get sorted out may vary in different legal jurisdictions.
- Cancer clusters may identify new sources of malignancy. One well-known cancer cluster was the identification of hemangiosarcoma of the liver among workers exposed to vinyl chloride. Another was the identification of small cell carcinoma among workers exposed to bis(chloromethyl)ether.

QUESTIONS

1. Regarding the mechanism of environmental and occupational carcinogenesis, most carcinogens

A. Act on products of oncogenes
B. Must be metabolically converted to active forms before damaging DNA
C. Require a threshold below which cancer does not occur
D. Have short latency periods
E. None of the above

2. Initiation can be defined as

A. A known repair mechanism that operates to correct DNA damage
B. Interactions that by themselves do not cause cancer but push forward the steps leading to cancer
C. Carcinogens that act epigenetically
D. An event in which an irreversible change in the cell's genetic material occurs
E. None of the above

3. The period of time between onset of exposure to a carcinogen and the clinical detection of cancer is

A. Synergism
B. Latency
C. Up to 2 to 5 years for hematologic cancers
D. Up to 10 to 50 years for solid tumors
E. B, C, and D

4. *Which of the following statements is (are) true about the IARC classification of chemical carcinogens?*

A. Group 1 chemicals are NOT human carcinogens.
B. Group 3 agents include probable human carcinogens.
C. Group 2 chemicals include possible human carcinogens.
D. Group 4 agents are definite human carcinogens.
E. All of the above.

5. *Refer to Tables 23.1 and 23.2. Examples of known or suspected carcinogens include which of the following*

A. Ethylene oxide
B. Epichlorhydrin
C. Styrene
D. Epoxide hydrolase
E. A, B, and C

=24=

Cardiovascular Disorders

OBJECTIVES

- Explain the impact of cardiovascular disease (CVD) in the workplace
- List risk factors for CVD
- Discuss methods used to assess work capability after a cardiac event
- Recall occupational agents that can cause or aggravate heart disease

OUTLINE

KEY POINTS

- CVD remains the predominant cause of morbidity and mortality in the United States. In 1997, CVD was the primary diagnosis for more than 6.1 million inpatients [1] and accounted for more than 45% of all deaths.
- Recent insights regarding the interconnections among CVDs now illuminate broader correlation between cardiac risk factors and a spectrum of CVDs [coronary heart disease (CHD), myocardial infarction (MI), peripheral arterial disease (PAD), cerebrovascular disease, heart failure, and arrhythmias].
- Cardiac risk factors have an aggregate effect on vascular performance, resulting in diminished endothelial synthesis of nitric oxide and related susceptibility to central vascular stiffening (translating into high afterload pressures), peripheral vascular stiffening (translating into high blood pressure), and the formation of unstable atherosclerotic lesions.
- Among a list of widely recognized modifiable risk factors are smoking, diabetes, hypertension, hypercholesterolemia, sedentary lifestyle, obesity, and excessive salt ingestion. Novel risk factors—hyperhomocysteinemia and low-grade systemic inflammatory states-are now well described.
- The occupational setting has often served as the base from which to provide preventive medical services. Benefits include ready access to large groups of people, greater ability to ensure follow-up study of abnormalities noted during screening measures, and financial and administrative support of the organization.
- Both diastolic and systolic hypertension are clearly associated with increased cardiovascular instability; risk increases as the degree of blood pressure elevation increases.
- Despite its severe consequences, hypertension is often undertreated. Of the estimated 50 million Americans with hypertension, almost one third evade diagnosis, and only one fourth receive effective treatment.
- Cigarette consumption constitutes the single most important modifiable risk factor for CVD and the leading preventable cause of death in the Unites States. It has been demonstrated that, compared with nonsmokers, those who consume 20 or more cigarettes daily have a twofold to threefold increase in total CHD.
- A causative role of low-density lipoprotein (LDL) cholesterol in the development of CHD has been recognized for many years. The impact of acute LDL cholesterol fluctuations and the swift benefits of cholesterol reductions have only recently become widely appreciated. Correspondingly, cholesterol reduction has become a growing health care priority.
- Physical fitness helps to reduce CVD. Even minimal increases in physical activity improves cardiovascular fitness among sedentary people and helps reinforce indirect cardiovascular benefits such as smoking cessation, blood pressure reduction, weight loss, and reduced arrhythmias. Although the precise amount of physical activity required to promote cardiovascular fitness is a matter of debate, sessions of 20- to 30-minute duration three times per week are routinely recommended [with the assumption that one exercises to about 75% of one's age-predicted maximal heart rate (220 − age in years) for the exercise period].

- Diabetes and insulin resistance are also particularly consequential cardiovascular risk factors. Three fourths of all deaths among diabetic patients result from CHD, and patients with diabetes have a three- to fivefold increase in future cardiovascular events compared with nondiabetics.
- Obesity itself is associated with substantially increased cardiovascular risk, independent of physical activity.
- Salt ingestion diminishes vascular endothelial production of nitrous oxide and normal vascular relaxation, which compounds risks of hypertension and results in high afterload pressures.
- A large series of cross-sectional and retrospective studies indicate a positive relationship between mild to moderate homocysteinemia and atherosclerosis; however, prospective studies exploring the relationship of elevated homocysteine and CHD have yielded mixed results. Benefits of homocysteine-lowering therapy remain controversial.
- Inflammation plays a key physiologic role in all phases of atherosclerosis; a cascade of proinflammatory cytokines (e.g., interleukin 1 and tumor necrosis factor) underlies the formation of fatty streaks and progression to more complex and unstable atherosclerotic lesions. Several markers of low-grade systemic inflammation have proven useful for cardiovascular risk prediction including the nonspecific acute phase reactants (C-reactive protein).
- Workers exposed to various sources of carbon monoxide may experience adverse health effects. Individuals with coronary artery disease (CAD) are especially sensitive to the effects of carboxyhemoglobin, the substance that is formed when carbon monoxide combines with hemoglobin, because it increases the likelihood of cardiac ischemia
- Solvents, including routine household products such as paint thinner, and industrial materials used in degreasing operations (e.g., trichloroethylene or methylene chloride) have been associated with cardiovascular risks including arrhythmias. Both halogenated and nonhalogenated compounds have been associated with sudden death.
- Carbon disulfide, a substance used in the viscose rayon industry, has been associated with increased rates of atherosclerosis and perhaps is related to a decrease in fibrinolytic activity.
- Occupational exposure to nitroglycerin and other aliphatic nitrates has been associated with angina-like pain, MI, and cardiovascular death in workers from the explosives industry.
- The major adverse medical prognosticators for failure to return to work after heart disease include left ventricular dysfunction and persistence of ischemia, but for most adults the ability to resume occupational activities depends more on comorbid, social, and psychologic factors (see Table 24.1). Nonmedical factors typically present the greatest impediment for people to resume occupational activities.
- Following a major cardiac event, and/or in a worker with multiple cardiac risk factors, the physician must make a thorough analysis of the patient. This requires a review of medical records and diagnostic studies and a related job analysis. The individual's current status is pertinent, with consideration of symptoms; physical findings; and laboratory testing, including an exercise stress test.
- A symptom-limited exercise ECG stress test is considered the most sensitive predictor of future reinfarction and death when the test is performed approximately 6 weeks after an acute MI. Cardiac rehabilitation attempts to improve physical capacity; psychosocial attributes; and lipoprotein patterns, with the goals of reduced cardiovascular complications, reduced risk factors in general, and improved health judgments.

• Occupational Safety and Health Administration (OSHA) reported that from 1991 to 1993, 15% of workplace deaths were due to sudden cardiac arrest usually from ventricular fibrillation. Without intervention, survival following sudden cardiac arrest decreases rapidly. Several studies have reported that for each minute of untreated cardiac arrest, the probability of successful rhythm conversion decreases by 7% to 10%. Conversely, survival rates as high as 90% have been reported when the collapse-to-defibrillation time is within 1 minute.

QUESTIONS

*1. Which of the following statements is **incorrect** regarding CVD?*

A. Modifiable risk factors are smoking, diabetes, hypertension, hypercholesterolemia, sedentary lifestyle, obesity, and excessive salt ingestion.
B. Both diastolic and systolic hypertension are clearly associated with increased cardiovascular instability, risk increases as the degree of blood pressure elevation increases.
C. Most Americans with hypertension receive effective treatment.
D. Cigarette consumption constitutes the single most important modifiable risk factor for CVD.

*2. Which of the following statements is **incorrect** regarding cardiovascular risk factors?*

A. Physical fitness helps to reduce CVD.
B. Minimal increases in physical activity do not improve cardiovascular fitness among sedentary people.
C. A causative role of LDL cholesterol in the development of CHD has been recognized for many years.
D. Obesity itself is associated with substantially increased cardiovascular risk, independent of physical activity.

3. Which of the following pairs of cardiac toxin and toxic effect is (are) correctly related?

A. Solvents/cardiac dysrhythmia
B. Carbon disulfide/increased atherosclerosis
C. Nitro compounds/rebound coronary spasm
D. Carbon monoxide/myocardial ischemia
E. All listed are correct

*4. Which of the following statements is **incorrect** regarding cardiac rehabilitation?*

A. The major medical predictors for failure to return to work include left ventricular dysfunction and persistence of ischemia.
B. Nonmedical factors rarely prevent patients from resuming occupational activities after MI.
C. A symptom-limited exercise ECG stress test is considered the most sensitive predictor of future reinfarction and death when the test is performed approximately 6 weeks after an acute MI.
D. Cardiac rehabilitation is intended to improve physical capacity, psychosocial attributes, and lipoprotein patterns.

25

Neurotoxic Disorders

OBJECTIVES

- Explain how hazardous materials may damage the nervous system
- Describe factors that may modify an individual response to toxic exposure
- Discuss methods of analysis used in the evaluation of nervous system disorders
- Describe the approach to determining a clinical diagnosis of neurotoxicity
- List the potential neurotoxic effects of commonly used hazardous materials

OUTLINE

KEY POINTS

- Clinical manifestations of neurotoxic effects vary with the region of the nervous system affected. The CNS is affected when metabolites of toxic chemicals cross the blood–brain barrier to reach particular neuronal systems. If access is prevented, effects are limited to the PNS. Clinical expressions of nervous system effects, such as damage to cell membranes, myelin sheaths, mitochondrial structures, or axonal transport mechanisms, may resemble those of common nontoxic neurologic syndromes.
- Coexistent systemic diseases, history of previous chemical exposures, individual susceptibility, duration of exposure, concentration of substance, and body burden are major factors to consider in *exposure assessment.*
- Confirmation of neurologic dysfunction related to toxic materials requires neurophysiologic, neuropsychologic, neuroimaging, neuropathologic, and biochemical methodologies. Clinical diagnosis, however, can be made based on subjective complaints (symptoms) and objective findings (signs) on neurologic examination.
- A systematic approach when making the diagnosis of a neurotoxic syndrome requires a thorough occupational and environmental history. Assessing all of the exposed individual's environmental and/or industrial hygiene data and biologic markers (e.g., urine or blood) helps to determine causal relationships between a specific exposure event and toxic effects.

- The Boston University Environmental Neurology Assessment (BUENA) is a systematic approach for the clinical assessment of those exposed to neurotoxic materials and/or suspected of having a neurotoxic disease. This protocol lists specific essential questions and uses an algorithm for documenting observations and detecting confounding variables to aid in reaching diagnostic conclusions.
- Motor weakness, sensory loss, altered mental status, ataxia, and tremor are some of the symptoms of neurologic dysfunction that are seen in both neurotoxic and nonneurotoxic syndromes. Triorthocresylphosphate poisoning can cause spinal cord lesions that mimic neurosyphilis, vitamin B_{12} deficiency, and multiple sclerosis. Ataxia and tremor seen in degenerative diseases of the cerebellum also result from exposure to toluene, mercury, and acrylamide. Parkinsonism can result from toxic effects of chemicals that act on neurons in the substantia nigra and striatum (e.g., carbon monoxide, carbon disulfide, manganese, and MPTP). Parkinsonian features such as bradykinesia, cogwheel rigidity, shuffling gait, tremor, and postural reflexes resemble those of idiopathic Parkinson's disease (PD). MPTP exposure is the only documented neurotoxicant that causes neuropathologic changes that are similar to idiopathic PD, but there is suspicion that PD may be caused by environmental agents. CNS symptoms include encephalopathy, headache, motor disturbances, altered consciousness, and mood changes.
- Encephalopathy is used to describe disturbances of brain function without exact localization of the damage. Toxic encephalopathies include cognitive disturbances, difficulty with problem solving and memory function, and psychotic-like behavior. Increased intracranial pressure from swelling (cerebral edema), elevated blood pressure, or chemical irritation can cause headache. It is usually associated with lightheadedness and/or dizziness. It may be seen with acute higher levels of exposures to metal fumes and solvent vapors.
- Peripheral neuropathies occur in patients with diabetes, as well as in those exposed to carbon disulfide, *n*-hexane, lead, arsenic, solvents, or organophosphate insecticides. Numbness, tingling, dysesthesia, weakness, and reduced reflexes are indicators of such damage.
- Neuropsychologic testing aids in assessing subtle effects of neurotoxicity. These tests have been validated, found reliable in research and clinical settings, and can be analyzed in terms of normative scores.
- EEG provides real-time electrophysiologic activity of the brain. It has been shown to have predictable patterns during normal waking, drowsing, and sleeping states. Abnormalities in normal symmetry, amplitude, frequencies, and patterns of the electroencephalogram are associated with brain function impairment.
- Evoked potentials are electrical cortical potentials produced by stimulation of specific afferent pathways; electrodes are used to record these potentials from the surface of the brain through the skull. The sensory evoked potentials include VEPs, BAEPs, and SSEPs. Nerve conduction studies and muscle activity measurements can be appropriately applied to help localize sites of impaired nerve, nerve root, plexus, or motor neurons of the PNS. The integrity of the motor neuron, its axon, and the muscle cell it supplies can be assessed by an EMG examination. EMG will detect a reduced number of motor units as evidence of denervation; as neuromuscular clinical signs emerge, greater electromyographic changes are recordable.
- Neuroimaging techniques provide objective data about the structural and functional integrity of the brain. Computed tomography (CT) scans can demarcate brain morphology as seen in cerebral edema associated with lead exposure. Magnetic resonance imaging (MRI) can provide hypointense or hyperintense signals depending on the

nature of the toxic exposure (e.g., the severity of cerebral white matter involvement following chronic toluene exposure) that correlates with changes in neuropsychologic performance. Other associations between MRI changes and exposure include those associated with organolead in gasoline and inorganic mercury. Single-photon emission computed tomography (SPECT) scans measure the regional cerebral blood flow (as seen in the described patient with exposure to manganese). Changes in glucose metabolism may be measured by positron emission tomography (PET) scan using 18-S-2-deoxyglucose. Such changes are described in persons exposed to tetrabromoethane who do not show abnormalities on CT or EEG.

- Biologic markers of exposure are indicators of alterations in cellular structure, biochemical processes, and/or nervous system functioning that can be measured in a biologic sample. Three types of biologic markers that are useful in making a diagnosis of neurotoxic illness are biologic markers of exposure, effect, and susceptibility.
- Table 25.1 best describes known chemical exposures and possible toxic effects.

QUESTIONS

*1. All of the following statements about neurotoxicity are true **except***

A. The anatomic site of the neurotoxic effect is the most important factor that determines how neurotoxicity is expressed as clinical symptoms.
B. The CNS is affected when toxic metabolites cross the blood–brain barrier.
C. Symptoms and signs of neurotoxic dysfunction are different from nontoxic neurologic syndromes.
D. Peripheral neuropathy associated with diabetes has symptoms that are similar to the symptoms seen in neuropathy resulting from lead poisoning.
E. Encephalopathy is used to describe brain dysfunction without exact localization of the damage.

2. A systematic approach when making the diagnosis of a neurotoxic syndrome may require which of the following?

A. A thorough occupational and environmental history
B. Ambient air samples and industrial hygiene monitoring data
C. Biologic markers of exposure such as urine or blood
D. The BUENA
E. All of the above

3. Which of the following statements is (are) correct concerning exposure to lead?

A. Acute and chronic encephalopathy may result from lead exposure.
B. Abdominal pain and constipation are not associated with lead exposure.
C. Sources of lead exposure include insecticides, lead-based paint, storage battery reclamation operation, and illicit whiskey.
D. Parkinsonism is a chronic manifestation of lead exposure.
E. Statements A and C are both correct.

4. Which of the following is (are) correct about neurologic studies?

A. Nerve conduction studies are appropriate to help localize sites of damage in the CNS.

B. SPECT scans use the metabolism of glucose to enhance areas of the brain that are damaged by neurotoxins.

C. MRIs can provide hyperintense signals in the white matter and, depending on the nature of the exposure, correlate with neuropsychologic performance.

D. Abnormal PET scan results due to neurotoxicity are expected only if the CT scan and/or EEG are abnormal.

E. All statements are correct.

5. *Biologic markers of exposure are methods of evaluating neurotoxic exposure. Which of the following statements is (are) correct?*

A. Biologic markers are indicators of alterations in cellular structure measured in samples taken from the exposed individual.

B. Nervous system function and biochemical processes can be measured using biologic markers of exposure such as urine or blood.

C. Exposure, effect, and susceptibility are three methods of determining biologic markers.

D. None of the above statements are true.

E. Statements A, B, and C are true.

26

Noise-Induced Hearing Loss

OBJECTIVES

- Explain how noise can cause hearing loss
- Identify the normal range of human hearing
- Discuss audiometry
- List types of hearing-protection devices (HPDs)
- Explain the components of a hearing conservation program

OUTLINE

KEY POINTS

- The National Institute for Occupational Safety and Health (NIOSH) estimates that 30 million people are exposed to noise levels in excess of 85 dB in their workplaces.

Losses of hearing associated with overexposures are called noise-induced, and such occurrences are mostly preventable. Noise-induced hearing loss is one of the 10 leading work-related disorders.

- Many industries expose workers to noise levels beyond the OSHA permissible exposure limit of 90 dB as an 8-hour time-weighted average.
- Noise-induced hearing loss is an insidious process, which occurs with chronic exposure to noise, without the worker being aware of the harm
- Many existing health conditions can predispose a worker to noise-induced hearing loss.
- Solvent exposures in the workplace may potentiate hearing loss from noise exposures.
- Audiometry, which measures hearing thresholds for different discrete pure-tone signals ranging from 500 to 6,000 or 8,000 hertz (Hz), furnishes valuable insight concerning the status of hearing. The lowest intensity level at which a sound (pure-tone signals) can be detected at a given test frequency is known as audiometric threshold, which is recorded in decibels (0 to 25 dB is considered to be the normal range).
- The most critical frequency range for human audition is between 500 through 2,000 or 3,000 Hz—the range indispensable for hearing and understanding normal conversational speech.
- Acute acoustic trauma may occur from unprotected exposure to very loud noise (about 140 dB), such as a ballistic blast or explosion. Clinical features may include vivid recall of the event, a sudden change in the status of hearing immediately following the encounter, possibly dizziness, and/or evidence of physical injury to the tympanic membrane.
- Excessive noise exposures damage the intricate microscopic structures within the inner ear, particularly those composing the organ of Corti.
- The physician's assessment of a patient's hearing impairment can be accomplished using several different testing mechanisms in addition to pure-tone audiometric testing.
- Observations of noise-induced hearing losses are classified into two categories: temporary and permanent. Noise-induced temporary threshold shifts (NITTS) are changes in hearing associated with transient overexposures to noise. Given an adequate period of auditory rest, hearing usually returns to preexposure levels. Noise-induced permanent threshold shifts (NIPTS) are irreversible conditions in which, despite a prolonged period of auditory rest, hearing does not return to normal.
- Determining the effects of noise on hearing can be accomplished by serial audiometry.
- The physician may be asked to evaluate hearing impairment in cases in which hearing loss is permanent and irreversible. The American Medical Association (AMA) guidelines assign a 1.5% impairment of monaural hearing for every decibel that the average hearing level in the speech range exceeds 25 dB. Impairment does not begin until an average hearing loss of 25 dB has been reached and is considered complete when the threshold average of 92 dB is reached.
- An occupational hearing conservation program should include (a) education, motivation, supervision, and discipline; (b) assessment of potentially hazardous noise exposures; (c) assessment at the ear of allowable exposures for those wearing HPDs; (d) monitoring audiometry; (e) personal hearing protection and noise control measures; (f) documentation of monitoring; and (g) disposition and follow-up activities.
- Hearing protectors consist of three basic types: insert (devices that insert into the ear canal proper), semiinsert (devices covering the entry into the ear canal and held in place by a band or other type of suspension device), and muffs (devices completely encapsulating the auricle or pinna).

QUESTIONS

1. Which frequency range is most important for comprehension of human speech?

A. 250 to 500 Hz
B. 500 to 3,000 Hz
C. 3,000 to 6,000 Hz
D. 6,000 to 8,000 Hz
E. 8,000 to 10,000 Hz

2. Which is the most effective and acceptable form of personal hearing protection?

A. Ear muffs
B. Foam earplugs
C. Ear caps
D. Molded plastic earplugs
E. Selection based on the worker's preference

*3. Which of the following is **not** required as part of a hearing conservation program?*

A. Noise surveys
B. Personal hearing protection
C. Annual audiometric evaluations
D. Record-keeping system
E. Supervision of the program by a physician

4. Most properly fitted hearing-protection devices provide how much attenuation?

A. The noise reduction rating (NRR) as it appears on the package
B. About 5 dB if worn according to instructions
C. About 15 to 30 dB
D. Protection depends on the intensity of ambient noise
E. Noise attenuated only in the speech range

27

Occupational Skin Diseases

OBJECTIVES

- Understand that skin conditions are a common cause of work-related illness
- Distinguish between irritant and allergic contact dermatitis
- Discuss the evaluation of occupational skin disorders
- Explain the importance of prevention as it relates to occupational skin disorders
- Discuss treatment of occupational skin disorders

OUTLINE

  I. Significance of occupational skin disease
 II. Causes and types of occupational skin disease
    A. Contact dermatitis
    B. Occupational and contact urticaria
    C. Acne and folliculitis
    D. Occupational vitiligo
    E. Granulomas
    F. Occupational skin neoplasms
    G. Physical injuries (Table 27.1)
    H. Occupational Raynaud's disease and vibration white finger
    I. Occupational skin infections (Table 27.2)
    J. Work-aggravated dermatitis
III. Evaluation of occupational skin disease
    A. History (Table 27.3)
    B. Physical examination
    C. Worksite evaluation
    D. Diagnostic testing for occupational skin disease
 IV. Preventive management
    A. Product or chemical substitution
    B. Engineering and hygienic controls
    C. Personal protective measures
    D. Personal hygiene
    E. Administrative controls and proactive management
  V. Treatment
 VI. Prognosis of occupational contact dermatitis

KEY POINTS

- Occupational skin diseases are those disorders of the skin caused, or made worse, by the workplace environment.
- Occupational skin diseases are among the most common of the occupational diseases with current annual incidence rate of 5 per 10,000 full-time workers.
- Contact dermatitis accounts for 90% of all occupational skin disease. Of all cases of contact dermatitis, irritant contact dermatitis accounts for 80%.
- Allergic and irritant skin reactions generally cannot be differentiated by their clinical expression.
- Irritant skin reactions are caused by substances that damage the skin at the site of contact by nonimmunologic mechanisms. Irritants cause injury to most individuals if given a sufficient concentration and time of exposure.
- Allergic contact reactions require a cell-mediated hypersensitivity mechanism, and generally, a smaller number of workers are affected.
- Ultraviolet (UV) radiation can react with certain chemicals on the skin to cause photosensitivity contact dermatitis.
- Urticarial reactions may occur as a result of allergy from prior sensitization or from direct contact with a substance that causes release of histamine and other vasoactive substances from mast cells.
- Heavy exposures to oils, greases, and other occlusive materials can cause or exacerbate acne-form lesions. Chloracne, a rare type of acne, is caused by exposure to certain chlorinated polycyclic hydrocarbons.
- Occupational vitiligo results from skin contact with depigmenting chemicals leading to localized areas of depigmentation.
- There are three principle types of skin cancer that can be caused by occupational exposures: squamous cell and basal cell carcinomas and malignant melanoma. All three types can be caused by sun exposure. In addition, both basal cell and squamous cell carcinomas can result from exposure to ionizing radiation and some chemicals.
- Physical and mechanical trauma to skin can result in a number of different lesions including blisters, calluses, and rashes (Table 27.1).
- Occupational Raynaud's disease and vibration white finger represent a complex of reversible vascular spasms in persons working with handheld vibrating tools. In more severe cases, neuromuscular and arthritic symptoms and bone degeneration may be present.
- Occupational skin infections may be caused by a number of different organisms (Table 27.2).
- Work-aggravated dermatitis occurs when a worker has a skin condition, such as psoriasis or eczematous dermatitis, that is exacerbated by exposure to irritants in the workplace.
- Evaluation of occupational skin disease should involve a complete history with special emphasis on workplace exposures and a physical examination (Table 27.3). If a chemical is involved, the Material Safety Data Sheets (MSDS) should be reviewed. A visit to the worksite may be helpful in identifying causes of skin disorders.
- In many instances, patch testing can be proof that sensitization, which has resulted in allergic contact dermatitis, has occurred. There is no scientific test to establish the presence of an irritant reaction.
- A number of methods are available to help the worker avoid exposure to the offending agent if it has been determined that either an allergic contact dermatitis or an irritant

contact reaction has occurred. These include engineering controls, personal protective measures, and administrative controls.
- Treatment options depend on the type of skin disorder and the severity. Topical steroids are a mainstay in the treatment of contact dermatitis.
- Severe occupational contact dermatitis has a poor prognosis. In some cases, a worker develops persistent postoccupational dermatitis in which the skin lesions continue despite the absence of ongoing exposure.

QUESTIONS

*1. Regarding occupational contact dermatitis, which statement is **false?***

A. It is the most common of the occupational skin diseases.
B. Patch testing is useful in determining allergic contact sensitization.
C. Allergic and irritant contact dermatitis cannot be differentiated by their clinical appearance.
D. Allergic contact dermatitis is more common than irritant contact dermatitis.
E. Phototoxic contact dermatitis is due to activation of an irritant by ultraviolet radiation.

2. Which of the following skin neoplasms is (are) associated with occupational exposure to sun exposure?

A. Malignant melanoma
B. Squamous cell carcinoma
C. Basal cell carcinoma
D. Both A and B
E. A, B, and C

*3. Which of the following statements about occupational Raynaud's disease and vibration white finger is **false?***

A. In addition to blanching, numbness and tingling may also occur.
B. Better tool design and selection can reduce the frequency of the disease.
C. Only those with underlying primary Raynaud's disease are affected.
D. Disease occurs in those working with handheld vibrating tools.
E. In more severe cases, the thumb may be involved.

*4. When evaluating a patient with suspected contact dermatitis from an occupational exposure, the physician should do all of the following **except***

A. Take a complete history, including an occupational history
B. Perform a skin biopsy to establish the work-relatedness
C. Tour the worksite if feasible
D. Perform a complete skin examination
E. Review the relevant MSDS

5. Reducing exposure to substances that cause allergic or irritant contact dermatitis may include

A. Substituting another chemical that is less irritating or allergenic

B. Improving ventilation in areas where airborne contact is the cause of contact dermatitis
C. Using protective clothing or gloves
D. Placing the worker where contact with the offending substance is avoided
E. All of the above

6. *Treatment options for occupational contact dermatitis include all of the following* ***except***

A. Use of topical steroids is recommended for localized acute contact dermatitis.
B. Systemic steroids should be routinely used for treatment of chronic contact dermatitis.
C. Lubricants should be used to decrease itching and to reduce scaling in chronic contact dermatitis.
D. Use of sedating antihistamines is appropriate in patients with itching that interferes with sleep.
E. Wet compresses and astringent application are recommended for acute weeping lesions.

=28=
Psychiatric Aspects of Occupational Medicine

OBJECTIVES

- Discuss the effects of life events on mental status
- Classify the major groups of psychiatric disorders
- Review diagnostic features of anxiety disorders
- Explain the time shift syndrome and preventive strategies

OUTLINE

E. Spread out life changes
F. Group stress management programs
XV. Shift work
   A. Acute time shift syndrome
   B. Chronic shift maladaptation syndrome
XVI. Violence in the workplace

KEY POINTS

- Normal emotions, behaviors, or routine social activities can all go awry in response to a multitude of stressors.
- Stressors may be internal (based on genetic composition or on internalized environmental stimuli from childhood) or external (e.g., a hazardous workplace, a troubled marriage, or a sick child).
- Most observed psychiatric symptoms can be divided into those affecting mood, anxiety level, or perception. Substance use can produce symptoms falling within any of these categories.
- The *mental status examination*, an assessment of a patient's mood, presentation, speech pattern, thought processes, and cognition, is the cornerstone of psychiatric evaluation and diagnosis.
- Substance use disorders are diagnosed independent of quantity or frequency of use but are based on whether the patient is harming himself or herself, aware that he or she is harming or placing himself or herself at substantial risk, and yet continues to use the substance despite that knowledge.
- If a substance use disorder is noted, it is of little value to attempt to determine if another primary psychiatric disorder is present. This may be determined after a significant period of sobriety has passed.
- Anxiety disorders seen in the workplace include panic disorder, generalized anxiety disorder, and posttraumatic stress disorder.
- Symptoms of *panic disorder* often include perceived tachycardia, diaphoresis, shortness of breath, and chest or abdominal discomfort. Agoraphobia (anxiety about being in a place from which escape or return home is difficult) often is present.
- *Generalized anxiety disorder (GAD)* is manifested by extended periods (over 6 months) of variable levels of worry and anxiety that significantly exceeds the level appropriate given the stressors. Symptoms generally include sleep difficulties, muscle tension, irritability, difficulty with concentration, fatigue, and restlessness (or a subset of these) and may be due to or worsened by substance use, medical illness, or workplace stress.
- *Posttraumatic stress disorder (PTSD)* refers recurrent episodes of "re-living" the trauma in which either a patient or a nearby individual was threatened (death or serious injury). The patient develops behavior in which he or she avoids certain places that remind him or her of the trauma. Motivation can drop off, and relationships with family and work colleagues can deteriorate. Symptoms must be present for greater than 1 month for the diagnosis to apply.
- *Mood disorders* can be divided into the unipolar group (depressive symptoms) and the bipolar group (experiencing both depressive and elevated symptoms).
- Depressive disorders include dysthymia (mild to moderate in severity, in which mood is found to be stable but low for years) and major depressive disorders, which generally start after adolescence, are cyclical in nature, and can sometimes be seen in combination with an ongoing dysthymia.

- Elevated symptoms include *manic* and *hypomanic disorders*. Manic episodes cause marked impairment in occupational or social functioning or include psychotic symptoms, whereas hypomanic episodes cause neither.
- *Psychotic symptoms* may result from bipolar disorder, depression, or substance use. They do not necessarily indicate the presence of a primary psychotic disorder such as schizophrenia. Paranoid and schizotypal personality traits may also be mistaken for signs of psychotic disorders. Psychotic symptoms are often divided into two groups: positive (all forms of hallucinations and delusions and acutely bizarre behavior and formal thought disorders) and negative (social inattention, poor grooming, lack of vocal inflections, and blocking of speech).
- *Adjustment disorders* describe difficulty coping with known stressors, which may be work-related or due to personal problems. They are described by the predominant symptoms (such as with depressed mood, with anxiety, and with mixed anxiety and depressed mood).
- Some personality types may be particularly sensitive to stressors. For example, a worker with an obsessive personality often has a rigid coping strategy for approaching new situations.
- *Somatoform disorders* refer to the presence of physical symptoms that suggest physical disorders but for which no organic basis can be established as the cause.
- Patients with factitious disorders have "voluntary" symptoms in that they are deliberate and purposeful but not in the sense that they can be controlled; there is a compulsive quality to the simulation of illness and no apparent goal other than to assume the patient role.
- *Malingering* patients are in voluntary control of the symptoms, but the goal is based on environmental circumstances (rather than the patient's psychology).
- Acute intoxication syndromes depend on the particular agent (e.g., solvents, pesticides, and heavy metals), but common symptoms include dizziness, light-headedness, and incoordination (see Chapter 25 in the textbook). In rare cases a florid psychosis may occur. Removal from exposure to the toxic substance usually clears the symptoms.
- Chronic neurotoxicant exposure can be divided into three types: mild, moderate, and severe. The *mildest* syndrome is an organic affective disorder, a reversible syndrome of depression identical to depression from other causes. With *moderate* severity, cognitive symptoms, such as short-term memory loss and psychomotor disturbances (slowness in response time, clumsy eye-hand coordination) may also occur. The most severe type resembles dementia, and withdrawal of the toxic substance is less likely to reverse the symptoms.
- Stress, in moderate amounts, can be motivating and is known as "eustress." If the duration or intensity of the stress overloads a person's ability to manage the stress, it can lead to "distress," a spiral of emotional and physical ills.
- Factors involved in causing stress can be divided into acute and chronic types. Dissatisfying interpersonal relationships are usually responsible for chronic stress. The mechanism whereby chronic stressors exert their damage is primarily due to the increase of corticotropin-releasing factor and other mediators, which increase levels of circulating corticosteroid and increase blood pressure and heart rate, as well as possibly impairing the immune response.
- Stress management techniques include time management, relaxation training, exercise, and avocational interests. It is helpful to spread out life changes (see Holmes-Rahe Schedule, Table 28.2 in the textbook). Group stress management programs are also useful.

- *Shift work* implies either long-term night work or work involving rotation between day, evening, and night shifts. Studies suggest that these workers, presumably because of a disruption in circadian rhythm, have increased morbidity and decreased work performance.
- Human circadian system can adapt to a phase delay of 2 hours or a phase advance of ½ hour without much disruption. Traveling westward across time zones (delay in time) has less potential for adverse effects than traveling eastward.
- Disturbance of the worker's "biologic clock" or circadian rhythms is responsible for a "shift maladaptation syndrome," which affects wakefulness, thermoregulation, and neuroendocrine regulation. The most common effects include gastrointestinal and cardiovascular disturbances and effects on level of alertness.
- Workplace violence, ranging from offensive language to homicide, is a common problem. Homicide itself is now the third leading cause of fatal occupational injury in the United States.
- The Occupational Safety and Health Administration (OSHA) has developed guidelines and recommendations to reduce worker exposures to the hazards of workplace violence. Four basic elements include (a) management commitment and employee involvement, (b) worksite analysis, (c) hazard prevention and control, and (d) training and education.
- Sexual harassment (unwelcome sexual advances, requests for sexual favors, and other verbal or physical conduct of a sexual nature when the response to this conduct might affect another individual's employment or work performance) may also be viewed as a workplace mental health hazard.

QUESTIONS

*1. Which of the following is **incorrect** about workplace stress?*

A. Stressors may be internal or external.
B. Stress, in moderate amounts, can be motivating.
C. Acute stress exerts its damage because of an increase of corticotropin-releasing factor.
D. Dissatisfying interpersonal relationships are usually responsible for chronic stress.
E. Stress management techniques include time management, relaxation training, exercise, and avocational interests.

*2. Which of the following is **incorrect** regarding shift work?*

A. Studies suggest that shift workers have decreased morbidity and increased work performance.
B. Traveling westward across time zones (delay in time) has less potential for adverse effects than traveling eastward.
C. The most common effects of shift work include gastrointestinal and cardiovascular disturbances and effects on level of alertness.
D. The human circadian system can adapt to a phase delay of 2 hours or a phase advance of ½ hour without much disruption.
E. The "shift maladaptation syndrome" affects wakefulness, thermoregulation, and neuroendocrine regulation.

3. *Which of the following statements is **incorrect?***

A. If a substance use disorder is noted, it is of little value to attempt to determine if another primary psychiatric disorder is present until a significant period of sobriety has passed.
B. Diagnosis of substance use is based on quantity or frequency of use.
C. Substance use can affect mood, anxiety level, or perception.
D. Use of alcohol does not speed resolution of jet lag symptoms.
E. Symptoms of generalized anxiety disorder may be due to or worsened by substance use, medical illness, or workplace stress.

4. *Which of these factors contribute most to a diagnosis of alcohol dependence?*

A. Frequency of use
B. Whether the patient drinks wine, beer, or hard liquor
C. Quantity of use
D. Consequences of alcohol use
E. Binge use of alcohol

5. *Initial treatment of anxiety disorder unresponsive to therapy alone should include*

A. A mood stabilizer such as lithium
B. An antidepressant such as sertraline
C. A sedative agent such as clonazepam
D. A psychotropic agent such as olanzapine
E. None of the above

6. *Which of the following does **not** lead to a higher risk of PTSD?*

A. Discussing the trauma in therapy shortly after the trauma takes place
B. Returning the worker to the site of the trauma soon after the initial event
C. Placing the worker in a different location where a similar trauma could take place
D. Exposing the worker to another traumatic situation or event
E. All of the above

7. *A patient with depressive symptoms may be suffering from*

A. Dysthymia
B. Adjustment disorder with depressed mood
C. Substance use disorder
D. Bipolar disorder, depressed
E. Any of the above

8. *Appropriate stress management techniques include*

A. Exercise
B. Avocational interests
C. Time management
D. Relaxation techniques
E. All of the above

29

Allergy and Immunology

OBJECTIVES

- Present a brief overview of the immune system
- List four types of hypersensitivity reactions
- Explain different manifestations of occupational asthma
- Discuss common types of occupational allergic diseases
- Explain the workup of the hypersensitive patient
- Review immunotoxicology
- Describe idiopathic environmental intolerance (IEI)

OUTLINE

KEY POINTS

- Occupational allergic illnesses include diseases of the skin, respiratory tract, and anaphylaxis. About 65,000 cases of occupational allergic respiratory disease are reported annually.
- Primary lymphoid organs are the thymus and bone marrow; secondary organs include the spleen, lymph nodes, and lymphoid tissue. Cellular elements arise from the bone marrow—T and B lymphocytes, plasma cells (from B lymphocytes), macrophages, mast cells, Langerhans' cells, polymorphonuclear leukocytes, natural killer (NK) cells, and other cells. Acellular immune system components include antibodies, complement, and cytokines.
- Hypersensitivity reactions are based on the presence or absence of humoral antibodies, the types of antibodies involved, whether or not complement is required to drive the reaction to completion, the target organ, and the cell types involved.
- Type I (allergic or anaphylactic) reactions require immunoglobulin E (IgE) antibody to be attached to mast cell receptors before antigen introduction. When an antigen cross links with a specific antibody, histamine, serotonin, and other vasoactive amines are released from mast cells. Leukotrienes and other inflammatory mediators are also released. These chemical mediators cause the allergic reactions seen in allergic rhinitis, asthma, and anaphylaxis
- Type II reactions usually require immunoglobulin G (IgG) antibodies directed against antigen located on target cell surfaces. Complement may be needed to drive the antigen-antibody reaction, resulting in target cell destruction (immune hemolytic anemia, transfusion reaction, and some types of autoimmune disease).
- Type III (immune complex) reactions occur when excessive antigen causes a precipitation of antigen-antibody complex along vascular endothelium, resulting in subsequent attraction of polymorphonuclear leukocytes that cause local damage. Complement is required in the chain of events. Examples of this type of reaction include HP and some autoimmune diseases.
- Type IV (delayed hypersensitivity) reactions require previously sensitized lymphocytes but no humoral antibodies or complement. Antigens stimulate the lymphocytes to cause the release of lymphokines (interleukins and interferons) that attract macrophages and leukocytes, resulting in allergic contact dermatitis or granulomatous diseases (e.g., tuberculosis).
- New research suggests that a type V (secretory) reaction exists.
- Sensitization occurs when an individual is originally exposed to antigen. It takes months to years for the specific IgE antibody to bind to mast cells. The shocking stage occurs on reexposure to the specific antigen and takes only seconds to minutes. A type I (allergic) reaction may occur immediately, or it may be delayed for several hours (late-phase allergic reaction). A delayed reaction can create confusion in evaluating the person with suspected occupational allergy.
- Laboratory studies are often inconclusive. The patient with asthma or eczema may have an elevated eosinophil count. The IgE level is not a good screening test for atopy. Skin

testing remains the gold standard in determining the presence of specific IgE antibody. The radioallergosorbent test (RAST) or enzyme-linked immunosorbent assay (ELISA) may be alternatives to skin tests.

- Occupational rhinitis and rhinosinusitis may be irritative or allergic in nature. Irritation may occur following exposure to a variety of physical or chemical agents. Allergic reactions may result from exposures to high or low molecular weight antigens. Most high molecular weight antigens are naturally occurring, such as dust mites, fungal spores, animal danders, or foods. Low molecular weight agents, including a variety of organic chemicals (isocyanates, acid anhydrides, aldehydes) and inorganic chemicals (chromium, platinum), cause allergy through IgE-IgG human serum albumin hapten complexes or by poorly understood mechanisms.

- Occupational rhinitis and rhinosinusitis may be irritative or allergic. Dusts, vapors, mists, and fumes in the workplace cause occupational asthma. Reactions may be immediate, isolated late, and dual. High molecular weight antigens frequently cause immediate reactions, whereas low molecular weight antigens cause more late phase reactions. High and low molecular weights cause both immediate and late phase (dual) reactions. High molecular weight antigens rarely cause isolated late reactions.

- In the evaluation of suspected occupational asthma, a complete history, physical examination, and routine laboratory workup are suggested. To establish the presence of an asthma, allergy, and workplace relationship: (a) evidence of airflow limitation is obtained, (b) hyperresponsiveness of the airways is detected, (c) the presence of atopy is evaluated, (d) the work-relatedness of asthma is suspected by a history of temporal association and prework and postwork or serial expiratory flow or peak flow rates, and (e) consideration is given to skin testing or *in vitro* measurements of specific IgE antibodies. Skin testing may be helpful in cases of high molecular weight sensitizing agents but not with low molecular weight agents. To establish bronchial hyperresponsiveness, either baseline spirometry should show an obstructive pattern or a methacholine challenge test should result in a 20% drop in forced expiratory volume in 1 second (FEV_1). In treatment of occupational asthma, it is important to remove the patient from the offending agent. With irritant asthma, personal protective equipment (PPE)—a National Institute for Occupational Safety and Health (NIOSH)-approved respirator—may be used, but with immunologic asthma, the worker must be permanently removed from exposure.

- HP (extrinsic allergic alveolitis) occurs when inhaled allergens in the home or work environment cause a type III immunologic inflammatory reaction in the bronchioles, alveoli, and lung interstitium. The most frequent allergens are the thermophilic actinomycetes, which are found in warm, humid environments. Other causes may include the isocyanates and trimellitic anhydride. The acute form appears as a flulike illness 4 to 6 hours after heavy exposure. Pulmonary function tests (PFTs) show restriction, and chest x-ray film may be normal or show granular or nodular infiltrates. In chronic disease, the chest x-ray film may show diffuse interstitial fibrosis. Although IgG antibodies to the offending agent may be helpful, the levels fall after exposure is terminated and severe HP may persist. There is no single test for HP.

- ABPA is severe asthma associated with an elevated serum IgE and total eosinophil count. The condition results from colonization of the lower respiratory tract with fungi, usually *Aspergillus fumigatus* spores. Skin testing usually shows an immediate reaction and IgG *Aspergillus* antibody is present. Long-term treatment with corticosteroids is required for control.

- Immediate and delayed hypersensitivity reactions to latex and natural rubber have been recently reported. Reactions can include eczema, urticaria, rhinitis, conjunctivitis, bronchospasm, and anaphylaxis. NRL antibodies in the serum can be measured, but there is a 25% false-negative response. Avoidance of the offending agent is important because premedication of sensitized individuals with steroids is questionable. Because total avoidance of NRL is very difficult, a latex safe environment is recommended, so that the ambient concentration of NRL protein is low.
- Chronic sinusitis may exacerbate asthma and may require long courses of antibiotics.
- Fungal diseases may cause all four types of hypersensitivity reactions. Mycotoxins in foods may cause disease.
- Anaphylaxis is a potentially life-threatening acute IgE-mediated reaction that results in the release of large amounts of inflammatory mediators. Reactions may be mild, moderate, or severe. Severe reactions are characterized by severe respiratory distress, cyanosis, hypotension, and loss of consciousness. Treatment is 1:1,000 epinephrine 0.3 to 0.5 mL subcutaneously and other supportive measures. Any patient who has had a generalized reaction should be referred for allergy evaluation and trained in the use of an emergency treatment kit containing epinephrine.
- Immunotoxicology is the study of toxic effects of xenobiotics on the cellular and humoral components of the immune system. Most immunotoxicant chemicals are suppressive, either dampening the whole immune apparatus or acting at specific points. Regarding immunostimulation, metals, such as nickel, platinum, and beryllium, and chemicals are capable of causing asthma and other types of hypersensitivity reactions.
- Because of the numbers of chemicals and the complexity of interactions, a logical system of testing is required. Tier I tests include measurement of humeral antibody, antibody titers, immunoglobulin levels, complete blood count with differential, lymphocyte enumeration and typing, and delayed-type hypersensitivity tests. Tier II tests are carried out in people with significant abnormalities in tier I testing and include induction of primary antibody response to injected protein or polysaccharide antigens, stimulation of lymphocyte proliferation with specific mitogens, additional T- and B-cell markers, and measurement of cytokines. Biopsy of lymphatic tissue, spleen, or bone marrow and tests for NK cell function are part of tier III testing; tier III testing is only done in people with significant abnormalities on tier II tests. Tier III testing should be performed by certified immunologists at well-established, university-recognized immunotoxicologic laboratories.
- IEI has displaced the use of the *term multiple chemical sensitivity* (MCS). Individual patients with IEI manifest a variety of symptoms triggered by extremely low-level exposure to environmental substances. There are no standard objective tests for this disorder. There is no objective evidence of hypersensitivity by immunologic parameters. The diagnosis is based on history alone and excludes patients with well-defined disease entities. The American Academy of Allergy and Immunology, the American College of Occupational Environmental Medicine, and the Council of Scientific Affairs of the American Medical Association have position statements to the effect that there are no well-controlled studies establishing a clear mechanism or cause for IEI (formerly MCS). Studies have demonstrated that many patients with IEI meet the criteria for diagnosis of depression, anxiety, or panic disorders. A general approach to individuals with IEI is (a) to listen with an open mind, (b) to do a complete initial examination, (c) to do sufficient standard testing to rule out any serious illness suggested by the history, (d) to treat with reassurance and appropriate medications, (e) to

encourage physical and social interaction, and (f) to refer to an appropriate specialist if needed.

QUESTIONS

1. Type II hypersensitivity reactions require which of the following?

A. Previously sensitized lymphocytes that release lymphokines resulting in illness.
B. IgE antibodies that crosslink with an antigen attached to mast cell receptors.
C. IgG antibodies directed against antigen located on target cell surfaces.
D. Immune complexes that precipitate along vascular endothelium.
E. None of the above.

2. Which of the following is (are) true about HP?

A. The acute form appears as a flulike illness 4 to 6 hours after the exposure.
B. IgG antibody levels may not be detectable in the chronic form of HP.
C. Skin testing is helpful in the confirmation of the diagnosis of HP.
D. The illness results from antigens that cause an immune complex reaction in the respiratory interstitium.
E. Only A, B, and D.

*3. According to the National Research Council's Committee on Biological Markers, which of the following is **not** a part of tier I immunotoxicologic testing?*

A. Measurements of antibodies
B. Blood counts with differentials
C. Isotope-specific antibody titration
D. Measurements of delayed-type hypersensitivity
E. Biopsy of lymphatic tissue

*4. All of the following are true regarding natural rubber latex (NRL) hypersensitivity **except***

A. Types of reactions may include bronchospasm and anaphylaxis.
B. NRL may be falsely negative in one fourth of the cases.
C. Low ambient concentration of NRL proteins is essential to ensure latex safe environment.
D. Premedication of sensitized individuals with steroids is highly recommended before significant NRL exposure.
E. The latex allergic person should be trained in the use of an injectable epinephrine kit.

*5. Regarding ABPA, which of the following is a **false** statement?*

A. It is a severe asthmatic condition associated with a significantly elevated serum IgE level.
B. *A. fumigatus* spores may colonize the lower respiratory tract.
C. Skin testing shows immediate skin reactivity to the fungal antigen.
D. IgE and IgG *Aspergillus* antibodies reactions cause damage through multiple mechanisms.
E. Use of corticosteroids is contraindicated in the management of ABPA.

=30=

Arm Pain in the Workplace

OBJECTIVES

- List common categories of musculoskeletal illness of the upper extremity
- Discuss systemic diseases that may cause arm pain
- Explain the similarities and differences between musculoskeletal disorders of the arm and cervical radiculopathies
- Explain the increasing incidence of soft tissue complaints in the upper extremity

OUTLINE

I. Regional musculoskeletal illness that can be ascribed to osteoarthritis
   A. Table 30.1: Upper-extremity symptoms and/or signs that suggest a systemic cause
II. The neuropathic syndromes
   A. Table 30.2: Classic clinical features of an entrapment neuropathy
III. Soft tissue regional musculoskeletal illness at the shoulder
   A. Soft tissue illness
   B. Regional musculoskeletal illness of the shoulder
   C. Regional musculoskeletal illness of the elbow
   D. Regional musculoskeletal illness of the wrist
   E. Regional musculoskeletal illness of the hand
IV. When is a regional musculoskeletal illness of the upper extremity an injury?

KEY POINTS

- Discomfort in the upper extremity is common. Regional musculoskeletal illness constitutes the majority of disorders of the upper extremity. There are three common categories of disorders in this region: illness that relates to osteoarthritis, illness as a consequence of neuropathy, and soft tissue illness.
- There are "red flags" associated with diseases (see Table 30.1) in which referral may be advisable.
- Osteoarthritis of the proximal joints of the upper extremity, the glenohumeral joint, and the elbow is unusual. Osteoarthritis of the hands is common. It may cause the development of osteophytes of the distal interphalangeal joints (Heberden's nodes), and the proximal interphalangeal joints may also be involved to a lesser degree (Bouchard's nodes).

- Arthritis of the first carpometacarpal joint is a common cause of pain at the base of the thumb, particularly in women beyond middle age. Forces of pinching are transduced during activities to the first carpometacarpal joint.
- Cervical radiculopathies are common and present with pain that, whether localized or radiating, is not exacerbated by limb motion.
- Entrapment neuropathies of the upper extremities are less frequent than cervical radiculopathies. They share features that are outlined in Table 30.2.
- The most common entrapment neuropathy of the upper extremity is carpal tunnel syndrome (CTS). If electrodiagnostic studies are used as the gold standard, the classical symptoms of CTS are useless as screening tools because of their low predictive value. With persistence of symptoms of CTS, and certainly with any hint of atrophy, the guidance of a perspicacious expert should be sought.
- Soft tissue illnesses represent the bulk of regional musculoskeletal disorders of the upper extremity. These patients have localized discomfort, tenderness, and often exacerbation with motion of the painful region. Their prognosis is excellent even though the symptoms can take months to remit. Acetaminophen is the analgesic with the most compelling benefit-to-risk ratio.
- The shoulder region is the most frequent target for regional illness of the upper extremity.
- Patients with elbow pain resulting from epicondylitis should be advised to avoid patterns of use that aggravates symptoms; improvement occurs in a matter of weeks.
- A trigger finger usually subsides spontaneously, although infiltration with corticosteroid preparations can be useful in persistent cases.

QUESTIONS

1. *A 55-year-old woman presents with the complaint of pain at the base of the right thumb when she pinches the burling tool. The likeliest diagnosis, by far, is which of the following?*

A. Early CTS
B. de Quervain's tenosynovitis
C. Osteoarthritis of the first carpometacarpal joint
D. Rheumatoid arthritis
E. Radial nerve entrapment

2. *A 38-year-old machinist presents with a painful left shoulder. Which physical finding suggests glenohumeral arthritis?*

A. Focal tenderness in the midbody of the deltoid muscle
B. Focal tenderness in the acromioclavicular joint
C. Exacerbation of pain when the arm is abducted and externally rotated
D. Restriction of internal rotation with the shoulder in a neutral position
E. A positive Adson's maneuver

3. *There have been a number of community epidemiologic surveys exploring the prevalence of the features of CTS. Which of the following statements regarding the results of these surveys is **false**?*

A. The prevalence of symptoms that suggest CTS approaches 20%.
B. Approximately 5% of adults have symptoms to suggest CTS and have prolonged median nerve conductivity.
C. Median distal motor latency correlates positively with body mass index and age.
D. Symptoms of CTS are intermittent regardless of median nerve conductivity.
E. Median nerve conductivity is more likely to be prolonged in the presence of symptoms of CTS.

4. *In the preponderance of epidemiologic studies, which of the following variables associates most closely with the complaint of disabling pain of the upper extremity?*

A. Measures of job satisfaction
B. Use of handheld vibrating tools
C. Physical demands of tasks
D. Repetitiveness of tasks
E. Monotony of tasks

31

Infectious Disease

OBJECTIVES

- List methods of disease transmission in the workplace
- List airborne pathogens
- Identify occupations at highest risk for work-related infection
- Discuss risks from blood-borne pathogens
- Recognize preventive measures to minimize transmission of infections

OUTLINE

KEY POINTS

- Any agent (bacterial, viral, fungal, protozoan, or helminth) that can be spread through the environment and that causes infection and clinical disease in an occupational setting is of concern. Transmission of infectious agents can occur through direct or indirect contact.
- Direct transmission can occur through three primary routes: (a) direct contact, such as skin-to-skin or skin-to-mucous membrane touching, or droplet spread of contaminated fluid onto the mucous membranes of the nose, mouth, or conjunctiva; (b) parental, which may take the form of percutaneous needle sticks or transfusion of contaminated fluid; and (c) exposure of susceptible skin to an infectious agent, such as through a bite, laceration, or compromised skin.
- Indirect routes include airborne (the most common; typically involves the dissemination of infectious agents through aerosols that enter a host through the respiratory tract), vector-borne transmission (disease carried by insects or animals), and vehicle-borne transmission (when an intermediate object transports an infectious agent into a suitable port of entry into the host).
- The potential of an infectious agent to pose an occupational risk is determined by the characteristics of the agent, its propensity to cause disease, the potential methods of transmission, and the ability of the agent to survive environmental conditions.
- The type of infections for which workers are at risk is largely dependent on the type of work that they do. Occupations at risk tend be those in which individuals have close or frequent contact with other humans and animals.
- Health care is one of the highest risk occupations for exposure to infectious disease.
- Blood-borne pathogens are typically spread through direct contact. Throughout the general population, many are spread through sexual contact or intravenous drug use, but exposure in the workplace typically occurs through percutaneous sticks, through spray of droplets onto mucous membranes or compromised skin, or via a parental route.
- **HIV** exposure is a definite risk for health care, laboratory, and home health care workers. Throughout the health care and research fields, universal precautions and personal protective equipment have minimized exposure to HIV. When an exposure occurs, post-exposure prophylaxis should be considered. The seroconversion rate following a needle stick with HIV-positive blood is generally estimated to be about 0.3%. The efficacy of zidovudine (AZT) in the reduction of risk of HIV in health care workers is about 80%.
- **HBV** was the first blood-borne disease recognized to pose an occupational risk through a preponderance of cases among pathologists, laboratory workers, and blood bank workers. Occupations at risk are those with exposure to blood or fluids.

- The risk of transmission is 1% to 6% with HBe antigen negative blood and is estimated to be 22% to 40% for HBe antigen positive blood. Since 1985, the rate of infection has decreased by 90% in health care workers because of the widespread adoption of preventive immunization, universal precaution, and personal protective equipment.
- **HCV** is responsible for most cases of transfusion-related hepatitis. Infection is spread primarily by parenteral exposure to blood and blood products. Health care workers are at risk for occupational exposure through percutaneous sticks or direct membrane exposure. The risk of HCV transmission from a needle stick has been found to be roughly 4% (using the anti-HCV test) or 10% using the more sensitive but less available ribonucleic acid (RNA) polymerase chain reaction (PCR) test for follow-up.
- Bacterial and viral pathogens can be carried by air, but they must be aerosolized, small (1 to 5 mm), and viable.
- **TB** is caused by *Mycobacterium tuberculosis.* Active TB presents with symptoms of cough, weight loss, and malaise. Diagnosis of TB can be made through a skin test or chest x-ray film. The skin test only indicates previous exposure; it does not designate active infection. If TB is suspected, a chest x-ray should be taken.
- The incidence of TB has increased significantly in the last decade because of laxity in public health measures and because of the acquired immunodeficiency syndrome (AIDS) epidemic. Health care workers and staff in institutional settings have the highest risk of exposure. Recent skin test converters should be evaluated for isoniazid (INH) prophylaxis after a chest x-ray is performed to rule out active disease. Multidrug resistant (MDR) strains of TB are of increasing concern.
- **Influenza** vaccination is recommended for health care workers, optimally given in mid-October to mid-November. Recent research has shown that the vaccine may reduce overall rates of respiratory illness and absenteeism compared with placebo, justifying its use on a cost-effectiveness basis even in healthy, low-risk workers.
- **Whooping cough** is due to *Bordetella pertussis.* Health care and childcare workers are at risk for exposure. The traditional pertussis vaccine for children is not used in adults because of frequent side effects. Specific testing is needed to diagnose adults with pertussis. After 5 days of treatment with antibiotics, the individual may return to work if asymptomatic.
- **Measles,** an acute viral disease, is transmitted by large airborne respiratory droplets and has an incubation period of 5 to 21 days. During an outbreak, vaccination within 72 hours after exposure without prior serologic testing is recommended to any adult who has not received two doses of vaccine, regardless of age or serologic status. The vaccine has an efficacy of 95% with one dose and 99% with two doses.
- Fecal-oral infections (e.g., *Salmonella, Shigella, Clostridium,* and a variety of *Enterococci*) may be transmitted via contaminated food or water. Occupations at risk include those who come in direct contact with an infected animals or contaminated water or food. Laundry workers, food handlers, and health care workers have been noted to be at increased risk. Prevention and control includes strict hygienic standards such as hand washing and appropriate personal protective equipment. Workers with acute gastrointestinal illness (i.e., vomiting, diarrhea, nausea, fever, and abdominal pain) should be excluded from work if it involves personal contact or contact with food.
- **HAV** is a common infection transmitted by the fecal-oral route. Many occupations are at risk for this infection, including military personnel, health care workers, day care workers, food handlers, staff workers in institutions for the developmentally delayed and/or handicapped, and those working in prisons and jails. HAV is one of most frequently reported vaccine-preventable diseases. Vaccination, which is 94% to 100%

effective, is recommended for persons at risk of occupational exposure and for those who travel abroad. Immune globulin given within 2 weeks of exposure is more than 85% effective in preventing symptomatic infection.

- Infections acquired by direct contact include infections of the skin, hair, or eyes and a variety of gastrointestinal disturbances. Direct contact may include actual skin-to-skin or skin-to-mucous membrane touching, contact with a contaminated fomite, or droplet spread. Blood-borne pathogens can also be transmitted through droplet spread. Skin breaks, lesions, and rashes, regardless of cause, may present an occupational health hazard.
- **Conjunctivitis** may result from many types of viruses or bacteria (e.g., *Hemophilus influenzae, Streptococcus pneumonia,* enterovirus, adenoviral pharyngitis, conjunctival fever, or chlamydia). EKC is spread by direct contact with infected eye secretions. Thorough hand washing and high-level disinfection can help prevent the spread of conjunctivitis.
- *Herpes simplex* **viruses (HSV I and II)** are transmitted through direct contact. Dentists and medical health care workers are at risk from oral secretions and can develop herpetic whitlow in the periungual skin of the hand. Treatment consists of both oral and topical acyclovir.
- **Varicella (chickenpox)** is an acute viral disease that is most severe in adults and is highly contagious, especially in the early stages of cutaneous eruption; an infected individual is contagious for 1 to 2 days before the rash. The Centers for Disease Control and Prevention (CDC) has recommended that individuals who have been exposed should not return to work for 10 to 21 days following exposure.
- *Herpes zoster* **(shingles)**, a localized outbreak of skin vesicles, results from reactivation of varicella virus following a dormant period of years after primary chickenpox infection. The virus is spread person-to-person by the airborne route or by direct contact with vesicular fluid or respiratory secretions or by articles freshly soiled with these fluids. *Herpes zoster* has a lower rate of transmission than varicella, but both can cause chickenpox in seronegative contacts.
- **Mumps** is a viral illness that is spread by contact with saliva or other respiratory secretions. Virus can be present in saliva for 6 to 7 days before observable parotitis, with an incubation period of 12 to 15 days. About one third of cases are asymptomatic. The vaccine is reported to be 95% effective.
- **Rubella (German measles)** is a mild febrile illness associated with a maculopapular rash. Transmission occurs through direct contact and nasopharyngeal droplets. Individuals are contagious during the rash eruption. A live attenuated virus vaccine elicits an antibody response in 98% to 99% of recipients. Rubella is most important because of its teratogenic effect on the developing fetus. Congenital rubella syndrome occurs in up to 90% of infants born to women infected during the first trimester.
- *Neisseria meningitidis* may lead to a wide spectrum of disease, including sepsis, meningitis, and pneumonia. Infection is ubiquitous, and disease occurs commonly in children and young adults, frequently among newly aggregated adults in crowded conditions. Infection transmission occurs by intimate, direct contact with oropharyngeal secretions of infected individuals.
- **Lice** (*Pediculus humanus, Pediculus capitis, Pediculus pubis,* or *Pediculus corporis*) and scabies (*Sarcoptes scabiei miti*) can be transmitted person-to-person. Scabies is a skin infection caused by a burrowing mite and usually involves the interdigital space of the hand and flexor surface of the wrists. Lice are ectoparasites that are transmitted from person-to-person by direct contact and with contact with clothing, where they can

live for up to a week. Diagnosis is confirmed by finding the adult lice or nits on hair or clothing of infested persons.

- Bite wounds from animals or humans can also lead to infections or blood-borne pathogen transmission. Treatment with broad-spectrum antibiotics covers most potential pathogens. Amoxicillin-clavulanate, clorfloxicin, or cloxacillin may be used for prophylaxis or treatment.

- **Zoonoses** diseases are naturally transmitted between vertebrate animals and humans. This definition is sometimes extended to include those diseases transmitted by insects, such as arboviruses. Occupations at risk include zoologic workers, farmers, veterinarians, research laboratory workers, and animal control workers.

- The most common zoonoses are brucellosis, rabies, Q fever, tularemia, Lyme disease, toxoplasmosis, cryptosporidiosis, and arboviruses causing encephalitis. A risk also exists for transmission of leptospirosis, anthrax, Hantavirus, viral hemorrhagic fevers, and spongiform encephalitis, although these are more rare. For illnesses transmitted via insect vectors, prevention of bites from ticks, flies, and fleas by use of appropriate repellents and personal protective clothing while working in endemic areas limits the acquisition of these illnesses.

- **Brucellosis** species (*Brucella suis, Brucella melitensis,* and *Brucella abortus*) can cause a wide array of syndromes that include nonspecific fever, rigor, malaise, anorexia, and arthralgia. Infections can be acquired through direct cutaneous contact, inhalation, conjunctival inoculation from animal tissue or placenta, or ingestion of unpasteurized milk products. A wide variety of animals harbor the organisms, including goats, sheep, camel, cattle, pigs, dogs, buffalo, and yaks.

- **Rabies** causes an acute viral encephalomyelopathy, which presents as headache, fever, malaise, and other localized sensory changes, that progresses to delirium, convulsions, and death. The route of infection is typically from saliva via a bite from a zoometric source or from person-to-person contact. The most common animal carriers include skunks, raccoons, rabbits, coyotes, bats, beavers, foxes, cattle, dogs, and cats. Rabies in the United States occurs infrequently, but is almost always fatal. Prophylaxis is highly recommended following a bite, scratch, or stick with potentially infected material or if mucous membranes or broken skin is splashed with infected fluid.

- **Q fever** is due to *Coxiella burnetii.* It may present as a nonspecific febrile illness, pneumonia, osteomyelitis, endocarditis, or hepatitis. Many animals are known to harbor the organism, but the most common animal reservoirs are cattle, goats, and sheep. The placentas of infected animals have large numbers of the organism. Other routes of infection include direct contact with infected animals, laboratory contact, or ingestion of contaminated milk.

- **Tularemia** is due to *Francisella tularensis.* Clinical disease may present in several syndromes and varies with the site of inoculation. Most of the time it is an ulcer at the site of inoculation with local lymphadenopathy. Disease transmission most commonly occurs because of direct contact with or a bite from an infected animal, inhalation, contact with infected animal tissue, or a bite from an infected insect. Insect vectors vary according to geographic locale, but ticks, biting flies, and mosquitoes may transit the organism. The disease may be transmitted by inhalation of aerosolized particle during slaughtering of infected animals or in the laboratory during routine microbiologic handling. Direct contact with contaminated water or mud may also transmit the disease.

- **Lyme disease** is caused by *Borrelia burgdorferi,* which is transmitted by a tick bite and causes a characteristic rash, fever, arthralgias, arthritis, carditis or neurologic abnormalities.

- **Toxoplasmosis** is caused by *Toxoplasma gondii* whose definitive host is the cat and whose intermediate hosts include birds, sheep, goat, swine, cattle, and chicken. The acute disease in humans may be asymptomatic or may produce a nonspecific mononucleosis-like illness with fever, lymphadenopathy, and lymphocytosis. In immunocompromised humans, it may result in chorioretinitis or cerebritis. Women who acquire the infection during pregnancy may pass the infection on to the fetus. Prevention involves meticulous attention to hand washing. Women who are pregnant should be advised to avoid cat litter boxes or cats with an unknown feeding history. Litter boxes should be changed daily.
- **Leptospirosis** is caused by a number of serovariants of spirochete such as *Leptospira interrogan*. The clinical symptoms are varied, but usually include nonspecific constitutional symptoms of fever, headache, myalgia, and nausea. Severe illness is characterized by conjunctivitis, jaundice, meningitis, and renal failure. The organism has been found in rodents, swine, dogs, cats, raccoons, and cattle. Human contact with contaminated food and inhalation of infectious aerosols has also been implicated as modes of transmission.
- **Anthrax** is caused by *Bacillus anthracis* and can result in a cutaneous or pulmonary infection. Cutaneous anthrax is characterized by a black eschar ulcer on the skin. Outbreaks have been described in industrialized countries resulting from the importation of contaminated animal products, especially goat hair. Reservoirs include large herbivores such as agricultural animals, and the bacteria may be found in contaminated soil where animal graze.
- Environmental infections may spread through contact with the environment. Agents can be inhaled or inoculated through the skin. Direct inoculation from different organisms can cause infection or illness. Such infections can occur from a bite or through breaks in the skin. Infection can be prevented through the appropriate use of personal protective equipment.
- Artificial or indoor environments may allow exposure to microbiologic aerosols. About one third of indoor air problems in buildings are related to contamination from fungi, bacteria, and viruses or toxins produced by them. These environmental infectious agents may cause hypersensitivity, inhalation fever, or infections (including legionellosis; TB; and various bacterial, viral, or fungal diseases).
- Infections may develop among individuals who travel domestically or internationally. They may knowingly or unknowingly become carriers. Persons from industrialized nations who travel to underdeveloped countries where a threat exists of acquiring infectious illnesses should take specific precautions.
- Many insurance companies in the United States do not provide medical coverage for care obtained outside of the country; however, some companies now have coverage for employees that travel abroad to foreign lands.
- The most common mode of disease transmission in travelers is through ingestion of contaminated food or water. Usually, these infections are self-limiting and last only 3 to 4 days.
- Insect bites are another common route of disease transmission in travelers. The most common are those caused by mosquito-borne transmission, such as yellow fever, malaria, and Japanese encephalitis.
- **Malaria** is a febrile flulike illness that can present in a 3- or 4-day cycle; it can also cause more severe disease, including cerebral, pulmonary, and renal failure. Precautions against malaria include preventive vaccination or treatment of the illness with mefloquine, primaquine, or chloroquine.
- Laboratory-related infections may be transmitted in academic, hospital, industrial, or government settings. Exposure can occur from agents or organisms being studied or

used in the course of research, recombinant viruses or organisms, hazards in human- or primate-derived materials, zoonoses, and shared equipment. The most commonly reported laboratory acquired infections are brucellosis, Q fever, typhoid, hepatitis, tularemia, chlamydia, TB, dermatomycosis, Venezuelan equine encephalitis, psittacosis, and coccidioidomycosis. A potential exists for transmission of simian immune deficiency virus, Hantavirus, Sabia virus, spongiform encephalopathies, and systemic lupus erythematosus, although these are rare.

QUESTIONS

*1. Which of the following is **not** an example of direct transmission of infection?*

A. Disease spread by skin-to-skin contact, such as scabies
B. Disease spread by transfusion, such as HCV
C. Disease spread insect bite, such as malaria
D. Disease spread by hands, such as conjunctivitis
E. Disease spread after a cut, such as cellulitis

*2. Which of the following statements is **least** correct about work-related infections?*

A. The type of infections for which workers are at risk is largely dependent on the type of work that they do.
B. Occupations at risk tend be those in which individuals have close or frequent contact with other humans and animals.
C. Health care is one of the highest risk occupations for exposure to infectious disease.
D. HIV exposure is a definite risk for health care, laboratory, and home health care workers.
E. The seroconversion rate after a needle stick with HIV-positive blood is estimated to be 30%.

*3. Which of the following statements concerning blood-borne disease is **incorrect**?*

A. Occupations with exposure to blood are at risk from HBV.
B. The risk of transmission is 1% to 6% with HBe antigen negative blood and is estimated to be 22% to 40% for HBe antigen positive blood.
C. Since 1985, the rate of infection has increased by 90% in health care workers.
D. HCV is responsible for most cases of transfusion-related hepatitis.
E. The risk of HCV transmission from a needle stick ranges from 4% to 10%.

*4. Which of the following statements is **least correct** regarding TB exposure?*

A. TB can be diagnosed through a skin test or chest x-ray film.
B. Recent skin test converters should be evaluated for INH prophylaxis.
C. The positive TB skin test designates active infection.
D. Health care workers and staff in institutional settings have the highest risk of exposure to TB.
E. MDR strains of TB are of increasing concern.

*5. Which of the following statements about immunization is **incorrect**?*

A. Influenza vaccination is recommended for health care workers, optimally given in mid-October to mid-November.

B. Pediatric vaccine for whooping cough is not used in adults because of frequent side effects.
C. During measles outbreak, vaccination of adults is contraindicated within 72 hours of exposure.
D. Measles vaccine has an efficacy of 95% with one dose and 99% with two doses.
E. Mumps vaccine is reported to be 95% effective.

6. *Which of the following statements about fecal-oral infections is **incorrect?***

A. Occupations at risk include those who come in direct contact with an infected animal or contaminated water or food.
B. Prevention and control includes strict hygienic standards such as hand washing and appropriate personal protective equipment.
C. Workers with acute gastrointestinal illness should be excluded from work if it involves personal contact or contact with food.
D. HAV vaccination is only 50% effective.
E. Immune globulin given within 2 weeks of exposure is more than 85% effective in preventing symptomatic infection from HAV.

7. *Which of the following statements regarding occupational infection is **incorrect?***

A. Dentists and medical health care workers exposed to oral secretions may develop herpetic whitlow in the periungual skin of the hand.
B. Health care workers exposed to chickenpox should not return to work for 10 to 21 days following exposure.
C. *Herpes zoster* (shingles) cannot cause chickenpox in seronegative contacts.
D. About one third of patients with mumps are asymptomatic.
E. Congenital rubella syndrome occurs in up to 90% of infants born to women infected during the first trimester of pregnancy.

8. *Which of the following is **least** correct regarding work-related infections?*

A. Scabies is a skin infection caused by a burrowing mite,
B. Prophylactic treatment of human or animal bite wounds with broad-spectrum antibiotics is rarely necessary.
C. Rabies is often carried by skunks, raccoons, or bats.
D. Rabies in the United States occurs infrequently but is almost always fatal.
E. Q fever is an example of a zoonosis.

9. *Which of the following statements regarding work-related infection is **not** correct?*

A. Anthrax (*B. anthracis*) outbreaks have been described in industrialized countries because of the importation of contaminated animal products, especially goat hair.
B. About one third of indoor air problems in buildings are related to contamination from fungi, bacteria, and viruses or toxins produced by any of these.
C. Toxoplasmosis is caused by *T. gondii* whose definitive host is the cat.
D. The most common mode of disease transmission in travelers is through ingestion of contaminated food or water.
E. Precautions against infection with Japanese encephalitis includes use of mefloquine, primaquine, or chloroquine.

32

Hepatic Disorders

OBJECTIVES

- Understand various detoxification functions of the liver
- Distinguish between various types of hepatotoxins
- List types of toxic liver disorders
- Recognize various tests used to detect liver disease

OUTLINE

   I. Role of the liver in detoxification of foreign substances
  II. Classification of hepatotoxins
       A. Table 32.1
       B. Intrinsic hepatotoxins
       C. Idiosyncratic hepatotoxins
 III. Hepatotoxic injuries
       A. Acute hepatotoxic injury
       B. Necrosis
       C. Steatosis
       D. Cholestasis
       E. Subacute hepatotoxic injury
       F. Chronic hepatotoxic injury
       G. Hepatoportal sclerosis
       H. Porphyria cutanea tarda
       I. Cancers of the liver
  IV. Occupational and environmental exposures to hepatotoxins
       A. Hepatotoxins in the workplace, environment, and home
       B. Table 32.2
       C. Inorganic compounds and metals
       D. Halogenated aliphatic organic compounds
       E. Halogenated aromatic compounds
       F. Organochlorine pesticides and chlorophenoxy herbicides
       G. Nitroaliphatic and nitroaromatic compounds
       H. Potentiation related to alcohol and other chemical interactions
   V. A practical guide the prevention of and medical surveillance for occupational
       liver disease
       A. Medical monitoring of workers exposed to hepatotoxins
       B. Biochemical tests
       C. Bilirubin

D. Synthetic liver function and clearance tests
E. Physical examination and structural studies

KEY POINTS

- Occupational liver diseases are caused by a variety of biologic, chemical, and physical agents. Biologic agents involved in occupation settings are primarily confined to the viral hepatitides. Physical agents include ionizing radiation, heat (e.g., heat stroke), and vibration. Chemical agents may also induce liver disease.
- The liver is the organ that is mainly responsible for the detoxification and elimination of foreign substances (i.e., xenobiotics) from the bloodstream. By virtue of the portal circulation, the liver is the initial site for action on ingested toxins. Those absorbed through inhalation and the skin also rapidly make their way to the liver through the hepatic artery.
- The liver has ability to detoxify chemicals and drugs through complex biochemical reactions, many times facilitated by enzyme systems that include mixed function oxidases (MFOs), also known as the cytochrome P450 enzyme systems.
- Phase I reactions make lipid-soluble compounds more polar through hydrolysis, oxidation, or reduction.
- Phase II reactions are those in which the foreign compound is conjugated with another functional group, usually resulting in a less toxic, more easily excreted compound.
- Most hepatotoxic agents produce liver injury only after biotransformation to an active metabolite through the action of these enzyme systems.
- Chemical hepatotoxins include two broad categories based on their presumed mechanism of action (Table 32.1 in the textbook).
- Intrinsic hepatotoxins are agents that are directly or indirectly toxic to the liver. Toxicity is a predictable and inherent property of the chemical structure of the compound or its metabolite and is generally dose dependent.
- Direct intrinsic hepatotoxins produce hepatic injury through the direct destructive action of the toxin on the hepatocyte. Direct toxic actions include peroxidation by free radicals and covalent binding of toxins or their metabolites to tissue molecules. Direct hepatotoxins most often lead to cell necrosis or steatosis.
- Indirect intrinsic hepatotoxins produce liver injury by disruption and interference with specific cellular metabolic processes or components responsible for cellular structural integrity or secretory activity. Hepatic injury by indirect hepatotoxins may result in necrosis, steatosis, or a combination of the two. They can also produce cholestatic injury through interference with bile excretion or bile duct injury.
- Idiosyncratic hepatotoxins produce injury as a result of an individual susceptibility (rather than an intrinsic property of the agent) by immunologic (allergic) response or as a result of a metabolic aberration.
- Hepatotoxic injuries vary in severity and may cause outcomes that range from mild transient elevation of liver enzymes to massive necrosis and death.
- Chronic exposures to toxins can result in subacute disease that may or may not progress to chronic disease.
- Acute hepatotoxic injuries usually result from a significant exposure occurring over a relatively short period, and most involve a cytotoxic injury.
- Necrosis of hepatocytes is thought to result from injury to plasma membranes and cellular organelles. It may occur in a zonal or nonzonal pattern. Zonal necrosis is identified by the zone of the liver lobule in which it occurs.

- Steatosis refers to fatty changes in the liver and is often an early indicator of hepato-toxicity.
- Cholestasis refers to cessation or alteration of bile flow, which can result from hepato-canalicular injury, canalicular injury, necrosis of bile ducts, or necrosis, and scaring of septal ducts. Cholestasis is suspected when tests reveal elevation of serum bilirubin or alkaline phosphates.
- Chronic hepatotoxic injury can result in cirrhosis, hepatoportal sclerosis, hepatic por-phyria, and neoplastic changes.
- Cirrhosis is a chronic, irreversible condition in which the normal hepatic architecture is replaced by fibrous tissue and regenerating nodules. It is most often seen as a sequela of long-standing alcohol abuse or chronic viral infection.
- Hepatoportal sclerosis is a fibrous lesion that causes obstruction of branches of the por-tal vein.
- Porphyria cutanea tarda is the most common type of porphyria in humans. It causes increased iron stores in the liver. It is characterized by chronic photosensitivity with resultant skin fragility and the appearance of lesions (i.e., vesicles and bullae) most fre-quently seen on the dorsum of the hands, forearms, and face.
- Cancers of the liver in humans have been described in association with a number of agents including chronic viral infections (e.g., hepatitis B and C), chronic alcohol ingestion, contraceptive steroids, aflatoxin B_1, inorganic arsenic, and vinyl chloride.
- Hepatic angiosarcoma is a rare form of liver cancer that has been associated with expo-sure to vinyl chloride and has been reported with long-term exposure to arsenicals.
- Exposure to hepatotoxins can occur in a variety of settings, including the workplace, home, and external environment. In the occupational setting, inhalation is the primary route of exposure, but many hepatotoxins are readily absorbed through the skin and can contribute substantially to total worker exposure (Table 32.2 in the textbook).
- A large number of agents commonly encountered in occupational settings can be toxic to the liver, including inorganic chemicals, halogenated aliphatic organic compounds, halogenated aromatic compounds, organochlorine pesticides and herbicides, and nitro-gen-bearing compounds (i.e., nitroaliphatic and nitroaromatic).
- Hepatotoxic environmental exposures most often occur through contamination of food and water. A large number of consumer products including medications (e.g., aceta-minophen, aspirin); pesticides; automotive products (e.g., antifreeze, carburetor clean-ers); painting products; adhesives; and cleaning products contain a variety of hepato-toxic chemicals.
- Halogenated aliphatic organic compounds are the most widely known group of hepa-totoxins. Carbon tetrachloride (CCl_4) is the prototype of this group. CCl_4 causes a char-acteristic zone 3 hepatic necrosis leading to rapid destruction of the hepatic parenchyma and causing liver failure.
- Ethanol, as well as isopropanol, methanol, 2-butanol, and acetone, potentiates the tox-icity of CCl_4. Alcoholics are more likely to develop hepatic injury after exposure to CCl_4 than nondrinkers. The likely mechanism for this potentiation is alcohol induction of hepatocyte cytochrome P450 systems with enhanced metabolic conversion of CCl_4 to its toxic metabolite.
- The first step in preventing occupational liver disease is to substitute and replace hepa-totoxic agents with nonhepatotoxic agents when possible. Engineering controls can also reduce exposure.
- When an individual presents with a possible work-related liver disorder, removal from exposure should be considered early on and may provide both preventative and diag-nostic benefits.

- The surveillance of workers with potential exposure to hepatotoxins presents a challenge. The ideal medical surveillance test would be one that has high sensitivity and high specificity. However, there is a lack of tests that meet this criterion and that are practical to implement.
- Biochemical tests most commonly used measures to detect liver disease include aspartate aminotransferase (AST), alanine aminotransferase (ALT), serum alkaline phosphatase (ALP), serum lactate dehydrogenase (LDH), and γ-glutamyltranspeptidase (GGT). Transaminases are released from hepatocytes after cell injury or death. These tests are more sensitive than then they are specific and may be useful in detecting early stages of toxic liver injury and nontoxic liver disease (e.g., viral hepatitis, extrahepatic obstructive conditions). Transaminase screening frequently identifies individuals with elevated transaminase levels that could be caused by a variety or combination of factors (e.g., medications, alcohol use).
- The serum bilirubin level is typically elevated when there is significant parenchymal liver injury. It is the pigment most likely to be elevated in patients with toxic liver injury. Nevertheless, compared with transaminases, it is considered an insensitive measure of chemical liver injury and therefore is of limited value in the occupational setting. Hyperbilirubinemia may be conjugated or unconjugated. Unconjugated hyperbilirubinemia is commonly seen in Gilbert's disease, hemolytic disorders, and congestive heart failure.
- Measurements of serum albumin levels and prothrombin time are commonly done to assess the liver's synthetic function. However, neither is a sensitive measure of liver injury. Such tests have little or no value in medical surveillance for exposure to hepatotoxins.
- Clearance tests measure the ability of the liver to excrete substances and can be sensitive and specific in the detection of liver disease. These tests can measure clearance of exogenous substances (e.g., indocyanine green, antipyrine) or endogenous substances (e.g., serum bile acids).
- Physical examination is useful in detecting hepatomegaly. However, hepatomegaly usually occurs after there has been a prolonged or significant hepatotoxic exposure. As such, physical examination is not a sensitive screening tool.
- Liver biopsy is the gold standard in establishing the most specific diagnosis possible. However, liver biopsy is highly invasive and carries significant risks of complications. It is never used as a screening tool and is reserved for cases in which a tissue diagnosis is required. Even with a biopsy-proven histologic diagnosis, the work relatedness of an individual's liver pathology may remain in question.

QUESTIONS

*1. Which of the following is **incorrect** concerning liver injury?*

A. By virtue of the portal circulation, the liver is the initial site for action on ingested toxins.

B. The liver has ability to detoxify chemicals and drugs through complex biochemical reactions, many times facilitated by enzyme systems that include MFOs.

C. Phase I reactions are those in which the foreign compound is conjugated with another functional group that usually result in a less toxic, more easily excreted compound.

D. Most hepatotoxic agents produce liver injury only after biotransformation to an active metabolite through the action of these enzyme systems.

E. Intrinsic hepatotoxins are agents that are directly or indirectly toxic to the liver.

2. *Which of the following is **least** correct concerning liver injury?*

A. Direct intrinsic hepatotoxins produce hepatic injury through the direct destructive action of the toxin on the hepatocyte.
B. Indirect intrinsic hepatotoxins produce liver injury by disruption and interference with specific cellular metabolic processes or components responsible for cellular structural integrity or secretory activity.
C. Idiosyncratic hepatotoxins produce injury as a result of an individual susceptibility.
D. Chronic exposures to toxins usually progress to chronic disease.
E. Zonal necrosis is identified by the zone of the liver lobule in which it occurs.

3. *Steatosis refers to*

A. Fatty changes in the liver
B. Cessation or alteration of bile flow caused by hepatocanalicular injury
C. Hepatoportal sclerosis
D. Hepatic porphyria
E. Fibrotic scarring of the liver

4. *Hepatic angiosarcoma has been associated with which of the following?*

A. Chronic hepatitis B infection
B. Chronic hepatitis C infection
C. Contraceptive steroids
D. Vinyl chloride
E. Aflatoxin B

5. *Which of the following is **least** correct?*

A. Halogenated aliphatic organic compounds are the most widely known group of hepatotoxins.
B. Ethanol and other alcohols (e.g., isopropanol, methanol, 2-butanol, acetone) reduce the toxicity of CCl_4.
C. The first step in preventing occupational liver disease is to substitute and replace hepatotoxic agents with nonhepatotoxic agents when possible.
D. Hepatotoxic environmental exposures most often occur through contamination of food and water.
E. Ideal medical surveillance tests for hepatotoxicity would have high sensitivity and high specificity.

6. *Which of the following is most useful to screen for occupational liver disease?*

A. AST and ALT
B. Unconjugated hyperbilirubinemia
C. Indocyanine green clearance
D. Physical examination to detect hepatomegaly
E. Liver biopsy

=33=
The Case Report: Discovery of Occupational Disease

OBJECTIVES

- Explain clinical tools used to identify occupational illness
- Describe the types of clinical observations that are appropriately published in a case report
- Describe how to prepare a case report of a new or unexpected disease association with a particular work setting

OUTLINE

KEY POINTS

- One goal is to prevent occupational illness. It is first necessary to identify the cause. Case reports of clusters of tumors of unusual type or at unusual anatomic sites have led to the identification of occupational carcinogens.

- The following three elements contribute to a valid and useful case report: an accurate diagnosis, a meticulous exposure history, and a literature review that supports the plausibility of a casual relationship. Likely alternative causes must be excluded.
- The occupational history should be sufficiently detailed to identify the type, intensity, and duration of exposure to materials.
- Some medical conditions may be more likely to be related to workplace factors. A *sentinel health event* is a condition already known to have occupational causes that contributes to unnecessary disease, disability, or untimely death.
- A review of current information in the literature concerning exposure may assist in the determination of causality.
- Characteristics of exposure, such as intensity, duration, and route, and personal characteristics, such as cigarette smoking, alcohol consumption, age, genetic susceptibility, intercurrent disease, and coexposures, may interact to influence the ultimate effect on health.
- Exposures may not always be safe simply because levels of exposure are below recommended standards.
- Work practices or personal habits may modify apparently harmless industrial processes.
- Exposures during hobby or home activity may be related to a condition that appears to be caused by workplace exposure.
- The diagnosis of occupational illness is often one of exclusion.
- Useful types of case reports include a new disease or condition, a new association between disease and stressor, and an unexpected development in a disease associated with an exposure, unusual circumstance of exposure, or new data to clarify pathophysiology.
- A typical format for case presentation is as follows: introduction, description of case, other considerations, and discussion.

QUESTIONS

1. *You are seeing a patient who has some health concerns that are attributed to work. In obtaining the occupational history, which of the following items of information is generally **least** helpful?*

A. Relationship of symptoms to periods away from work
B. Direct communication with the patient's attorney
C. Description of other activities such as hobbies
D. Description of past work history
E. Inquiring about job satisfaction

2. *Which of the following resources is most accurately paired with the type of information available from the resource?*

A. Agency for Toxic Substances and Disease Registry (ATSDR) Case Series in Environmental Medicine/Description of a case followed by overview of key considerations
B. A regional office of National Institute for Occupational Safety and Health (NIOSH)/How to distinguish different causes of chest pain
C. The manufacturer of the chemical/Search of medical literature

D. Computerized databases such as MEDLINE and TOXLINE/Chemical formulations and toxicity of particular products used in industry
E. MSDS/Potential health effects of combined exposures

3. *You are evaluating a young man complaining about inability to conceive a child with his wife. The workup reveals a low sperm count. Occupational factors most likely to contribute to this condition would be*

A. Work in asbestos abatement
B. Supervising vinyl chloride polymerization process
C. Exposure to the nematocide dibromochloropropane
D. Manufacture of ion exchange resins
E. Removing old paint with solvents

4. *Each of the following could be presented as a case report in the field of occupational medicine* **except**

A. Unique occupational illness
B. Previously unrecognized effect of a chemical material
C. Unexpected course of an occupational illness
D. Description of the biochemical pathways of a chemical substance
E. Unusual occurrence of exposure

Occupational Ophthalmology

OBJECTIVES

- Identify the causes of "red eye"
- Discuss the occupational physician's approach to the evaluation of eye complaints
- List methods of analysis of visual requirements for jobs
- Describe materials that cause eye injury
- Summarize preventive efforts to reduce eye complaints or injuries

OUTLINE

2. Table 34.6: Differential diagnosis of red eye
  E. Slit lamp biomicroscopy
  F. Laboratory diagnosis
 IX. Treatment
  A. Blepharitis
  B. Stye and chalazion
  C. Subconjunctival hemorrhage
  D. Foreign bodies of the cornea and conjunctiva
 X. Occupational eye infections
  A. Epidemic keratoconjunctivitis
  B. Blood-borne pathogens
 XI. Screening for eye disorders in the workplace
  A. How to evaluate vision for various jobs
  B. Visual standards
   1. Observational methods
   2. Statistical methods
  C. Table 34.7: Visual job family: clerical and administrative profile
  D. Table 34.8: Visual job family: inspection and close machine work profile
  E. Table 34.9: Visual job family: operator of mobile equipment profile
  F. Table 34.10: Visual job family: machines operators profile
  G. Table 34.11: Visual job family: laborers profile
  H. Table 34.12: Visual job family: mechanics and skilled tradesmen profile
 XII. Environmental surveillance programs
 XIII. Americans with Disabilities Act issues: performance of essential functions with or without accommodation
 XIV. The role of ergonomics
 XV. Prevention and control
  A. Preventive strategies and tactics
  B. Beyond prevention: promotion
 XVI. General requirements for personal protective equipment (PPE)
  A. Static shielding of equipment
  B. Static shielding of personnel
 XVII. Contact lenses at work
 XVIII. Developing a PPE program
  A. Hazard assessment guidelines
   1. Dusts, powders, and fumes
   2. Flying objects or particles
   3. Injurious gases, vapors, and liquids
   4. Splashing metal
   5. Thermal and radiation hazards
   6. Lasers
   7. Electrical hazards
  B. Identification of personal eye and face protection equipment
  C. Efficacy
  D. Types of hazards versus PPE
 XIX. Special purposes lenses
  A. General
  B. Photochromic lenses
  C. Limitations

KEY POINTS

- An estimated 2.4 million people suffer eye injuries each year, and between 40,000 and 60,000 of these injuries are associated with severe vision loss. Millions more visit physicians in emergency rooms or clinics each year for less serious acute eye conditions, such as a nonpurulent conjunctivitis.
- The physician's most important responsibility is to distinguish between vision-threatening conditions and those that are minor. Serious disorders require early recognition and prompt referral to an ophthalmologist for ideal management.
- Work-related eye complaints can be safely and effectively handled by occupational or primary care providers in the absence of "red flags," which are defined as signs or symptoms of a potentially serious condition indicating a need for further consultation, support, or specialized treatment.
- The specific work activity may provide clues about the extent of damage. Hammering or welding activities, for example, may suggest a penetrating wound to the globe.
- If chemical exposure was involved, all available information should be obtained, including the identification of the chemical and consideration of caustic effects. Material Safety Data Sheets may be of great assistance.
- A systematic approach to the examination of the eye should be used, beginning with the inspection of the face, orbital area, and lids and ending with a close view of the eyeball. The preferred method for examination of the eyeball includes the use of the slit lamp biomicroscope and the ophthalmoscope.
- A new standardized classification of ocular trauma (i.e., BETT) has been endorsed by numerous organizations and is reasonably expected to become the international descriptor of ocular trauma.
- *Red eye* refers to hyperemia of the superficially visible vessels of the conjunctiva, episclera, or sclera that can be caused by disorders of these structures or of adjoining structures, including the cornea, iris, ciliary body, and ocular adnexa.
- The patient's complaints may reveal the cause of the red eye. A *scratchy or burning sensation* suggests lid, conjunctival, or corneal disorders, including foreign bodies, in-turning eyelashes, and dry eyes. *Localized lid pain* or tenderness is a common presenting complaint of a stye or an acute chalazion of the lid. *Deep, intense aching pain* is not localized but may reflect corneal abrasions, iritis, keratitis, ulcer, iridocyclitis, or acute glaucoma, as well as sinusitis or tension headaches. *A halo effect* around lights is commonly reported in acute glaucoma. *Blurred vision* often indicates serious ocular disease. *Photophobia* is an abnormal sensitivity to light. *Exudation* is a typical result of conjunctival or eyelid inflammation and does not occur with iridocyclitis or glaucoma. A *corneal ulcer* is a serious condition that may or may not be accompanied by an exudate. *Itching* is a nonspecific symptom but usually indicates allergic conjunctivitis. Acute onset of spots, floaters, or flashes of light or a *curtain drawn across the eye* suggests retinal detachment.
- *Conjunctivitis* is manifested by hyperemia of the conjunctival blood vessels; the cause may be bacterial, viral, allergic, or irritative; the condition is common and often not

serious. *Scleritis* is an inflammation (localized or diffuse) of the sclera. It is uncommon, often protracted, and is usually accompanied by pain. It may indicate serious systemic disease such as a collagen-vascular disorder that is potentially serious to the eye. *Subconjunctival hemorrhage* is an accumulation of blood in the potential space between the conjunctiva and the sclera and is rarely serious. A *pterygium* is an abnormal growth consisting of a triangular fold of tissue that advances progressively over the cornea, usually from the nasal side. *Herpes simplex keratitis* is an inflammation of the cornea caused by a virus, which is a common, potentially serious problem that can lead to corneal ulceration.

- *Reduced visual* acuity suggests serious ocular disease, such as an inflamed cornea, iridocyclitis, or glaucoma. *Corneal opacification* in a patient with a red eye always denotes disease. These opacities may be detected by direct illumination with a penlight, or they may be seen with a direct ophthalmoscope outlined against the red fundus reflex. *Corneal epithelial disruption* occurs in corneal inflammations and trauma. It can be detected with topical application of fluorescein to the eye. Areas denuded of epithelium stain a bright green with a blue filter. *A pupillary abnormality* may be noted in an eye with iridocyclitis. Typically, the affected pupil is somewhat smaller than that of the other eye due to reflex spasm of the iris sphincter muscle.
- Inspection of the *anterior chamber* in terms of its depth and the contents of the anterior chamber is extremely important. With narrow angle glaucoma, the edema of the cornea is associated with an *iris bombe*, in which the anterior surface of the iris almost touches the cornea and the anterior chamber is extremely shallow. An ancillary finding in these cases is an increase in intraocular pressure averaging 40 to 60 Hg. The content of the anterior chamber is significant. In cases of a uveitis (e.g., purulent cyclitis), the presence of protein and cells in the anterior chamber is classic, and a *hypopyon* may be present. A *hyphema* is an accumulation of red blood cells caused by trauma to the anterior chamber. *Shallow anterior chamber depth* in a red eye (especially related to acute ocular pain, nausea, and sometimes vomiting) should always suggest acute angle-closure glaucoma.
- *Proptosis*, a forward displacement of the globe, suggests serious trauma, orbital infection, or tumor when it is of sudden onset. The most common cause of chronic proptosis is thyroid disease. Acute orbital proptosis caused by trauma is an ophthalmologic emergency because it causes severe pressure on the eyeball with markedly elevated intraocular pressure, which can lead to central retinal artery occlusion. Pressure must be relieved within 10 minutes, or the patient may have no light perception because of the lack of blood supply through the central retinal artery.
- *Discharge* may be an important clue to the cause of conjunctivitis. Preauricular node enlargement can be a prominent feature of some unusual varieties of chronic granulomatous conjunctivitis, known collectively as Parinaud's virus oculoglandular syndrome and conjunctivitis.
- The red eye can be generally categorized in four classes: conjunctivitis, iritis, keratitis (i.e., corneal inflammation or foreign body), and acute glaucoma. The changes in vision, type of discharge, presence or absence of pain, pupillary size, presence of conjunctival injection, pupillary response to light, intraocular pressure, appearance of the cornea, and the anterior chamber depth assist in the determination of the diagnosis.
- The slit lamp examination is a standard of practice when examining the eye. The use of the slit lamp biomicroscope has been established as a competency for occupational health physicians by the American College of Occupational and Environmental Medicine (ACOEM).

- Conditions that require no treatment or may be appropriately treated by most occupational physicians include blepharitis, stye and chalazion, subconjunctival hemorrhage, conjunctivitis, and superficial corneal and conjunctival foreign body. Cases requiring prolonged treatment or those in which the expected response to treatment does not occur promptly should be referred to an ophthalmologist.
- *Blepharitis*, or inflammation of the eyelid, responds slowly to treatment, and relapses are common. The mainstays of treatment include eradication of staphylococcal infection with frequent applications of appropriate ophthalmic antibiotics, treatment of scalp seborrhea with antidandruff shampoos, and cleansing of the lids to alleviate seborrheic blepharitis.
- A *stye, or hordeolum*, is an acute inflammation of the eyelid that may be characterized as an external swelling. An external hordeolum occurs on the surface of the skin at the edge of the lid. An internal hordeolum manifests on the conjunctival surface of the lid. A *chalazion* is a chronic granulomatous inflammation of a meibomian or hair follicle gland. Styes are initially treated with hot compresses and topical antibiotics. Because most chalazia are sterile, antibiotic therapy is of no value, but hot compresses may be useful for early lesions.
- *Subconjunctival hemorrhage* in the absence of blunt trauma requires no treatment and, unless recurrent, no evaluation. Causes include a sudden increase in ocular venous pressure, such as occurs with coughing, sneezing, vomiting, or vigorous rubbing of the eye. Many subconjunctival hemorrhages occur during sleep.
- *Bacterial conjunctivitis* is treated with frequent antibiotic eye drops and antibiotic ointment applied at bedtime. There is no specific medicinal treatment for viral conjunctivitis. Corticosteroids have no place in the treatment of infectious conjunctivitis. Eye drops containing a combination of antibiotics and corticosteroids are seldom indicated for the treatment of ocular inflammation and should be prescribed only by the ophthalmologist.
- *Foreign bodies* of the cornea or conjunctiva are best removed using a slit lamp. An attempt should be made to remove the object with wet (sterile saline) cotton swab, and if unsatisfactory, the physician can use a tuberculosis syringe and a 25-gauge needle or "eye spud." If unable to remove the object, the patient should be referred to an ophthalmologist. If treatment is satisfactory, a broad-spectrum ophthalmic antibiotic should be applied.
- *Epidemic keratoconjunctivitis* is common in the Far East. The disease periodically affects a considerable portion of workers. Outbreaks appear from time to time in hospitals, families, and ophthalmologic clinics, perhaps because of the use of unsterilized equipment or by finger-to-eye transmission. *Blood-borne pathogens* may be acquired if the eye, other mucous membranes, or nonintact skin is exposed to blood or other potentially infectious materials. A contaminated instrument may transmit the virus.
- Visual skills are one of the most universal and frequent factors affecting job performance. Visual standards are established by observational methods that outline types of testing to be used and levels of performance required for specific jobs based on direct and expert observation of the task or by statistical methods evaluating facts that determine which tests and what minimum levels of test performance most adequately identify the worker who is potentially better on a specific job.
- Analysis of workplace visual requirements requires a broad knowledge of visual abilities and limitations (e.g., problems of accommodation, convergence, presbyopia, coordination, muscle balance); lighting; physical factors; and the host of eye hazards of a particular operation. The visual survey is best accomplished as a cooperative venture

between the occupational physician, a consulting eye specialist, and plant management representatives.

- Visual job "families" were developed on statistical basis after large numbers of employees, assigned to diverse jobs and exhibiting all degrees of ability and achievement, were tested and classified on the basis of job success into categories that ranged from "definitely superior" to "definitely inferior." Visual demands for most industrial jobs fall into one of six job families.

- Graduated visual stimuli should be employed to allow quantitative determination of acuity (e.g., Snellen chart). Screening tests may also determine contrast sensitivity, ocular alignment, color vision, and visual fields. Common methods of ocular (vision) testing include the use of test batteries.

- The significance of any test depends on job requirements. Individual correlation is necessary. Careful diagnostic appraisal of near vision (e.g., near point acuity, near point accommodation, near point of convergence, lateral and vertical phorias) is important for job applicants requiring exact visual perception when working at distances of 16 inches or less. This is especially true for employees older than 40 years of age. In some jobs, speed of vision and recovery from glare may be important.

- Eye complaints occur in 50% to 90% of workers who use video display terminals (VDTs). Such problems result from visual inefficiencies or from eye-related symptoms caused by a combination of individual visual abnormalities and poor visual ergonomics. Visual symptoms can usually be resolved with ergonomic modification and the provision of appropriate visual care to the worker.

- The primary prevention of work-related disorders depends on the reduction or elimination of exposure to causal factors. Emphasis has been placed on physical risk factors (e.g., lighting, terminal design, posture), but other issues, such as workers' job satisfaction and interpersonal relations with supervisors, have a strong relationship to visual and ergonomic complaints. Secondary prevention involves a partnership with the worker, including two-way communication, exploration of myths and misconceptions, management of expectations, bilateral or trilateral planning, and management of the episode or situation. Tertiary prevention efforts require evaluation of job tasks and the person-job fit.

- Occupational Safety and Health Administration (OSHA) 29 CFR 1910.132 has listed general requirements for PPE. The use of PPE should not substitute for engineering out hazards or for work practice or administrative controls. *Static shielding of equipment*, such as barrier or deflector screens of transparent plastics, can provide a clear view of a work process while protecting workers from grinding fragments, accidental sprays, or specific optical irradiations. Booths that protect against heat and accidental splashes can provide *static shielding of personnel*. Static shielding may be suspended from the ceiling, mounted on the floor, or constructed as a separate control area.

- Individuals should not be disqualified from a job because of contact lens use. Such lenses may be used under a full-face respirator.

- To assess the need for eye and face protective equipment, the practitioner should conduct a walkthrough survey of the area to identify sources of hazards to the eyes and faces of workers. General hygiene and compliance with rules about the use of PPE, such as safety glasses, can be noted. The OSHA log can give valuable information about eye injury patterns. Safety equipment, such as eye wash booths, can be inspected.

- Appropriate protective equipment for the eye and face is required by OSHA (29 CFR 1910.133). Eye and face protection is required where there is reasonable probability of preventing injury with such equipment. Other standards (ANSI Z136.1 and Z136.3) address the prevention of laser burns using similar engineering controls or personal protective goggles.

- A 1980 Bureau of Labor Statistics Study found that about 60% of workers who suffered eye injuries were not wearing eye protective equipment. When asked why they were not wearing face protection at the time of the accident, workers indicated that face protection was not normally used for practice in their type of work or was not required for the type of work performed at the time of the accident.
- Selection of safety glasses is especially critical for individuals with a loss of accommodation (i.e., presbyopia) or for those who must use contact lenses in the workplace. A presbyopic lens should provide for the lack of accommodation so the user can perform visual tasks efficiently and effectively.

QUESTIONS

1. *Which of the following statements is most correct regarding eye injury?*

A. The physician's most important responsibility is to distinguish between vision threatening conditions and those that are minor.
B. Work-related eye complaints should always be seen by an ophthalmologist.
C. BETT has been rejected by most organizations.
D. The specific work activity may provide clues about the extent of damage. Hammering or welding activities, for example, may lead to bacterial conjunctivitis.

2. *Which of the following symptoms is most suggestive of eyelid, conjunctival, or corneal disorder?*

A. Sudden curtain drawn across the eye
B. Halo effect around lights
C. Scratchy or burning sensation
D. Blurred vision

3. *Which of the following conditions is associated with uveitis (i.e., purulent cyclitis)?*

A. An *iris bombe*
B. Hypopyon
C. Hyphema
D. Pterygium

4. *Which of the following treatments for blepharitis is **least likely** to be indicated?*

A. Frequent applications of ophthalmic antibiotics
B. Corticosteroid eye drops
C. Treatment of scalp seborrhea with antidandruff shampoos
D. Cleansing of the lids

5. *Which of the following statements is **incorrect** regarding visual standards?*

A. Visual standards are typically established by observational methods or statistical methods
B. Analysis of workplace visual requirements requires a broad knowledge of visual abilities and limitations.

C. The visual survey is best accomplished plant management.

D. Visual job families were developed on statistical basis after large numbers of employees assigned to diverse jobs were tested and classified on the basis of job success.

6. *Which of the following statements regarding VDTs is **incorrect**?*

A. Eye complaints occur in 50% to 90% of workers who use them.

B. Problems result from visual inefficiencies or from eye-related symptoms caused by a combination of individual visual abnormalities and poor visual ergonomics.

C. Visual symptoms can rarely be resolved with ergonomic modification.

D. Workers' job satisfaction and interpersonal relations with supervisors have a strong relationship to ergonomic complaints.

7. *Which of the following statements regarding eye protective equipment is **incorrect**?*

A. About 60% of workers who suffered eye injuries were not wearing eye protective equipment.

B. PPE should not be used as a substitute for engineering out hazards or for work practice or administrative controls.

C. Static shielding of equipment, such as barrier or deflector screens of transparent plastics, can provide a clear view of a work process while protecting workers

D. Individuals who have to use contact lenses must be disqualified from a job if they must wear a full-face respirator.

Not needed

35

Use of Molecular Genetics in Occupational Medicine

OBJECTIVES

- Understand the principles, methods, and terminology of molecular genetics
- Explain uses of the polymerase chain reaction (PCR)
- Describe other molecular genetic assays used to evaluate potential susceptibility, risk, or damage in workers
- Discuss the basis for molecular genetic assays and their clinical application
- Explain the ethical, legal, and social implications related to the use of genetic testing in the workplace

OUTLINE

I. Introduction
  A. Figure 35.1: Biomarker of exposure and effect
  B. Table 35.1: Clinical applications of genetic tests in occupational medicine
II. Background
III. Molecular genetic assays
  A. Table 35.2: Selected examples of molecular genetic assays
  B. PCR amplification
  C. Applications using PCR
    1. Restriction enzymes for genetic mutations and polymorphisms
    2. Genotyping
    3. DNA sequencing
  D. Carcinogen-DNA adduct detection
  E. Cytogenetic assays
  F. Microarray technology
IV. Clinical applications of genetic testing-selected applications
V. Implications for genetic testing in the workplace

KEY POINTS

- The genetic basis for disease and disease risk is the focus of many research laboratories. It is expected to have wide-ranging clinical importance as it is introduced into the workplace. The lessons learned through molecular genetics will impact medical decision-making, worker protection, risk assessment processes, and other areas of occupational medicine practice.

- Genetic biomarkers are being developed that reflect a spectrum of effects, from internal exposure to disease and prognosis. The ethical, legal, and social implications of genetic testing are profound, with significant efforts being made to ensure the proper uses of such testing. Many potential problems are only now being elucidated.
- Genetic biomarkers may allow the physician to predict which workers are at risk for specific diseases (e.g., polymorphism); to identify those who need additional workplace protection; and to suggest maximal allowable exposures, ethical, legal, and social issues notwithstanding.
- Genetic biomarkers may also be used to find an occupational cause for a disease in an individual worker or to provide prognostic information. The primary goal for biomarkers, however, is to prevent disease and secondarily to allow the early detection of disease.
- Molecular genetics is the study of genes and gene structure. There are more than 100,000 human genes located on 46 chromosomes. An important property of DNA is that it is double-stranded and that these strands bind to complementary copies of each other. The genetic language that codes for the amino acid sequence in proteins is organized in triplets called codons. Exons are parts of genes that are transcribed; introns are parts that are not.
- Diversity in cellular functions and characteristics are controlled through variations in gene sequences. Any variation that occurs in more than 1% of the population is considered a polymorphism. It is estimated that genetic polymorphisms occur in approximately every 500 bases.
- Diseases in every organ and body system may be caused by genetic dysfunction due to point mutations, gene deletions, or gross chromosomal aberrations. Mutations and hypermethylation in genes may result in a decrease in necessary protein production or altered gene transcription that can lead to a variety of diseases, including cancer, hormonal disturbances, and rheumatologic problems.
- Exogenous exposures, such as to viruses and chemicals, may cause mutations and hypermethylation in genes. Genetic dysfunction can also be acquired through endogenous mutational mechanisms, such as oxidative damage by chemicals released from neutrophils, errors during cell replication, and others. Endogenous mutations are estimated to occur millions of times each day in any one person but are efficiently repaired by the body.
- Several recently developed genetic tests can (a) detect mutations, (b) determine susceptibilities through genetic polymorphism detection, (c) detect carcinogens bound to DNA, and (d) measure abnormal or altered gene products. Many of these techniques are based on the PCR, a technique for the amplification of DNA or RNA. The detection of mutations or polymorphisms, along with genotyping and DNA sequences, can all be conducted using PCR techniques. Other molecular genetic assays include DNA adduct detection, cytogenetic assays, and the detection of DNA damage by observations of micronuclei.
- The newest genetic assays use microarray technology. These methods begin with PCR, followed by enzymatic fragmentation of the PCR product and fluorescent labeling. The labeled product is hybridized to a microarray chip. The fragmented PCR products that have the identical sequence to the permanently bound sequence bind to the chip. The chip is then scanned with a fluorescent reader, which informs the investigator about the amount of binding and, hence, the amount of labeled product. These technologies, because of the large amount of information that can be obtained, pose formidable data handling and bioinformatics issues.
- The use of genetic assays for polymorphisms in individuals and populations offers the physician an opportunity to assess individual worker's risk to chronic diseases. For

example, the assessment of α_1-antitrypsin phenotype can be useful in the evaluation of premature emphysema. The assessment of acetylator phenotype and its impact on the detoxification of aromatic amines and bladder cancer has been well documented.

- Studies have shown that DNA "fingerprints" can be developed that may help identify individuals at high risk to cancer after exposure to xenobiotic agents.
- Many of the genetic assays are still in the research phase but are emerging for consideration and use by the occupational health physician.
- The ethical, legal, and social implications for the use of genetic assays have stimulated much debate. Employers and medical providers are required to avoid discriminatory practices, as addressed in part by the Americans with Disabilities Act. Other forms of discrimination, such as can occur in the insurance industry, remain to be adequately addressed.
- The use of genetic testing for evaluation of disease risk, diagnosis, and prognosis will be incorporated into many parts of our lives. The prevalence of genetic disease is not increasing, in contrast to diseases caused by infectious agents. Genetic testing should not have a negative economic impact on society. There may be a reduction in the cost of health care and a positive influence on the workforce if preventable genetic diseases are appropriately addressed.

QUESTIONS

1. A polymorphism is defined as an inheritable trait that occurs in at least what percentage of the population?

A. 1%
B. 5%
C. 10%
D. 50%

*2. PCR can be used in all of the following applications **except***

A. Identify gene mutations
B. Detect carcinogen-DNA adducts
C. Conduct genotyping
D. Perform DNA sequencing

3. Microarray technology coupled with PCR can be used for

A. DNA nucleotide sequence detection
B. Assessment of cellular damage from xenobiotic exposure
C. Assessment of phenotypes for polymorphic enzymes
D. Detection of alternations in microtubules after exposure to cadmium

*4. Clinical applications of genetic testing should include all of the following **except***

A. Prediction of susceptibility to premature emphysema by assessment of the polymorphic enzyme, $\alpha_1$antitrypsin.
B. Prediction of susceptibility for bladder cancer by assessment of the polymorphic enzyme *N*-acetyltransferase
C. Assessment of genetic profile to determine suitability for employment
D. Development of DNA fingerprinting to help understand the cause of cancer

=36=

The Human Genome Project and Occupational Medicine Practice

OBJECTIVES

- Understand the history and accomplishments of the Human Genome Project (HGP)
- Review emerging technologies related to molecular genetics
- Identify the clinical applications of these new technologies
- Recognize the potential impact of the HGP on the practice of occupational medicine

OUTLINE

   I. Introduction
  II. Background of the HGP
 III. History of the HGP
 IV. Recent findings of the HGP
  V. New genomic technologies and the status of the HGP
     A. DNA microarrays
     B. Expression profiles
     C. Protein arrays
     D. Informatics
 VI. Clinical medicine and the potential impact of the HGP
     A. Primary screening
     B. Genomic surveillance in primary care medicine
     C. Diagnosis, prognosis, and pharmacogenetics
 VII. Occupational medicine and the impact of the HGP
     A. Preemployment screening
     B. Genomic surveillance and occupational medicine monitoring
     C. The HGP and the diagnosis and treatment of occupational diseases
VIII. The HGP and occupational epidemiology
 IX. The HGP and ethical, legal, and social issues in the workplace
  X. The HGP and implications for the future

KEY POINTS

- The HGP has published a nearly complete, validated, publicly accessible sequence of the human genome, and it has produced complete genomic sequences of a number of nonhuman species (with enormous research value), a rapidly expanding library of human polymorphisms, and new technologies that will carry genetics and medicine into new frontiers.

- The HGP is built on previous landmark discoveries such as the structure of DNA, concepts and details of RNA transcription from DNA templates, protein translation from messenger RNA templates, and the recombinant DNA molecule. Later, sequencing efforts were propelled by dideoxy chain termination, restriction endonuclease digestion, and mapping techniques. Automation of DNA sequencing techniques and the development of polymerase chain reaction accelerated the ability to identify, replicate, and sequence substantial lengths of DNA.

- The first Five-Year Plan of the HGP, published in 1990, included the following goals: developing preliminary genetic maps of the human genome, developing physical maps of the chromosomes, mapping and fully sequencing simple laboratory organisms, investing in sequencing technologies, and proactively researching potential ethical, legal, and social issues expected to arise from the project.

- By the year 2000, two groups announced working drafts of the human genome. The total number of human genes appears to be only about 30,000, which is one third of that previously estimated. The average human gene is 3,000 base pairs long but may range to more than 2 million base pairs. Humans apparently generate most translation products through "alternative splicing" of mRNA, so that the number of protein products actually is in the range of 100,000. Function is currently known for only one half of the human genes that have been sequenced.

- Existing research strategies, such as gene amplification, DNA sequencing, probing for specific sequences with blot techniques, investigation of nonhuman homologs of human genes, and elucidation of DNA adduct formation and repair, will continue to be used to explore the human genome.

- New research technologies for humans and nonhuman species are fueling *genetic research* (i.e., elucidation of the structure, control, and products of individual genes) and *functional genomic research* (i.e., study of gene function in the context of the other genes, gene products, and regulatory processes that affect expression and variation).

- DNA microarrays (i.e., DNA "chips") are fields of single-stranded DNA that may comprise tens or hundreds of thousands of oligonucleotides or cDNA strands. The chips are small wafers, usually glass, and the DNA fragments bound to them can be "downloaded" in arrays based on known sequence, so that each tethered DNA probe sits in a defined location. This array is then bathed in a solution of the labeled nucleic acid mixture that is to be probed.

- The nucleic acids being assayed can be derived from diverse sources, such as a clone of tumor cells, an uncharacterized infectious pathogen, or the blood of a patient seeking information on inherited disease susceptibility. The nucleic acid fragments in solution are labeled with fluorescent or radioactive tags that can be read by standardized instruments after washout of nonhybridized material. The location of the labeled sequences on the microarray after hybridization identifies gene fragments or transcripts as homologous to known probes.

- DNA microarrays can qualitatively identify specific sequences. More than 2 million single nucleotide polymorphisms (SNPs) have been mapped across the human genome. Most genetic variation in humans appears to be caused by SNPs, and many are probably associated with specific diseases. Microarrays can rapidly identify individual SNPs or other structural alleles known to cause inherited illnesses (e.g., sickle cell disease, cystic fibrosis).

- DNA microarrays are ideally suited for identifying multiple target sequences or patterns of genes. They can also identify markers known to increase the risk of diseases of multigene origin (e.g., diabetes, certain malignancies, coronary artery disease, Alzheimer's disease) and be used for rapid identification of pathogens, screening for drug-resistance plasmids, and identification of clones of tumor markers associated with differential responses to chemotherapy agents.
- Expression profiles (i.e., quantitative measurements of mRNAs or cDNA copies of mRNAs from tissue samples) can be performed with this technology, allowing an understanding of regulatory pathways and functional genomics. The levels and pattern of mRNA production for specific genes and gene groups give a snapshot of cellular function at a single point in time. Such levels and patterns can be followed sequentially to study developmental and disease states.
- Expression profiles can also be used to study drug responses or the effects of lifestyle interventions at the level of the genome in different individuals or populations.
- Protein arrays or protein "chips" consisting of defined arrays of antibodies embedded in small surfaces can be used to probe for protein products (just as DNA arrays can be used to probe for oligonucleotides, mRNAs, or cDNAs). Proteins reflect the regulation and transcription of mRNAs, but they may be even more diverse and potentially easier to study. Protein arrays could be used to look for multiple protein products, coexpressed protein products, and protein synthesis responses to drugs, toxins, or diseases.
- The exponentially proliferating data on gene sequences, products, functions, and regulation pose a huge bioinformational challenge. The HGP leadership has committed to immediate public access to data, although privately generated data may be restricted to various degrees. Clinicians, as well as researchers, will have stay continuously educated regarding the basic science; clinical applications; and ethical, legal, and social issues of the HGP.
- Numerous human diseases have Mendelian inheritance consistent with single-gene etiologies. Most of these are relatively rare, and many might have conveyed a selective advantage to heterozygotes (e.g., thalassemias, cystic fibrosis, spinal muscular atrophy, muscular dystrophy, sickle cell anemia, retinoblastoma, hemochromatosis, phenylketonuria). Prenatal and neonatal genetic screening for gene carriage is routinely available for screening and diagnosis of these conditions. More common, adult-onset conditions (e.g., diabetes, hypertension, vascular disease, emphysema, allergy) that have more complex polygenic causes are beginning to be amenable to genomic testing.
- Most adult diseases are the result of complex interactions between lifetime environmental exposures and genes or gene combinations that confer an increased risk. Genomic screening is being studied for many diseases with such complex causes (e.g., early-onset Alzheimer's disease, some breast cancers, nonmelanoma skin cancers, lung cancer, diabetes).
- Screening for *gene products*, as with lipid profiles or HLA screening, is already used for many common adult-onset diseases. The ability to screen patients directly for genes that convey increased risk for these diseases will give clinicians and their patients the earliest opportunities to intervene with treatment such as dietary change, lifestyle modification, and drug therapy. Patients or populations with genomic risk for specific diseases may also benefit from increased surveillance to allow early diagnosis and treatment.
- Tests resulting from HGP efforts may also enable clinicians to monitor for genomic changes that indicate early disease in patients or populations at risk to facilitate sec-

ondary prevention (e.g., early detection of colon cancer, lung cancer, mutation loads due to environmental carcinogens). DNA microarray technology will likely increase the sensitivity of surveillance.

- Some of the most widely used genomic tests are those used to characterize malignancies with respect to expression profiles that define specific diagnoses even in atypical presentations and identify tumors with good or poor prognoses.
- Expression profiling (i.e., fingerprinting) can also identify patients who will benefit most from specific therapies or who will be most at risk for adverse drug reactions from specific therapies. This new field is called *pharmacogenetics*, and it will likely dominate drug development and drug response monitoring in coming decades.
- Occupational medicine practice includes (a) screening for susceptibility to occupational injury and illness, (b) surveillance or monitoring for exposure, (c) designing and implementing interventions to minimize hazardous exposures, (d) early diagnosis of occupational syndromes, and (e) treatment of occupational illnesses. All of these are likely to expand as a result of genomic testing and pharmacogenetics evolution.
- Employers provide most health insurance in the United States. They have an interest in identifying genetic risk factors for disease and injury. The employer may hope to decrease costs by encouraging risk-reduction interventions or by excluding high-risk persons from insurance or even employment.
- Preemployment health screening has been recommended for many years to improve workers' health, to decrease their risk of chronic disease, and to decrease employer costs. The range, sophistication, and predictive value of genetic and genomic testing for the workplace will increase in the future.
- Occupational medicine physicians will need to maintain up-to-date knowledge of (a) the biologic bases of these tests, (b) whether the tests have actually been linked to susceptibility phenotypes, (c) whether workplace screening is likely to decrease adverse medical outcomes, and (d) whether and which interventions are available to protect susceptible workers.
- The HGP is likely have its greatest immediate impact on primary care by genomic testing (i.e., multigenic profiling and expression profiling) to identify risks for common polygenic diseases such as coronary artery disease, diabetes, and hypertension.
- It is likely to have its greatest immediate impact on occupational medicine screening by testing for enhanced susceptibility for common polygenetic conditions such as occupational allergies, occupational asthma, DNA-repair deficiencies, and connective tissue variants linked to musculoskeletal injuries.
- Genetic testing can be used like other biomarkers to screen for damage from hazardous exposures before the development of symptoms or disease states. The HGP will enhance this capability by furthering our understanding of clinically relevant sequence changes and DNA adduct formation. For example, the *KRAS* oncogene mutation occurs after occupational exposure to asbestos in patients who go on to develop lung cancer. This occurs independently of asbestos-related fibrotic changes. This *KRAS* mutation could potentially serve as a surveillance tool in high-risk workers and may eventually replace radiologic surveillance.
- DNA adducts have the potential to serve as surveillance tools. They are likely to become more useful as HGP sequence and microarray data enable us to understand which adducts are most reliably linked to adverse clinical outcomes.
- The HGP will also allow researchers, and eventually clinicians, to detect expression profiles and protein profile techniques to monitor individual reactions to toxins and

perhaps infectious agents. These techniques may also allow early diagnosis of occupational malignancies (e.g., bladder cancer, lung cancer, skin cancer) and nonmalignant occupational diseases, including fibrosing lung diseases, hepatotoxicity, and allergies.

- Occupational epidemiology can now address molecular genetics. Discoveries resulting from the application of these new techniques and more specifically from the application of HGP discoveries will allow workers to be stratified into risk groups based on their genomic makeup and the hazards to which they are exposed. Tests will allow the identification of genetic traits that may be associated with increased susceptibility to toxic exposures.

- In 2000, the National Institute of Environmental Health Sciences (NIEHS) launched an Environmental Genome Project focused on common sequence variations in environmental-response genes. Certain genetic polymorphisms affect drug and xenobiotic metabolism and have important implications for human health. Knowledge about these relationships is important to understand disease causation and to allow effective disease prevention strategies.

- Optimal use of HGP data in occupational medicine research and practice will require links between genomic information, exposure history, and outcome. Defining exposures and outcomes for a study population has always been problematic in occupational epidemiology. Diverse confounding exposures and multiple sources of potential bias complicate histories. Outcomes (e.g., absences, decreased productivity, exacerbation of preexisting diseases, injuries and illnesses to self or others) may be difficult to quantitate.

- Potential exists for abuse of genomic technology, especially for workers. Genetic information may result in denial of employment or insurance because of genetic susceptibility to an occupational agent. Worker selection and job placement could supplant protective environmental controls and stricter standards for permissible exposure limits.

- Workers may decline genetic testing for fear of employment discrimination, loss of primary medical insurance, and lack of privacy in the workplace. Legislative and regulatory strategies are needed to address these concerns, particularly when health insurance and employment are intertwined.

- The Americans with Disabilities Act (ADA) and Health Insurance Portability and Accountability Act (HIPAA) of 1996 offer limited protection from discrimination but do not prohibit employers and insurers from gaining access to genetic information. HIPPA provides that genetic information should not be used as a "preexisting condition" in absence of medical diagnoses of the conditions related to such information.

- The ADA potentially offers protection from discrimination. Although the ADA prevents employers from making preemployment medical inquiries, it does not prevent employers from obtaining medical information, including genetic information, after a conditional offer of employment.

- Employers can require a preplacement medical examination, which may include a physical examination and blood tests (including genetic tests). There is no uniform protection against the use of, misuse of, and access to genetic information in the workplace.

- HGP research is likely to advance our understanding of disease mechanisms and lead to the availability of safer, more effective therapeutics. There will be potential for mass genetic screening with identification of workplace susceptibilities and predisposition to disease in essentially healthy people.

QUESTIONS

*1. Which of the following is **not** one of the goals of the Five-Year Plan of the HGP?*

A. Developing preliminary genetic maps of the human genome
B. Developing physical maps of the chromosomes
C. Understanding RNA transcription from DNA templates
D. Proactively researching potential ethical, legal, and social issues

*2. Which of the following is **incorrect** regarding DNA microarrays?*

A. DNA microarrays (i.e., DNA chips) are fields of single-stranded DNA that may comprise tens or hundreds of thousands of oligonucleotides or cDNA strands.
B. DNA microarrays are small wafers, usually glass; DNA fragments bound to them can be downloaded in arrays based on known sequence, so that each tethered DNA probe sits in a defined location.
C. Nucleic acids being assayed may be from diverse sources (e.g., clone of tumor cells, uncharacterized infectious pathogen, blood of a patient seeking information on inherited disease susceptibility).
D. DNA microarrays are unable to identify SNPs.

3. Based on the findings of the HGP, which of the following is correct about human genome structure and function?

A. The total number of genes appears to be about 300,000
B. The human genome consists of more than 3 billion base pairs, but only 2% appears to code for proteins.
C. The average human gene contains 3 million base pairs.
D. Humans generate most translation products through alternative splicing of mRNA, so that there are millions of different protein products.

*4. Which of the following is **least** desirable as an application of the HGP?*

A. Identify markers known to increase the risk of diseases of multigene origin (e.g., diabetes, certain malignancies, coronary artery disease)
B. Screen patients directly for genes that convey increased risk for diseases
C. Identify patients who can benefit most from specific therapies or be most at risk for adverse drug reactions from specific therapies
D. Denial of employment or insurance because of genetic susceptibility to disease

5. Which of the following is correct concerning genetic testing?

A. Legislative and regulatory strategies currently and adequately address concerns about genetic testing by health insurance companies and employers.
B. The ADA and HIPAA offer protection from discrimination and prohibit employers and insurers from gaining access to genetic information.
C. HIPPA provides that genetic information should not be used as a preexisting condition in absence of diagnosis of the condition related to such information.
D. ADA prevents employers from making preemployment medical inquiries and from obtaining medical information, including genetic information, after a conditional offer of employment.

Answers to Chapters 20–36

CHAPTER 20 ANSWERS

1. The answer is A. (Ref: p. 280)

Clinicians have an important role to play in identifying potential workplace risks and possible work-related health problems in their patients. One obstacle to physicians' recognition of job-related health problems is insufficient education. A survey in 1983 showed that 50% of medical schools taught courses in occupational health, but the average curriculum time was only 4 hours. The Institute of Medicine has suggested how to foster the role and education of the primary care physician in environmental and occupational medicine, and there are now many resources available. Another impediment to the recognition of work-related illness is a lack of uniqueness in the clinical manifestations of many occupational illnesses. A long latency, or the period from initial exposure to presentation of disease, is another factor that leads to underrecognition of some occupational diseases. Despite these obstacles, physicians can enhance their recognition of occupational disease by taking a good occupational and environmental history using an organized approach.

2. The answer is C. (Ref: p. 281)

To detect cases of occupational disease, an occupational and environmental history, even if brief, should be obtained for every patient. With this in mind, the first step in the occupational and environmental history is a brief survey of all patients that may include (a) a list of current and longest held jobs and a current job description; (b) attention to the chief complaint (or diagnosis) for clues suggesting a temporal relationship to activities at work or at home; (c) a review-of-systems–type question about exposures to fumes, dusts, chemicals, loud noise, radiation, or musculoskeletal stresses; and (d) observance of the presence of other triggers that prompt further inquiry, such as a sentinel health event diagnosis, disease in an unlikely person, symptoms with unknown origins, and patient concerns about exposures.

3. The answer is E. (Ref: Fig. 20-1, p. 281)

See answer to question 2.

4. The answer is C. (Ref: p. 281)

In the case of allergic reactions, it may take months of exposure before sensitization and clinical allergy develops. Symptoms related to current exposures may initially improve on nonwork days or vacations, but prolonged exposure can lead to the persistence of symptoms beyond the workday. Exposure to occupational or environmental substances can also aggravate underlying medical conditions. Other triggers may prompt the need for further inquiry, such as the presence of a "sentinel health event (occupational)" diagnosis; a disease, disability, or untimely death that is occupationally related and whose occurrence may provide the impetus for evaluations (e.g., epidemiologic studies, industrial hygiene evaluations); and interventions to prevent future cases.

5. The answer is E. (Ref: p. 282)

See answer to question 4.

6. The answer is B. (Ref: p. 281)

Something elicited in the occupational and environmental history survey questions may raise the practitioner's suspicion that the patient's condition is related to an environmental or work exposure, prompting further questioning and gathering of information about work and home exposures. This may require a detailed evaluation of the work history regarding jobs held, places of employment, and description of operations performed and including (a) an inquiry about illnesses in other workers on relevant jobs; (b) content, type, and manner of handling substances; (c) personal protective equipment used; and (d) mode of entry (e.g., ingestion, inhalation, skin absorption). To obtain this information, the practitioner can ask the worker or manufacturer for the Material Safety Data Sheets (MSDS) that usually list the product's ingredients, physical properties, and some environmental protection information. It is frequently useful to obtain and review any industrial hygiene or air quality evaluations that may have already been performed.

7. The answer is E. (Ref: p. 290)

The routine survey questions may suggest that the symptoms are related to hazardous materials or conditions in the home. Possible sources of hazards in the home environment include internal sources, such as use of household chemicals and pesticides; performance of certain hobbies; presence of biologic contamination; faulty heating system; water and food contamination; and transport of toxic dust or chemicals into the home on work clothes.

8. The answer is D. (Ref: p. 291)

After potential exposures have been identified, the next question is whether exposure has actually occurred and, if so, to what degree. Documenting and quantifying exposures can involve performing biologic monitoring tests of the affected person, as well as evaluating the work or environmental site. Within the office setting, the patient can be tested for evidence of exposure in body fluids (i.e., biologic monitoring) or of adverse health effects on target organs.

The practitioner must know what agent to look for, the desirable test medium (e.g., urine, blood, hair, tissue), appropriate timing, and influences on test results. For example, blood carboxyhemoglobin, a measure of exposure to carbon monoxide, should be performed as soon as possible after exposure because the half-life of carbon monoxide in the body is approximately 4 hours when breathing room air. Urine arsenic is a good marker for recent (but not past) exposure because arsenic is excreted rapidly in the urine within a few days.

With exposure data in hand, the clinician can go on to determine if the symptoms and medical findings in the particular patient are consistent with the health effects and time course of toxicity associated with a particular hazardous exposure. In some cases, the correlation between exposure levels (in the environment or the body) and health effects is good, and in other cases, it is poor.

CHAPTER 21 ANSWERS

1. The answer is D. (Ref: p. 295)

Occupational lung disorders include pneumoconioses, asthmatic responses, irritant reactions, and hypersensitivity reactions. Paraneoplastic syndromes are not a major category of occupational lung disease.

2. The answer is E. (Ref: p. 296)

The principal sites in the respiratory tract where different agents have the greatest effect are determined by their water solubility and particle size. Highly soluble agents dissolve readily in the secretions of the eyes, upper respiratory tract (e.g., nose, pharynx), and airways; less-soluble agents exert their main effects in the peripheral small airways and in the lung parenchyma. Particles greater than 10 μm tend to settle out in the upper respiratory tract, those 3 to 10 μm settle mainly in the airways, and those less than 3 μm deposit mainly in the lung parenchyma and small airways. Irritant agents that are relatively insoluble in water produce few upper respiratory or airway symptoms and manifest more insidiously.

3. The answer is C. (Ref: pp. 309–310)

Hypersensitivity pneumonitis is not mediated by immunoglobulin E (IgE). The pathogenesis of this group of disorders is thought to involve a type IV T-lymphocyte response to inhaled antigens.

Patients with hypersensitivity pneumonitis typically present with recurring episodes of fever, cough, headache, breathlessness, and general malaise that mimic acute infectious disease. During the acute illness, the white blood cell count is elevated and generally shows a left shift; the sedimentation rate and serum immunoglobulins are also increased. With repeated acute episodes, however, there may be progression to lung fibrosis with a restrictive ventilatory defect and a decreased diffusing capacity for carbon monoxide.

The outlook for most patients with extrinsic allergic alveolitis is good if they present before lung fibrosis is extensive and if they cease being exposed to the offending agents. Corticosteroid therapy may help accelerate recovery.

4. The answer is D. (Ref: pp. 301–304)

The risk of pulmonary tuberculosis is increased in patients with silicosis, not decreased. Silicosis is the most common pneumoconiosis worldwide. Workers in mines, blasting, drilling operations, foundries, and sandblasting are at risk of silicosis. Workers in pottery, porcelain, glass, and granite cutting operations are also at risk of inhaling silica particles. Although pleural thickening may result from inhalation of asbestos particles, the term *asbestosis* refers only to interstitial lung disease.

5. The answer is E. (Ref: p. 297)

The International Labor Office (ILO) classification was developed by the World Health Organization for epidemiologic study of occupational lung disease. The standard technique that ILO-certified "B-readers" use to evaluate chest films is a semiquantitative method for determining the nature, size, and extent of radiographic opacities observed in the lung fields. Additions to the ILO criteria also allow grading of pleural shadows. An important feature of the ILO system is the provision of a standard series of graded radiographs against which a B-reader judges the degree of abnormality present. This approach can be used to classify radiographic changes at a single point in time or to quantify changes that occur over time.

The intraobserver and interobserver variability of B-readers in reading chest films has been established. When presented with the same films on separate occasions, most B-readers show high agreement in their readings at different times; greatest intraobserver variability is seen in cases of mild abnormalities, particularly with respect to pleural changes and small, irregular parenchymal densities. When the same chest radiographs are read by different B-readers, it is apparent that the experts can disagree substantially. As expected, interobserver variability is also greatest for films showing minimal parenchymal or mild pleural changes.

Although chest radiographs can demonstrate radiodense opacities in the lungs, such opacities may not indicate appreciable impairment of lung function or disability of the patient.

6. The answer is E. (Ref: pp. 306–309)

Some forms of occupational asthma share characteristics with atopic or extrinsic asthma (i.e., IgE-mediated asthma), but other forms resemble nonatopic or intrinsic asthma (i.e., independent of an IgE-mediated immune mechanism). Intrinsic asthma is mediated by activated T lymphocytes and is accompanied by increased numbers of eosinophils and metachromatic cells in the bronchial mucosa (23). In general, asthma associated with high-molecular-weight compounds often has an IgE-mediated response, but this is less common with low-molecular-weight compounds where T-cell–mediated responses may be more important.

Although many patients experience typical recurrent episodes of wheezing and breathlessness on exposure to allergens, in some, the onset of symptoms may develop more insidiously and may not be obviously work related. A sizable fraction of workers with occupational asthma experience their symptoms mainly in the evenings or at night. After exposures to some occupational causes of asthma (e.g., western red cedar, toluene diisocyanate), the recovery period may take several days or weeks. Asthma may be precipitated in some cases by minute levels of the responsible agents.

CHAPTER 22 ANSWERS

1. The answer is E. (Ref. p. 314–315)

Significant risk factors for disabling back injury include previous back injury claims; job dissatisfaction; poor ratings from supervisors; repetitive, boring tasks; younger age and shorter duration of employment; smoking; and a history of nonback injury claims.

2. The answer is D. (Ref. p. 327–328)

National Institute for Occupational Safety and Health (NIOSH) criteria for diagnosis of work-related carpal tunnel syndrome include (a) symptoms suggestive of carpal tunnel syndrome; (b) objective findings, which can include a positive Tinel's or Phalen's sign, decreased sensation in the distribution of the median nerve, or abnormal electrodiagnostic findings of the median nerve across the carpal tunnel; and (c) evidence of work-relatedness, such as frequent, repetitive, or forceful hand work on affected side, prolonged pressure over the wrist or palm, or use of vibrating tools.

3. The answer is A. (Ref. p. 316–317)

Plain films of the lumbosacral spine have not been found effective in the identification of individuals predisposed to back injury. They are of limited value in the diagnosis of acute back pain, unless there is clinical suspicion of vertebral fracture, primary or metastatic cancer, or infection (e.g., osteomyelitis).

4. The answer is E. (Ref. p. 323)

An effective program for prevention of back injuries depends on proper selection and placement of employees, appropriate job design, maintenance of health through education, and physical fitness. Back belts and education regarding lifting techniques have not been shown to be effective in preventing back injuries.

CHAPTER 23 ANSWERS

1. The answer is B. (Ref: pp. 332–333)

Most carcinogens require metabolic activation by enzymes. Some carcinogens, such as bis(chloromethyl)ether, can damage DNA directly, but most require metabolic activation by enzymes. The enzymes primarily responsible for this activation are those of the cytochrome P450 system. Others include *N*-acetyltransferase, epoxide hydrolase, and glutathione *S*-transferase. The primary function of these enzymes is to render xenobiotics more polar and therefore more readily excretable. However, their products are often reactive electrophiles, which can bond with DNA to cause adducts and result in mutations.

Some RNA viruses that code genetic sequences were found to cause malignant transformation when inserted into host genomes. The result is an oncogene.

Whether safe thresholds exist below which cancer does not occur is controversial. It is thought a single-cell mutation may lead to cancer. However, several arguments in support of thresholds have been advanced. There are known repair mechanisms that correct DNA damage, at least at low levels of exposure. Certain empiric data have been interpreted to be consistent with the existence of thresholds.

2. The answer is D. (Ref: p. 333)

Initiation is an event in which an irreversible change in the cell's genetic material occurs. Promotion consists of subsequent interactions that do not by themselves cause cancer, but push forward the process leading to cancer after initiation

3. The answer is E. (Ref: p. 334)

Latency refers to the period between onset of exposure to a carcinogen and the clinical detection of a cancer.

4. The answer is C. (Ref: pp. 335–336)

Group 2 of the International Agency for Research on Cancer (IARC) classification system includes agents that are probably (group 2A) or possibly (group 2B) carcinogenic to humans. Group 1 agents are definite human carcinogens, group 3 are agents not classified, and group 4 are agents probably not carcinogenic. The IARC has evaluated approximately 750 chemicals, industrial processes, and personal habits. More than 50 chemicals have been placed in group 1.

5. The answer is E. (Ref: pp. 336–337)

Ethylene oxide, epichlorhydrin, and styrene are all strongly suspected human occupational carcinogens (IARC group 2A).

CHAPTER 24 ANSWERS

1. The answer is C. (Ref: p. 343)

Diastolic and systolic hypertension are clearly associated with increased cardiovascular instability, with the risk increasing with the extent of blood pressure elevations. Despite its severe consequences, hypertension is often undertreated. Of the estimated 50 million Americans with hypertension, almost one third evade diagnosis, and only one fourth receive effective treatment. Among a list of widely recognized modifiable risk factors are smoking, diabetes, hypertension, hypercholesterolemia, sedentary lifestyle, obesity, and excessive salt ingestion.

2. The answer is B. (Ref: pp. 344, 347)

Physical fitness helps to reduce cardiovascular disease. Even minimal increases in physical activity improves cardiovascular fitness among sedentary people and helps reinforce indirect cardiovascular benefits such as smoking cessation, blood pressure reduction, weight loss, and reduced arrhythmias.

Although the precise amount of physical activity required to promote cardiovascular fitness is a matter of debate, sessions of 20- to 30-minute duration three times per week are routinely recommended (with the assumption that a person exercises to about 75% of one's age-predicted maximal heart rate [220 – age in years] for the exercise period).

3. The answer is E. (Ref: pp. 349–350)

Carbon monoxide can cause headaches, lightheadedness, and dizziness, as well as chest pain from myocardial ischemia. The major cardiovascular risk of solvents appears to be dysrhythmias.

Carbon disulfide, a substance used in the viscose rayon industry, has been associated with increasing the rate of atherosclerosis. Occupational exposure to nitroglycerin and other aliphatic nitrates has been associated with angina-like pain, myocardial infarction, and cardiovascular death. This manifestation is presumed to be caused by rebound coronary spasm as a result of withdrawal of nitrates.

4. The answer is B. (Ref: pp. 352–353)

The major adverse medical "prognosticators" for failure to return to work include left ventricular dysfunction and persistence of ischemia, but for most adults, the ability to resume occupational activities depends more on comorbid, social, and psychologic factors (Table 24.1). Nonmedical factors typically present the greatest impediment for people to resume occupational activities.

CHAPTER 25 ANSWERS

1. The answer is C. (Ref: pp. 360–361)

Clinical manifestations of neurologic dysfunction caused by toxic exposure generally resemble those of primary nontoxic neurologic disorders.

2. The answer is E. (Ref: p. 358)

All of these statements are true.

3. The answer is E. (Ref: p. 373)

Statements A and C are true. Lead toxicity is not characterized by parkinsonism or parkinsonian symptoms (Table 25.1). Parkinsonism is a feature of manganese and carbon disulfide toxicity. Abdominal pain and constipation are clinical features associated with acute lead poisoning.

4. The answer is C. (Ref: pp. 369 and 371)

Nerve conduction studies are used to evaluate peripheral nervous system (PNS) disturbances. Positron emission tomography (PET) scans measure the metabolism of glucose to determine areas of damaged brain tissue. A PET scan may be abnormal because of the neurotoxic effects of chemicals, whereas the computed tomography (CT) scan and electroencephalographic results may be normal.

5. The answer is E. (Ref: p. 372)

Biologic markers of exposure are indicators of alterations in cellular structure, biochemical processes, or nervous system functioning that can be measured in a biologic sample. Three types of biologic markers useful in making a diagnosis of neurotoxic illness are biologic markers of exposure, effect, and susceptibility.

TABLE 25.1. *Neurotoxic chemicals: sources of exposure and clinical features*

Neurotoxic chemical	Sources of exposure	Clinical features
Metals		
Arsenic	Pesticides, pigments, antifouling paints, electroplating industry, seafood, smelters, semiconductors	*Acute*: encephalopathy, Mee's lines, seizures, renal failure *Chronic*: peripheral neuropathy, encephalopathy, hyperkeratosis
Lead	Solder, lead and bullets, illicit whiskey, insecticides, calcium supplements, autobody industry, storage battery manufacturing and reclamation, foundries, smelters, lead-based paints, lead water pipes	*Acute*: encephalopathy, constipation, abdominal pain, porphyria *Chronic*: encephalopathy and peripheral neuropathy
Manganese	Iron, steel industry, welding rods, metal-finishing operations, fertilizers, manufacturers of fireworks, matches, manufacturers of dry cell batteries	*Acute*: mood changes, hallucinations, emotional lability *Chronic*: parkinsonism
Mercury	Scientific instruments, electrical equipment, amalgams, electroplating industry, photography, felt making	*Acute*: headache, emotional lability, nausea, respiratory tract irritation, fever, tremor, renal failure *Chronic*: ataxia, tremor, encephalopathy, social withdrawal, peripheral neuropathy, gingivitis
Tin	Canning industry, solder, electronic components, polyvinyl plastics, fungicides	*Acute*: memory defects, seizures, disorientation *Chronic*: encephalomyelopathy
Solvents		
Carbon disulfide	Manufacturers of viscose rayon, preservatives, textiles, rubber cement, varnishes, electroplating industry	*Acute*: encephalopathy *Chronic*: peripheral neuropathy, parkinsonism
n-Hexane and Methyl-*N*-butyl ketone	Paints, lacquers, varnishes, metal-cleaning compounds, quick-drying inks, paint removers, glues, adhesives	*Acute*: narcosis *Chronic*: peripheral neuropathy
Perchloroethylene	Paint removers, degreasers, oil extraction agents, dry cleaning industry, textile industry	*Acute*: narcosis *Chronic*: peripheral neuropathy, encephalopathy
Toluene	Rubber solvents, cleaning agents, glues, paints, paint thinners, lacquers, gasoline, aviation fuel	*Acute*: narcosis *Chronic*: ataxia, encephalopathy
Trichloroethylene	Degreasers, varnishes, electronics manufacturing industry, spot removers, process of caffeine extraction, dry cleaning industry	*Acute*: narcosis *Chronic*: encephalopathy, cranial (trigeminal and facial nerve) neuropathy
Insecticides		
Organophosphates	Agricultural industry, chemical manufacturing	*Acute*: cholinergic crisis *Chronic*: ataxia, paralysis, peripheral neuropathy
Carbamates	Agricultural industry, chemical manufacturing, flea powders, home gardening products (e.g., Sevin)	*Acute*: cholinergic crisis characterized by sweating, lacrimation, urinary retention *Chronic*: tremor, peripheral neuropathy

Modified from Feldman, 1999, with permission.

CHAPTER 26 ANSWERS

1. The answer is B. (Ref: p. 386)

The most critical frequency range for human audition is between 500 and 2,000 to 3,000 Hz—the range indispensable for hearing and understanding normal conversational speech.

2. The answer is E. (Ref: p. 392)

No single type is best for all users, and many factors affect overall functional compatibility and effectiveness. The Occupational Safety and Health Administration (OSHA) and others recommend that employees be allowed to make selections from two or more types of appropriate devices.

3. The answer is E. (Ref: pp. 390–393)

An occupational hearing conservation program (OHCP) should contain specific and well-defined functional elements: (a) education, motivation, supervision, and discipline; (b) assessment of potentially hazardous noise exposures; (c) assessing at-the-ear allowable exposures for those wearing hearing-protective devices (HPDs); (d) monitoring audiometry; (e) personal hearing and protection and noise control measures; (f) documentation of OHCP monitoring; and (g) disposition and follow-up actions.

4. The answer is C. (Ref: p. 392)

Actual efficacy of HPDs in the workplace depends on many variables. The attenuation provided under normal work conditions may be 25% to 75% of the labeled noise reduction rating (NRR).

CHAPTER 27 ANSWERS

1. The answer is D. (Ref: pp. 395–396)

Occupational contact dermatitis is the most common type of occupational skin disease, with approximately 80% due to irritant contact dermatitis. Allergic and irritant contact dermatitis cannot be distinguished by their clinical appearance. Ultraviolet (UV) radiation can cause contact dermatitis by activation of an irritant. Patch testing is useful only in determining the presence of allergic contact sensitization.

2. The answer is E. (Ref: pp. 397–398)

All three types of skin neoplasms can be caused by exposure to UV radiation. Both basal cell and squamous cell carcinomas are associated with certain chemical exposures. There is no known chemical exposure associated with the development of malignant melanoma.

3. The answer is C. (Ref: p. 398)

Occupational Raynaud's disease and vibration white finger consist of a complex of reversible vascular spasm that also manifests with numbness and tingling in the fingers. In more severe cases, the thumbs may also be affected, and the individual may develop neuromuscular and arthritic symptoms. The disease is seen in workers that use hand-held vibrating tools such as chain saws and jackhammers. Improved tool design has reduced the frequency of occurrence. Primary Raynaud's disease is a separate entity caused by other factors and is not the cause of occupational Raynaud's disease and vibration white finger.

4. The answer is B. (Ref: p. 406)

Taking a complete history is important in the evaluation of the patient with an occupational skin disorder. In addition to the occupational history, it is useful to seek answers to the other questions listed in Table 27.3. A complete skin examination helps to characterize the illness and can provide other clues that assist in the diagnosis. Visiting the worksite and reviewing information contained in an MSDS can provide the physician with useful information on the exposure and how this relates to the skin disorder. Skin biopsies are not generally useful in the diagnosis or management of contact dermatitis, although they may be useful in diagnosis of other types of occupational skin disease.

5. The answer is E. (Ref: p. 407)

There are many ways to reduce exposure to chemicals in the workplace that cause occupational skin diseases. Substituting another chemical may eliminate the problem. If substitution cannot be accomplished, reducing the exposure of the worker can be done in other ways, including improved ventilation, better housekeeping, or use of protective clothing. Improving personal hygiene and avoiding smoking, eating, and drinking at the workstation can further reduce exposure. Worker assignment may need to be altered, and in some cases, removal of the worker from the workplace may be necessary to eliminate the exposure.

6. The answer is B. (Ref: p. 408)

Use of topical steroids is the mainstay of treatment for acute contact dermatitis. Lubricants and emollients are helpful in reducing dryness and scaling that further aggravate itching and rashes associated with contact dermatitis. Antihistamines that are sedating help the patient sleep. When acute weeping lesions are present, astringent solutions and wet compresses are helpful. Systemic steroids are not routinely recommended for use in chronic contact dermatitis because of the difficulty of discontinuing the steroids, which is often followed by recurrence of the dermatitis.

CHAPTER 28 ANSWERS

1. The answer is C. (Ref: pp. 417–418)

Acute stress results in an immediate release of epinephrine (i.e., the "adrenaline rush") causing the familiar fight or flight response that increases heart rate, blood pressure, and respiratory rate.

The mechanism whereby chronic stressors exert their damage is primarily the increase of corticotropin-releasing factor and other mediators, which increase levels of circulating corticosteroid and increase blood pressure and heart rate, as well as possibly impairing immune response.

2. The answer is A. (Ref: pp. 419–420)

Shift work implies long-term night work or work involving rotation between day, evening, and night shifts. Studies suggest that these workers, presumably because of a disruption in circadian rhythm, have increased morbidity and decreased work performance. It is true that traveling westward across time zones (i.e., delay in time) has less potential for adverse effects than traveling eastward.

3. The answer is B. (Ref: pp. 411–412)

Addictive disease does not depend on quantity of use or frequency of use, but rather more on reason for use. If a substance use disorder is identified, it is of little value to attempt to determine if another primary psychiatric disorder is present. This may instead be determined after a significant period of sobriety has passed.

4. The answer is D. (Ref: p. 411)

Although binge use may indicate the presence of alcohol dependence, it is also the typical form of use among certain age groups. Unless there are significant consequences of use (e.g., occupational, educational, marital), alcohol dependence is likely not present.

5. The answer is B. (Ref: p. 412)

Sedatives should be avoided because of their potential for significant side effects. Antidepressants have been shown to be efficacious for anxiety disorders. Buspirone may also be considered as a nonaddictive antianxiety agent.

6. The answer is A. (Ref: pp. 412–413)

Literature indicates that the more rapidly the trauma is addressed in therapy, the less likely posttraumatic stress disorder (PTSD) symptoms are to develop. A quick return to the original site of the trauma or to a site where a similar event can conceivably occur or the occurrence of an additional traumatic event can all lead to higher likelihood of PTSD symptoms developing.

7. The answer is E. (Ref: p. 413)

It is also possible that the patient has appropriate brief depressive symptoms in response to psychosocial stressors, in which case there may be no psychiatric diagnosis at all.

8. The answer is E. (Ref: p. 419)

Stress management techniques include:

Time management
Relaxation training
Exercise
Avocational interests
Spread-out life changes

CHAPTER 29 ANSWERS

1. The answer is C. (Ref: p. 424)

The Gell and Coombs classification of hypersensitivity reactions remains the standard guide for types of immune responses. The four types of reactions are based on the presence or absence of humoral antibodies, the type of antibodies involved, whether complement is required to drive the reaction to completion, the target organ, and the cell types involved.

Type I is the allergic reaction seen in allergic rhinitis, asthma, and anaphylaxis; antigen crosslinks with immunoglobulin E (IgE) antibodies attached to mast cells.

Type II results in target cell destruction (i.e., immune hemolytic anemia, transfusion reaction, and some types of autoimmune disease); IgG antibodies are directed against antigen on target cell surfaces.

Type III: examples of this type of reaction are hypersensitivity pneumonitis and some autoimmune diseases; antigen-antibody immune complexes (usually IgG or IgM) deposit on vascular endothelium, causing the attraction of inflammatory leukocytes.

Type IV results in allergic contact dermatitis; previously sensitized lymphocytes release lymphokines that attract macrophages and leukocytes.

2. The answer is E. (Ref: p. 430)

Hypersensitivity pneumonitis does occur when inhaled antigens in the home or work environment cause a type III (immune complex) immunologic inflammatory reaction. In the acute phase, flulike illness may result. Antibody levels begin to fall once exposure to the antigen is terminated. Patients with severe chronic hypersensitivity pneumonitis may have no detectable precipitating antibodies. Skin testing detects only IgE antibodies, which is not helpful in confirming the diagnosis.

3. The answer is E. (Ref: pp. 434–435)

The subcommittee on immunotoxicology of the National Research Council's Committee on Biological Markers has proposed a tiered testing approach. Biopsy of lymphatic tissue, spleen, or bone marrow and tests for natural killer (NK) cell function are part of tier III testing, which is done only in people with significant abnormalities identified on tier II tests. Measurement of antibody, immunoglobulin, complete blood cell counts, and delayed-type hypersensitivity tests are all tier I tests. Lymphocyte enumeration and typing also are tier I tests. Tier II tests are carried out in people with significant abnormalities identified in tier I testing and include induction of primary antibody response to injected protein or polysaccharide antigens, stimulation of lymphocyte proliferation with specific mitogens, additional T- and B-cell marker determinations, and measurement of cytokines.

4. The answer is D. (Ref: pp. 431–432)

Premedication of sensitized individuals with steroids is questionable before significant natural rubber latex (NRL) exposure such as surgery. Avoidance of NRL is the best method of protection against significant allergic reactions.

5. The answer is E. (Ref: p. 431)

Long-term use of corticosteroids is generally required for control of acute bronchopulmonary aspergillosis (ABPA).

CHAPTER 30 ANSWERS

1. The answer is C. (Ref: p. 439)

Osteoarthritis of the hands, however, is common. The process afflicts all of us as we age but is most frequent and more advanced in the postmenopausal woman. The principal occupationally related compromise to which these women are at risk is related to power pinch. Osteoarthritis of the first carpometacarpal joint is a far more common cause of discomfort at the base of the thumb tunnel syndrome or tendonitis in women beyond middle age.

2. The answer is D. (Ref: p. 441)

The diagnostic maneuver is to have the patient stand with the arm dependent and the elbow flexed. Passive internal rotation isolates the glenohumeral joint and should be gliding and pain free.

3. The answer is E. (Ref: pp. 439–440)

There are two community-based surveys that quantify the prevalence of symptoms suggestive of carpal tunnel syndrome and the coincident prevalence of electrodiagnostic abnormalities. In both surveys, nearly 20% of the adults had recently experienced or were experiencing symptoms that were classic for carpal tunnel syndrome. Of these, almost 20% had delayed median conductivity. Can it be that 5% of people are suffering from carpal tunnel syndrome and only 1 in 50 of them find their way to diagnostic labeling each year? Some have argued so, but I doubt it. Rather, numbness, even nocturnal numbness, is yet another one of the intermittent and remittent symptomatic regional musculoskeletal disorders with which we must all cope if we are to remain well.

Electrodiagnostic studies leave much to be desired in that they are difficult to perform well, are uncomfortable, and are of limited sensitivity for radiculopathies and for all entrapment neuropathies other than carpal tunnel syndrome. Even when carpal tunnel syndrome is the issue, the clinician needs to be wary of minimal conduction delay as a basis for diagnosis because of the considerable variability in the normal population. Conductivity by the median nerve is inversely proportional to age and body mass index, particularly in women, further compromising the specificity of the finding of a conduction delay.

4. The answer is A. (Ref: p. 440)

If all that is sought is an association between the physical demands of tasks and the disabling arm pain, that is all that can be found, although anything but consistently and seldom is the association robust. Fortunately, modern science is no longer bound to this preconception. If the physician seeks associations with the physical demands of tasks and with aspects of the psychosocial context of work, the former pales next to the latter. The cutting edge of clinical investigation is probing the elements of the psychosocial context of work that compromise a person's ability to cope with the next episode of regional musculoskeletal pain.

CHAPTER 31 ANSWERS

1. The answer is C. (Ref: p. 445)

Direct transmission can occur through three primary routes: (a) direct contact, such as skin-to-skin or skin-to-mucous membrane touching, or droplet spread of contaminated fluid onto the mucous membranes of the nose or mouth or the conjunctiva; (b) parental spread, which may take the form of percutaneous needle sticks or transfusion of contaminated fluid; (c) exposure of susceptible skin to an infectious agent, such as through a bite, laceration, or compromised skin.

Indirect routes include airborne (the most common route, typically involving the dissemination of infectious agents through aerosols that enter a host through the respiratory tract); vector-borne (disease carried by insects or animals); and vehicle-borne transmission (when an intermediate object transports an infectious agent into a suitable port of entry into the host).

2. The answer is E. (Ref: pp. 445–448)

Human immunodeficiency virus (HIV) exposure is a definite risk for health care, laboratory, and home health care workers (Table 31.1.). Throughout the health care and

TABLE 31.1. *Occupations at risk for infectious disease*

Agricultural workers
Miners
Animal handlers
Packinghouse workers
Animal husbandry workers
Personal care workers
Butchers
Pest control workers
Cannery workers
Primate handlers
Cattle breeders
Public safety and emergency response workers
Construction workers
Ranchers
Dairy farmers
Research laboratory workers
Day care workers
Sewer workers
Excavators
Sheepherders
Fishermen
Slaughterhouse workers
Forestry workers
Stockyard workers
Geologists
Trappers
Health care workers
Travelers
Hunters
Veterinarians
Livestock handlers
Weavers
Lumberjacks
Zookeepers
Meat and poultry workers

research fields, universal precautions and personal protective equipment have minimized exposure to HIV. When an exposure occurs, postexposure prophylaxis should be considered. The seroconversion rate after a needle stick with HIV-positive blood is estimated to be about 0.3%. The efficacy of AZT in the reduction of risk of HIV in health care workers is about 80%.

3. The answer is C. (Ref: p. 448)

Hepatitis B virus was the first blood-borne disease recognized to pose an occupational risk through a preponderance of cases among pathologists, laboratory workers, and blood bank workers. Occupations at risk are those with exposure to blood or fluids. The risk of transmission is 1% to 6% with HBe antigen–negative blood and is estimated to be 22% to 40% for HBe antigen–positive blood. Since 1985, the rate of infection has decreased by 90% among health care workers because of the widespread adoption of preventive immunization, universal precautions, and personal protective equipment. Hepatitis C virus is responsible for most cases of transfusion-related hepatitis (Table 31.2).

4. The answer is C. (Ref: pp. 449–450)

The skin test indicates only previous exposure; it does not designate active infection. If active tuberculosis is suspected, a chest radiograph should be taken. Active tuberculosis presents with symptoms of cough, weight loss, and malaise.

The incidence of tuberculosis has increased significantly in the last decade because of laxity in public health measures and the acquired immunodeficiency syndrome (AIDS) epidemic. Health care workers and staff in institutional settings have the highest risk of exposure. Recent skin test converters should be evaluated for isoniazid (INH) prophylaxis after a chest radiograph is performed to rule out active disease.

TABLE 31.2. *Vaccine preventable diseases*

Cholera
Plague
Diphtheria
Pneumococcal disease
Hepatitis A
Polio
Hepatitis B
Rabies
Influenza
Rubella
Japanese encephalitis
Tetanus
Lyme disease
Tick-borne encephalitis
Malaria
Typhoid
Measles
Typhus
Meningococcal disease
Varicella
Mumps
Yellow fever
Pertussis

5. The answer is C. (Ref: pp. 450–451)

Measles, an acute viral disease, is transmitted by large, airborne respiratory droplets and has an incubation period of 5 to 21 days. During an outbreak, vaccination within 72 hours after exposure without prior serologic testing is recommended for any adult who has not received two doses of vaccine, regardless of age or serologic status. The vaccine has an efficacy of 95% with one dose and 99% with two doses.

6. The answer is D. (Ref: pp. 451–452)

Hepatitis A virus is one of most frequently reported vaccine-preventable diseases. Vaccination, which is 94% to 100% effective, is recommended for persons at risk of occupational exposure and for those who travel abroad. Immune globulin given within 2 weeks of exposure is more than 85% effective in preventing symptomatic infection.

7. The answer is C. (Ref: p. 452)

Herpes zoster (i.e., shingles), a localized outbreak of skin vesicles, results from reactivation of varicella virus after a dormant period of years after primary chickenpox infection. The virus is spread from person to person by the airborne route, by direct contact with vesicular fluid or respiratory secretions, or by contact with articles freshly soiled with these fluids. Herpes zoster has a lower rate of transmission than varicella, but both can cause chickenpox in seronegative contacts.

8. The answer is B. (Ref: pp. 453–454)

Bite wounds from animals or humans can lead to infections or blood-borne pathogen transmission. Treatment with broad-spectrum antibiotics covers most potential pathogens. Amoxicillin-clavulanate, clorfloxicin, or cloxacillin may be used for prophylaxis or treatment.

9. The answer is E. (Ref: pp. 455–457)

Mosquitoes transmit diseases such as yellow fever, malaria, and Japanese encephalitis. Japanese encephalitis virus can occur in Southeast Asia and the Indian subcontinent. Those at risk should obtain a three-dose series of inactivated vaccine before travel.

Malaria is a febrile, flulike illness that can manifest in a 3- or 4- day cycle or that can cause more severe disease, including cerebral, pulmonary, and renal failure. Precautions against malaria include preventive vaccination or treatment of the illness with mefloquine, primaquine, or chloroquine.

CHAPTER 32 ANSWERS

1. The answer is C (Ref: p. 459)

Phase I reactions make lipid-soluble compounds more polar through hydrolysis, oxidation, or reduction. Phase II reactions are those in which the foreign compound is conjugated with another functional group, usually resulting in a less toxic, more easily excreted compound.

Most hepatotoxic agents produce liver injury only after biotransformation to an active metabolite through the action of these enzyme systems. Intrinsic hepatotoxins are agents that are directly or indirectly toxic to the liver. Toxicity is a predictable and inherent property of the chemical structure of the compound or its metabolite and usually is dose dependent (Table 32.1).

2. The answer is D (Ref: pp. 458–460)

Chronic exposures to toxins can result in subacute disease that may or may not progress to chronic disease.

3. The answer is A. (Ref: p. 459)

Steatosis refers to fatty changes in the liver and is often an early indicator of hepatotoxicity. Cholestasis refers to cessation or alteration of bile flow, which can result from hepatocanalicular injury, canalicular injury, necrosis of bile ducts, or necrosis, and scaring of septal ducts. Hepatoportal sclerosis is a fibrous lesion that causes obstruction of branches of the portal vein. Porphyria cutanea tarda is the most common type of porphyria in humans. Cirrhosis is a chronic, irreversible condition in which the normal hepatic architecture is replaced by fibrous tissue and regenerating nodules.

4. The answer is D. (Ref: p. 460)

Cancers of the liver in humans have been described in association with a number of agents, including chronic viral infections (e.g., hepatitis B and C), chronic alcohol ingestion, contraceptive steroids, aflatoxin B_1, inorganic arsenic, and vinyl chloride. Hepatic angiosarcoma (HAS) is a rare form of liver cancer that has been associated with exposure to vinyl chloride and has also been reported with long-term exposure to arsenicals.

5. The answer is B. (Ref: p. 461)

Ethanol, as well as isopropanol, methanol, 2-butanol, and acetone, potentiates the toxicity of carbon tetrachloride (CCl_4). Alcoholics are more likely to develop hepatic injury after exposure to CCl_4 than nondrinkers (23). The likely mechanism for this potentiation

TABLE 32.1 *Classification of hepatotoxins*

Type of hepatotoxin	Compounds
Intrinsic direct hepatotoxins	Carbon tetrachloride, 1,1,2,2-tetrachloroethane, paraquat, white phosphorous
Intrinsic indirect hepatotoxins	Aflatoxin B_1, ethanol, bromobenzene, methylenedianiline, acetaminophen
Idiosyncratic (immunologic)	Halothane, phenytoin
Idiosyncratic (metabolic)	Isoniazid, valproate

is alcohol induction of hepatocyte cytochrome P450 systems, with enhanced metabolic conversion of CCl$_4$ to its toxic metabolite.

6. The answer is A. (Ref: pp. 463–464)

The surveillance of workers with potential exposure to hepatotoxins presents a challenge. The ideal medical surveillance test would be one that has high sensitivity and high specificity. Biochemical tests most commonly used measures to detect liver disease include those for aspartate aminotransferase (AST), alanine aminotransferase (ALT), serum alkaline phosphatase (ALP), serum lactate dehydrogenase (LDH), and γ-glutamyltranspeptidase (GGT). These tests are more sensitive than they are specific and may be useful in detecting early stages of toxic liver injury and nontoxic liver disease.

Hyperbilirubinemia may be conjugated or unconjugated. Unconjugated hyperbilirubinemia is commonly seen in Gilbert's disease, hemolytic disorders, and congestive heart failure.

Measurements of serum albumin and prothrombin time have little or no value in medical surveillance for exposure to hepatotoxins.

Clearance tests measure the ability of the liver to excrete substances and can be sensitive and specific in the detection of liver disease. These tests can measure clearance of exogenous substances (e.g., indocyanine green, antipyrine) or endogenous substances (e.g., serum bile acids).

Physical examination is useful in detecting hepatomegaly, but this usually occurs after there has been a prolonged or significant hepatotoxic exposure. As such, physical examination is not a sensitive screening tool.

Liver biopsy is the gold standard in establishing the most specific diagnosis possible but is highly invasive and carries significant risks of complications. It is never used as a screening tool and is reserved for cases in which tissue diagnosis is required.

CHAPTER 33 ANSWERS

1. The answer is B. (Ref: p. 467)

The occupational history is the clinical tool used to elicit and organize information about the workplace for any thorough diagnostic evaluation. A basic occupational history includes the following:

1. Description of current and recent work, including longest held job and years worked in each position (Answer D).
2. Report of any exposure to chemicals, dusts, or fumes, including type, intensity, and duration; and information from manufacturers, employers, and MSDS.
3. Relationship of symptoms to periods away from work (e.g., weekends, holidays, vacations, other absence) and to changes in work schedule (Answer A).
4. Description of any change in work activities, production quotas, work processes, or other work routine preceding or coinciding with the development of symptoms.
5. Occurrence of similar symptoms or illness in coworkers.
6. The patient's opinion regarding the relationship of the illness to work and reasons supporting the opinion.
7. History of use of substances in avocational activities and their relationship to symptoms or illness (Answer C).
8. Contact with workplace of worksite visit.

The acronym WHACS also can be used. The S stands for job satisfaction, which is critical in the presentation, course, prognosis, and employee perceptions about their condition (Answer E).
Answer B is incorrect. It is not listed in the text.

2. The answer is A. (Ref: p. 470)

The correct pairing for Answers B through E would be

B. A regional office of the NIOSH: current information on commercial substances and their health effects
C. The manufacturer of the chemical: chemical formulations and toxicity of particular products used in industry
D. Computerized databases such as MEDLINE and TOXLINE: computerized search of medical literature
E. MSDS: description of a material and its toxicity

3. The answer is C. (Ref: p. 469)

Clusters of people with unusual illness (e.g., aspermia in workers exposed to the nematocide dibromochloropropane) in groups sharing work experiences have led to case reports of new relationships between exposure and disease. The other answer options are related to health effects other than aspermia.

4. The answer is D. (Ref: pp. 472–473)

See Table 33.2 and the text on guidelines for preparing the case report. Answer D falls under basic science research, whereas a case report usually deals with a disease in a person.

CHAPTER 34 ANSWERS

1. The answer is A. (Ref: pp. 477, 481–482)

Work-related eye complaints can be safely and effectively handled by occupational or primary care providers in the absence of "red flags," which are defined as signs or symptoms of a potentially serious condition, indicating need for further consultation, support, or specialized treatment.

2. The answer is C (Ref: p. 484)

The patient's complaints may reveal the cause of the red eye. A *scratchy or burning sensation* suggests lid, conjunctival, or corneal disorders, including foreign bodies, in-turning eyelashes, and dry eyes.

A *halo effect* around lights is commonly reported in acute glaucoma. *Blurred vision* often indicates serious ocular disease. *Photophobia* is an abnormal sensitivity to light. Acute onset of spots, floaters, or flashes of light or a sensation of a *curtain drawn across the eye* suggests retinal detachment.

3. The answer is B. (Ref: p. 486)

In cases of a uveitis (i.e., purulent cyclitis), the presence of protein and cells in the anterior chamber is classic, and a hypopyon may be present. A *hyphema* is an accumulation of red blood cells caused by trauma to the anterior chamber. A *pterygium* is an abnormal growth consisting of a triangular fold of tissue that advances progressively over the cornea, usually from the nasal side.

4. The answer is B. (Ref: p. 488)

Blepharitis responds slowly to treatment and relapses are common. The mainstays of treatment include eradication of staphylococcal infection with frequent applications of appropriate ophthalmic antibiotics; treatment of scalp seborrhea with antidandruff shampoos; and cleansing of the lids to alleviate seborrheic blepharitis.

5. The answer is C. (Ref: pp. 490–493)

The visual survey is best accomplished as a cooperative venture between the occupational physician, a consulting eye specialist, and plant management representatives.

Analysis of workplace visual requirements requires a broad knowledge of visual abilities and limitations (e.g., problems of accommodation, convergence, presbyopia, coordination, muscle balance); lighting; physical factors; and the host of eye hazards of a particular operation.

Visual job "families" were developed on statistical basis after large numbers of employees, assigned to diverse jobs and exhibiting all degrees of ability and achievement, were tested and classified on the basis of job success into categories that ranged from "definitely superior" to "definitely inferior." Visual demands for most industrial jobs fall into one of six job families.

6. The answer is C. (Ref: p. 493)

Eye complaints occur in 50% to 90% of workers who use video display terminals (VDTs). Such problems result from visual inefficiencies or from eye-related symptoms caused by a combination of individual visual abnormalities and poor visual ergonomics. Visual symptoms can usually be resolved with ergonomic modification and the provision of appropriate visual care to the worker.

7. The answer is D. (Ref: p. 496)

Individuals should not be disqualified from a job because of contact lens use. Such lenses may be used under a full-face respirator.

A 1980 Bureau of Labor Statistics study found that about 60% of workers who suffered eye injuries were not wearing eye protective equipment (PPE). The use of PPE should not substitute for engineering out hazards or for work practice or administrative controls. *Static shielding of equipment*, such as barrier or deflector screens of transparent plastics, can provide a clear view of a work process while protecting workers from grinding fragments, accidental sprays, or specific optical irradiations. Booths that protect against heat and accidental splashes can provide *static shielding of personnel*. Static shielding may be suspended from the ceiling, mounted on the floor, or constructed as a separate control area.

CHAPTER 35 ANSWERS

1. The answer is A. (Ref: p. 511)

Genes are the basic building blocks of heredity, controlling diverse body cellular functions such as determining hair color, height, and facial characteristics. This diversity is controlled through variations in DNA sequence. Any variation that occurs in more than 1% of the population is considered a polymorphism. Genetic polymorphisms may result in only one base change that fundamentally alters structure (i.e., sickle cell disease), or they may be reflected in all or part of a gene being deleted. It is estimated that genetic polymorphisms occur approximately every 500 bases.

2. The answer is B. (Ref: p. 513)

Other applications involve the identification of single-base mutations or genetic polymorphisms by designing primers that anneal only if matched to the unique sequence (e.g., oligospecific polymerase chain reaction [PCR] for the identification of polymorphisms in the *N*-acetyl transferase gene predictive of cancer risk in workers exposed to aromatic amines). Genotyping to determine genetic variation (e.g., color of hair, metabolic activity, DNA repair) can be done by using different types of detection methods after PCR.

Several methods are currently available for the measurement of DNA adducts, although all remain research tools. These include the ^{32}P-postlabeling assay, an assay that uses hydrolytic enzymes to reduce DNA to individual nucleotides and then uses another enzyme to radiolabel the nucleotides. Any adducts that are present are then resolved chromatographically and quantitated by measuring the radioactivity incorporated into the nucleotide. This assay can be used as a screening method to detect unknown adducts or can be combined with purification techniques to identify specific compounds such as adducts formed from polycyclic aromatic hydrocarbons and *N*-nitrosamines. Several important immunologic methods are available for the detection of DNA adducts. Using procedures such as enzyme-linked immunoadsorbent assays (ELISAs) or radioimmunoassays, adducts for polycyclic aromatic hydrocarbons can be measured. Newer methods use improved mass spectroscopy methods and fluorescence detection. DNA adducts are not analyzed using PCR.

DNA sequencing can be used to determine the actual genetic code. This may be used for identifying an inherited code (i.e., sequence of entire gene or single nucleotide polymorphisms [SNPs]) or mutations in tumors. The dideoxy-mediated chain termination method was among the first established and allows for the determination of a nucleic acid sequence of a gene. For example, a PCR fragment is amplified, and four dideoxy reactions are carried out for each of the four nucleotides.

3. The answer is A. (Ref: pp. 512–514)

Microarray technology can be used for nucleotide sequence detection, SNP analysis, and aberrant gene expression using RNA. These methodologies begin with PCR, followed by enzymatic fragmentation of the PCR product and fluorescent labeling.

4. The answer is C. (Ref: pp. 515–516)

A potentially important clinical application of genetic testing will be the prediction of occupational lung disease in persons with decreased production of α_1-antitrypsin. Absence of two functional copies of this gene leads to the development of premature emphysema, which is worsened by concurrent exposure to tobacco smoke. The absence of one of two copies may lead to a partial deficiency and an inability for natural lung defense mechanisms to work properly when challenged by pulmonary irritants, allergens, or inflammatory agents. This gene is polymorphic, with more than 7% of the population carrying a defective gene. The presence of an inheritable abnormality is demonstrable by PCR and oligonucleotide hybridization. If studies identify an increased genetic risk, industrial hygiene and medical surveillance may change.

Several genetic polymorphisms for drug and carcinogen metabolism have suggested that some workers might be at increased risk for occupational cancers. For example, the *N*-acetyltransferase enzyme is responsible for activating and detoxifying aromatic amines and heterocyclic amines, depending on the organ and compound, and may place workers at increased risk for bladder cancer.

The ethical, legal, and social implications for the use of genetic assays has stimulated much debate, especially in the workplace. Employers and medical providers are mandated to avoid discriminatory practices, as addressed in part by the Americans with Disabilities Act (ADA). Additional legislation related to inherited risks may be required. Other forms of discrimination, such as may occur in the insurance industry, remains to be adequately addressed. The odds of never developing a disease despite having a specific genetic trait must be considered in the context of other commonly used actuarial predictors (e.g., cholesterol level, hypertension). Separately, the stigmatization of having a specific genotype needs to be addressed in a number of different forums. Providing results of genetic testing can avoid wrongful stigmatization if accurate risks are presented clearly. Because of the large diversity in human genotypes (i.e., polymorphisms of individual nucleotides occurs approximately every 500 bases), there can no longer be one genotype that is considered "normal"; instead, there are common and less common types. The potential harmful effects of genetic testing must be considered in light of the many potential benefits.

Recent advances in PCR amplification and DNA sequencing have led to findings that chemicals can cause specific point mutations in DNA that may be "fingerprints" of that exposure (i.e., mutational spectra). This type of testing may be useful in learning the cause of cancer in an individual.

CHAPTER 36 ANSWERS

1. The answer is C. (Ref: pp. 519–520)

The first Five-Year Plan of the Human Genome Project (HGP), published in 1990, included the following goals: (a) developing preliminary genetic maps of the human genome; (b) developing physical maps of the chromosomes; (c) mapping and fully sequencing simple laboratory organisms; (d) investing in sequencing technologies; and (e) proactively researching potential ethical, legal, and social issues expected to arise from the project (Table 36.1).

2. The answer is D. (Ref: p. 521)

DNA microarrays (i.e., DNA "chips") are fields of single-stranded DNA that may comprise tens or hundreds of thousands of oligonucleotides or cDNA strands. The chips are small wafers, usually glass, and the DNA fragments bound to them can be "downloaded" in arrays based on known sequence, so that each tethered DNA probe sits in a defined location. This array is then bathed in a solution of the labeled nucleic acid mixture that is to be probed. The nucleic acids being assayed can be derived from diverse sources (e.g., a clone of tumor cells, an uncharacterized infectious pathogen, the blood of a patient seeking information on inherited disease susceptibility). The nucleic acid fragments in solution are labeled with fluorescent or radioactive tags that can be read by standardized instruments after washout of nonhybridized material. The location of the labeled sequences on the microarray after hybridization identifies gene fragments or transcripts as homologous to known probes.

DNA microarrays can qualitatively identify specific sequences. More than 2 million SNPs have been mapped across the human genome. Most genetic variation in humans appears to be caused by SNPs, and many are probably associated with specific diseases. Microarrays can rapidly identify individual SNPs or other structural alleles known to cause inherited illnesses (e.g., sickle cell disease, cystic fibrosis).

3. The answer is B. (Ref: p. 520)

The HGP has yielded a plethora of insights into human genome structure and function. The total number of genes appears to be only about 30,000. Although the genome consists of more than 3 billion base pairs, only 2% appears to code for proteins, and more than 50% consists of highly repetitive "junk DNA," sequences that do not have regulatory or coding function. Humans apparently generate most translation products through "alternative splicing" of mRNA, so that the number of protein products actually is in the range of 100,000. The average human gene is 3,000 base pairs long, but it may range to more than 2 million base pairs

4. The answer is D. (Ref: pp. 526–527)

Prenatal and neonatal genetic screening for gene carriage is routinely available for screening and diagnosis of these conditions. More common, adult-onset conditions (e.g., diabetes, hypertension, vascular disease, emphysema, allergy) that have more complex polygenic causes are beginning to be amenable to genomic testing.

There is potential for abuse of genomic technology, especially for workers. Genetic information may result in denial of employment or insurance because of genetic susceptibility to an occupational agent. Worker selection and job placement may supplant pro-

TABLE 36.1. *Examples of genetic and genomic screening tests in occupational medicine*

Marker(s)	Susceptibility hazard	Disease	Validated yet in workplace	Reference
HLA-DpbetaGlu69	Beryllium	Berylliosis (chronic beryllium disease)	No	43,44
Vitamin D receptor (VDR-B)	Lead	Hypertension	No	45
Delta-aminolevulinic acid dehydratase (ALAD1, ALAD2)	Lead	Hypertension, heme synthesis	No	45,46
Alpha1 antitrypsin (A1AT)	Particulates	Chronic obstructive pulmonary disease	No	47
Glucose-6-phosphate dehydrogenase (G6PD)	Environmental oxidants	Hemolysis	No	48
Pseudocholinesterase variants	Organophosphates	Organophosphate toxicity	No	40
Cytochome P450 polymorphisms	Aromatic hydrocarbons, and others	Hepatic injury	No	48
Peripheral myelin protein (PMP-22)	Ergonomic stresses	Carpal tunnel syndrome	No	49

tective environmental controls and stricter standards for permissible exposure levels (PELs).

5. The answer is C. (Ref: p. 526)

The Americans with Disabilities Act (ADA) and Health Insurance Portability and Accountability Act (HIPAA) of 1996 offer limited protection from discrimination but do not prohibit employers and insurers from gaining access to genetic information. HIPPA provides that genetic information should not be used as a "preexisting condition" in absence of diagnosis of the condition related to such information. Legislative and regulatory strategies are needed to address these concerns, particularly when health insurance and employment are intertwined.

The ADA potentially offers protection from discrimination. Although ADA prevents employers from making preemployment medical inquiries, it does not prevent employers from obtaining medical information, including genetic information, after a conditional offer of employment.

═══37═══
Industrial Hygiene

OBJECTIVES

- Identify ways that industrial hygienists help physicians consider health risks
- State the goals of industrial hygiene
- Distinguish categories of hazards found in the workplace
- List types, methods, and expressions of results of monitoring
- Explain sources of exposure guidelines
- Identify specialized sampling methods for exposure assessment
- Identify sources of industrial hygiene services

OUTLINE

I. Types of hazards
   A. Gases and vapors
   B. Dusts
   C. Fumes and mists
   D. Physical agents
   E. Biologic agents
II. Monitoring
   A. Figure 37.1: A passive dosimeter badge
   B Figure 37.2: Air sampling pump (i.e., personal sampling)
   C. Gases and vapors
      1. Figure 37.3: Colorimetric detector tubes
      2. Figure 37.4: Direct-reading instrument for hazardous atmospheres
      3. Figure 37.5: Confined space sampling
   D. Dusts
   E Fumes and mists
   F. Physical agents
      1. Figure 37.6: Noise dosimeters
   G. Biologic agents
      1. Figure 37.7: Biologic sampling device (i.e., spore trap)
      2. Figure 37.8: Liquid sampler for bioaerosols
III. Occupational exposure limits
   A. Table 37.1: Recognized occupational exposure guidelines
   B. Table 37.2: Regulatory (occupational exposure) limits
   C. Table 37.3: Community-based exposure limits
   D. Evaluating exposures (i.e., mixture equation)

IV. Industrial hygiene services

KEY POINTS

- The profession of industrial hygiene has as its main goal the anticipation, recognition, evaluation, and control of workplace health hazards.

1. Anticipation implies that facts about previous exposures in the workplace may be applied to similar operations and substances.
2. Recognition of a hazard requires knowledge of the processes and the materials used in the processes.
3. Evaluation is the process of determining the level of worker exposure in day-to-day duties.
4. Control measures are prescribed to remove the worker from exposure, to lower the exposure, or to replace the hazardous agent with a less dangerous substitute.

- The hazards found in the workplace can generally be divided into five categories: gases or vapors, dusts, fumes or mists, physical agents, and biologic agents.
- Gases are substances that are normally in the gaseous state at room temperature; vapors are the gaseous state of substances that are normally in the liquid state at room temperature. The main route of entry into the body for gases and vapors is through inhalation.
- A variety of dusts may be found in the workplace, including nuisance-type dusts, toxic dusts, and pneumoconiosis-producing dusts.
- A fume is a solid that has been vaporized and subsequently condenses. In welding steel, for example, iron oxide fume is produced. A mist is a liquid that has been dispersed into the air as fine droplets.
- Dusts, fumes, and mists are collectively considered particulate hazards (i.e., aerosols), and the particle size is important in determining the exposure severity and the health effect.
- Physical agents encountered in the workplace may include noise, vibration, temperature (cold and heat), and radiation (nonionizing and ionizing)
- Biologic agents, including bacteria, viruses, and fungi, are being evaluated by industrial hygienists.
- The evaluations of bioaerosols in the environment have become important in assessing an individual's exposure to potentially infectious or irritative agents.
- The industrial hygienist monitors employee exposure to air contaminants. This can be done by obtaining personal or area samples. Personal samples are obtained by placing the sampling device or equipment on the worker. In area sampling, the apparatus is placed in the vicinity of the worker performing the job.
- Organic gases and vapors can be collected with an absorbing material, such as silica gel or activated charcoal. The concentration is determined based on the time the device was exposed to air and the amount of contaminant. Dusts may be monitored by a variety of instruments. Although the most common method is to collect the dust on a filter medium, real-time particle counters are being used to establish exposures immediately during the work operations. Like dusts, fumes and mists are collected on filters and analyzed in a laboratory.

- For chemical substances that are present in workplace air and suspensions of solid particles or droplets (i.e., aerosols), the particle size and the mass concentration can affect the health hazard presented by the contaminant. The size of the particle determines the level of deposition within the respiratory tract and may help to explain why certain occupational diseases are associated with particular regions of the respiratory tract. The use of particle size–selective sampling provides information about the most probable deposition location in three general categories: inhalable particulate mass (0 to 100 μm), thoracic particulate mass (0 to 25 μm), and respirable particulate mass (0 to 10 μm).
- Physical agents such as noise, radiation, or microwaves are measured with electronic instruments that respond to the energy field of the agent.
- There are several guidelines that are used by the industrial hygienist to evaluate the significance of exposure levels to air contaminants. The American Conference of Governmental Industrial Hygienists (ACGIH) publishes threshold limit values (TLVs) annually. These are meant to protect nearly all workers from adverse effects when they are repeatedly exposed to an agent 8 hours per day, 5 days each week, for a working lifetime. Other organizations also publish exposure guidelines that may assist the practitioner in evaluating an exposure. The physician cannot necessarily conclude that a worker's exposure is safe simply because the exposure is below guidelines. Symptoms may or may not be related to such exposure.
- *biologic exposure indices* The BEIs, also published by ACGIH, are warning levels of biologic response to a chemical or its metabolite. They are concentrations of a chemical or its metabolite, usually in blood or urine, that appear to reflect levels that are safe to human health.
- The Occupational Safety and Health Administration (OSHA)–permissible exposure limits (PELs) are published in the Code of Federal Regulations and are regarded as the "legal" limits for workplace exposures.
- Although most exposure limits are defined as 8-hour, time-weighted averages, other values refer to ceiling limits. Ceiling values, which should never be exceeded, are usually assigned to strong irritants, cardiac sensitizers, and carcinogens. Another limit value is the short-term exposure limit. It is typically calculated over a 15-minute exposure period.
- If a patient has symptoms of an illness that are suspected to be caused by the workplace, industrial hygiene data should be reviewed, if available. Such data may be available from many sources. OSHA offices, workers' compensation insurance carriers, or others may have conducted investigations of facilities and have monitoring data.

Amer. IH Ass. (AIHA) publishes Workplace Environment Exposure Limit (WEEL)

QUESTIONS

*1. Which one of the following is **not** a goal of industrial hygiene?*

A. Recognition of potential hazards in the workplace
B. Evaluation of potential hazards in the workplace
C. Evaluation of workers exposed to potential hazards in the workplace
D. Control of potential hazards in the workplace
E. Anticipation of potential hazards in the workplace

2. Burning is a common task in the fabrication of metal products. In burning, a hot flame from an oxygen-acetylene (oxyacetylene) torch is used to cut metal. Which one of the following is correct?

A. Acetylene and oxygen are vapors.
B. Metal oxides are gases.

C. Metal oxides are mists.

D. Metal oxides are fumes.

E. Metal oxides are dusts.

3. *Which of the following is **incorrect**?*

A. The ACGIH publishes TLVs.

B. OSHA publishes PELs.

C. The National Institute for Occupational Safety and Health publishes recommended exposure limits.

D. The American Industrial Hygiene Association publishes BEIs.

E. Even though the individual airborne concentrations of a mixture of chemicals do not exceed recommended guidelines (TLVs or PELs), it is possible that the equivalent exposure for the mixture may suggest overexposure.

4. *What is a permissible exposure limit (PEL)?*

A. An air contaminant concentration level used by the Environmental Protection Agency (EPA)

B. An air contaminant concentration level that is the same as a TLV

C. An air contaminant concentration level used by OSHA that is the upper limit of employee exposure acceptability

D. An air contaminant concentration level used to determine the acceptability of chemical emissions to the atmosphere

E. An air contaminant concentration level that is considered safe to exceed

5. *What is an occupational exposure limit designated as a "ceiling"?*

A. The concentration of a contaminant at the upper levels of a work environment to protect workers that must work on elevated platforms

B. The concentration of a contaminant at which a worker may be exposed for up to 30 minutes

C. The concentration used as an emergency exposure level

D. The concentration of a contaminant that should never be exceeded

E. The concentration of a contaminant below the regulatory limit, requiring action by the employer

6. *Which of the following best describes how industrial hygienists are involved in occupational health?*

A. They manage workers' compensation claims.

B. They are like physician's assistants.

C. They recognize, evaluate, and control sanitation problems in the workplace.

D. They recognize, evaluate, and control health hazards in the workplace.

E. They do stack testing for industrial emissions to determine compliance with EPA regulations.

7. *An industrial hygienist informs you that an overexposure to lead is occurring in the machining area. Which one of the following control strategies should be taken immediately?*

A. Open all windows and doors to dilute the lead dust in the air.

B. Shut down the operation until a long-term control strategy can be devised.
C. Tell the company to stop using lead.
D. Hire another industrial hygienist for a second opinion.
E. Shut down the operation until the employees are provided with the appropriate respiratory protection.

8. *What is the BEI?*

A. A warning level of biologic response to a chemical or metabolite
B. The OSHA exposure limit for employee exposure to air contaminants in the workplace
C. The same as a TLV
D. An exposure index used to evaluate a work group's biologic response to a chemical
E. An exposure index used by industrial hygienists to evaluate an employee's exposure to microbiologic contaminants in the workplace air

✓

9. *During an industrial hygiene review, a worker's exposures to ethyl alcohol and ethyl acetate are determined to be 600 ppm and 280 ppm, respectively. If the permissible exposure level for ethyl alcohol is 1,000 ppm and the PEL for the ethyl acetate is 400 ppm, how would you evaluate the mixture as an equivalent exposure?*

A. Worker is overexposed, equivalent exposure 880
B. Worker is overexposed, equivalent exposure 1.3
C. Worker is overexposed, equivalent exposure 1.5
D. Worker is not overexposed, equivalent exposure 0.6
E. Both exposures are below the PEL, so the worker is not overexposed

10. *Particle size–selective exposure limits consider the size of the contaminant particle to evaluate the hazard because*

A. The health effects of a particle may vary depending on the level at which it is deposited in the lungs.
B. Smaller-sized particles are more difficult to capture and could under represent the health hazard to the workers.
C. Larger particles settle out of the air faster and should only considered a hazard during active operations.
D. Smaller particles are cleared from the lungs easier, so their hazard potential is considered lower.
E. Particle size has no effect on the health hazard consideration.

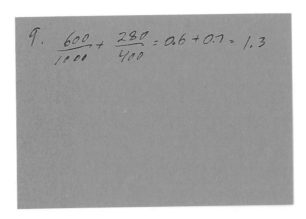

9. $\dfrac{600}{1000} + \dfrac{280}{400} = 0.6 + 0.7 = 1.3$

══════38══════
Workplace Safety

OBJECTIVES

- Describe the physician's role in the prevention of work-related injury and illnesses.
- Identify the responsibilities of safety personnel in industry
- Summarize common safety programs implemented to address specific hazards
- Determine the Occupational Safety and Health Administration (OSHA) requirements for safety programs
- Identify programs designed to evaluate and prioritize occupational hazards.
- Discuss the physician's role in injury and illness evaluation, recording, and long-term management of work injury limitations
- Explain advantages of the occupational health and safety management system
- Identify levels of "safety culture" and key characteristics for integration into a workplace

OUTLINE

KEY POINTS

- Physicians can participate and contribute to the workplace safety practices of an employer.

- Each year, a significant number of workplace related injuries and illnesses occur despite the implementation of federal regulations that mandate a safe and healthful workplace.
- The safety responsibilities should be designated to a safety professional or safety department. This department is responsible for organizing the safety program, responding to injuries and illnesses, and providing management with specific ways to reduce injuries and illnesses.
- Safety programs work best *when* what the management and workforce take ownership of the issue of safety and the reduction of injuries and illnesses.

QUESTIONS

1. The primary purpose of the safety professional is the following:

A. Anticipate regulations
B. Assist management in reducing the risk of work-related injury and illness
C. Provide information for occupational physicians
D. Provide regulatory compliance
E. Control costs associated with worker injuries

2. OSHA developed the VPP in 1980 to do the following:

A. Reward compliant employers
B. Increase penalties for those workplaces found in noncompliance
C. Supplement the chronically understaffed inspection and enforcement approach
D. Require minimum standards for workplace safety
E. None of the above

3. Which of the following organizations has a resource available to investigate unexplained clusters of illness or exposures?

A. OSHA
B. American College of Occupational and Environmental Medicine
C. Environmental Protection Agency
D. NIOSH
E. NORA

4. A worker's injury triggers OSHA recordability in which of the following circumstances?

A. The injury occurs while in the performance of job duties
B. An employee loses a day of work due to the injury
C. An employee has work restrictions imposed as a result of the injury
D. A and B
E. B and C

5. The determination of a "safety-sensitive job" is the responsibility of

A. Health care professional or physician
B. Management or employer
C. Patient or worker
D. All of the above
E. None of the above

39

Toxicology

OBJECTIVES

- Review general toxicologic principles
- List the factors that characterize exposure
- Describe how the shape and slope of a dose-response curve can be used in the clinical evaluation of a patient with chemical exposure
- Explain factors that affect the absorption and distribution of toxicants
- Identify two major types of chemical transformations and factors that affect them
- Explain how physiologically based pharmacokinetics modeling is used to predict the fate of a chemical in humans
- Explain factors that affect the excretion of toxicants
- Identify standard animal toxicity testing methods (including the Environmental Protection Agency Harmonized Test Guidelines)
- Review advantages and precautions to be considered in the application of animal toxicity tests to clinical situations
- Discuss the use of Material Safety Data Sheets (MSDS) to obtain toxicologic information

OUTLINE

     B. Dermal irritation and sensitization
     C. Eye irritation
     D. Subchronic exposure
     E. Chronic exposure and cancer bioassays
     F. *In vitro* assays
VIII. Advice to clinicians
  IX. Appendix: MSDSs

KEY POINTS

- Toxicology is the scientific study of the mechanisms of action and effects of exposure caused by chemical agents in living organisms. Toxicologists identify the nature of health damage that may be produced by a chemical substance and the range of doses in which damage is produced.
- It is important to differentiate the toxicity of an agent (i.e., inherent property of a chemical) from the hazards (i.e., product of the toxicity and the conditions of use and exposure).
- The basic laws of toxicology include the following: Paracelsus—the dose makes the poison; Paré—chemicals produce specific effects; and biology—humans are animals and share some of the toxicity seen in animals.
- The major routes by which toxic agents gain access to the body are by inhalation (through the lungs); absorption (through the skin); or ingestion (through the gastrointestinal tract). The rate of absorption varies by route of exposure, with inhalation being the most rapid and dermal being the slowest.
- The amount or dose needed to produce an adverse effect varies considerably among materials. Key elements in assessing the degree of human risk for any given chemical are the amount and route of exposure, the absorption, and the metabolism of the substance.
- Toxic effects of a chemical agent in humans or animal models are not produced unless the agent or its metabolites reach appropriate receptors in the body at a concentration and for a length of time sufficient to initiate the toxic manifestations. The most important factors influencing this critical event are the physical properties of the agent, the route of exposure, the dose, and the duration of exposure.
- Dose-response curves have three characteristics important for the understanding of the potential health effects of a chemical agent: (a) the shape of the curve, which determines how an animal responds; (b) the slope, which determines the potency, measured in terms of increased response rate per unit increase in dose; and (c) the threshold, if any, which determines if a safe level of exposure can occur.
- Chronic exposures generally produce more toxic or cumulative toxicity than single exposures.
- Factors that influence the concentration of toxic materials that reach a receptor site include the rate and amount of chemical absorbed; the distribution of the toxicant within the body; the rate of metabolism or biochemical transformation, if any; and the rate of excretion of the toxicant or its metabolites.
- After absorption, the distribution of a chemical toxicant occurs through the bloodstream. Distribution depends principally on the ability of the chemical to pass through the cell membranes of the various tissues of the body and the affinity of the various tissues for the chemical.

- The blood-brain barrier limits the number of lipid-soluble, non–protein-bound, non-ionized molecules. The fetus is more susceptible because of an undeveloped blood-brain barrier. The fetus is also more susceptible to chemicals that freely pass through the placenta.
- Metabolism or chemical transformation of compounds occurs through two basic mechanisms: phase I reactions, which are catalyzed by mitochondrial cytochrome P450 enzymes that introduce oxygen into the chemical through oxidation, reduction, or hydrolysis, and phase II reactions, which are driven by soluble enzymes that produce a variety of conjugates, including sulfates, acetates, glucuronides, and glutathione.
- A number of factors influence the rate of biotransformation. These include differences in age, nutritional status, sex, species, and strain of animal and whether there is an underlying disease.
- Toxicants are primarily eliminated from the body through the kidney, but the liver and biliary systems, the lungs, sweat, tears, and even breast milk can excrete chemicals from the body.
- Two fundamental assumptions underlie all animal toxicity testing: (a) effects produced by the compound in laboratory animals are often the same as the effects observed in humans and (b) the rate of adverse health effects increases as the dose or exposure increases. There are many exceptions to these assumptions.
- Acute animal toxicity studies are used to determine the median lethal dose (LD_{50}) for a chemical. Table 39.1 shows a relative toxicity rating based on the LD_{50}.
- Subchronic exposure studies are used to evaluate and characterize the potential toxicity of a compound when administered to experimental animal on a daily basis over a period of 3 to 4 months.
- *In vitro* toxicology assays use cell cultures and bacterial systems outside the living animal. These assays provide a rapid and relatively inexpensive means of identifying mutagenicity and a material's ability to damage DNA. The most widely used bacterial test system for identifying mutagenicity is the *Salmonella typhimurium* microsome test, commonly called the Ames assay. Other *in vitro* assays include mouse lymphoma (L5178Y), the Chinese hamster ovary (CHO), and the hamster fibroblast (V70) tests.
- An understanding of toxicologic principles and testing methods can assist the physician in the evaluation of patients who have symptoms or illness that are possibly caused by an occupational exposure. A detailed occupational history helps assess the degree and nature of the individual's exposure, as well as the agent, the degree of exposure, and the duration of exposure. The MSDS, if available, can provide important information.

QUESTIONS

*1. Which one of the following is **incorrect**?*

A. Toxicology is the scientific study of mechanisms of action and effects of exposure caused by chemical agents in living organisms.

B. The main objective of toxicology is to characterize the potential hazards of exposure to specific agents and to estimate the probability of adverse effects at a specified dose.

C. Toxic effects seen in animal studies serve as models for human health effects and are predictive of human health effects in almost all cases.

D. That the dose makes the poison and agents produce specific effects are two of the most important laws or concepts in toxicology.

2. Which one of the following is **incorrect?**

A. Lipid-soluble chemicals are more readily absorbed across membranes than water-soluble or ionized chemicals.
B. The stratum corneum is the primary anatomic barrier to dermal absorption.
C. The fetus has a well-developed blood-brain barrier protecting it from absorbing toxic chemicals through the placenta.
D. The most common routes of exposure in the workplace are inhalation, followed by dermal absorption, followed by ingestion.

3. Which one of the following statements about animal toxicity tests is **incorrect?**

A. Acute toxicity tests can determine acute toxic effects, as well as the concentration or dose likely to be lethal to 50% of animals.
B. Subchronic toxicity tests usually involve administering a test chemical, usually for several months.
C. Chronic toxicity tests involve exposing the test animals to the test compound for their lifetime (usually at least 2 years).
D. *In vitro* assays are slow and relatively expensive ways to determine mutagenicity.

4. Identify the **incorrect** characteristic of dose-response curves

A. Characteristics are independent of the test animal and the route of exposure.
B. The shape of the curve
C. The slope of the curve
D. The presence of a threshold

5. Identify the **incorrect** statement

A. An inhalation dose can be calculated as a product of the concentration of the airborne agent times the exposure duration times the ventilation or breathing rate.
B. Detoxification reactions always transform a toxic agent to a less toxic, water-soluble metabolite.
C. The rate of excretion of an ionized urinary metabolite is affected by the urine pH.
D. The most important thing that a clinician can do when evaluating a potential toxic condition in a worker is to ask the questions "Where do you work?" and "What is your job?"

=40=
Epidemiology and Biostatistics

OBJECTIVES

- State the characteristics of epidemiology that distinguish it from other perspectives
- Discuss the shortcomings of epidemiology
- Explain the characteristics of the major observational epidemiologic study designs
- Discuss the application of biostatistics in epidemiologic studies
- Discuss major factors that affect interpretation of epidemiologic studies, including causation

OUTLINE

KEY POINTS

- Epidemiology is the study of distribution and determinants of disease in human populations. The fundamental goal of these investigations is to obtain valid and reasonably precise estimates of exposure-disease associations in groups.
- Epidemiologic studies measure the risk of disease directly in human populations. There is no need to rely on questionable extrapolations across animal species to estimate the impact of an exposure in humans. It is possible in epidemiology to examine the consequences of an occupational or environmental exposure in the manner in which it actually occurs in humans, not the artificial manner in which laboratory studies of animals are done. The issues of dose, route of exposure, concomitant exposures, and host factors are also directly assessed.
- Shortcomings of the epidemiologic method include the following: (a) low-level risks are difficult to detect; (b) the long latency period of most chronic diseases make detection of exposure-disease associations quite difficult and render timely evaluation of new agents virtually impossible; (c) there are often many concurrent exposures, which can be difficult to disentangle; and (d) there is an inability to control for unknown confounding in the data.
- The most common type of study in occupational epidemiology is the *cohort study*, in which information on exposure to a factor or factors of interest is collected in a defined population that is followed over time for the occurrence of a disease (or diseases). The disease rate among those exposed is compared with the rate among nonexposed to assess if there is an association between the study factor and disease.
- The *prospective* study takes a long time to complete because investigators have to wait sometimes for years before acquiring enough cases of disease or death. A *retrospective* cohort study may be used to eliminate this long follow-up period. Past records of individuals are used to characterize the exposure status of the study subjects, and the disease status is determined until a particular date.
- The major methodologic advantage of the cohort design is that information on exposure is recorded before the development of disease. This eliminates recall bias.
- The *case-control* study examines two groups. One group consists of people with a particular disease, and the other consists of those from the source population or study base without the disease. From each person in the two groups, information regarding past exposures and habits is obtained. If a larger proportion of cases than controls report the exposure of interest, an association between the exposure and disease can be said to exist. Case-control studies are more efficient and suitable for the study of rare diseases and diseases with long latency periods.
- In a *cross-sectional* study, people are selected regardless of exposure or disease status. Often, this study design is called a survey or prevalence study.
- The number of subjects needed to assess the potential exposure-disease relationship is a fundamental issue when planning a study. The larger the sample size, the greater the power to detect a specified difference in risk. The *power* of a study is the probability of finding an association of a given magnitude between an exposure and a disease when, in fact, it exists.
- *Chance variation* refers to the natural variation in health outcomes observed among similarly exposed individuals. Two statistical tools used for assessing the role of chance are the *p* value and the *confidence interval*. The *p* value is the probability of obtaining by chance alone a difference in disease rates between the exposed and unexposed as large as or more extreme than what was observed. A *p* value of .005 means that the

[handwritten margin notes:]
RR (Relative Risk) can be calculated
(Odds Ratio) OR can be calculated (OR estimates the RR for a rare disease)
Randomized study

probability of obtaining by chance alone an exposure effect as large as or more extreme than what was observed is only 5 per 1,000. Small p values (below .05) are sometimes referred to as statistically significant. The <u>confidence interval</u> gives the plausible values for the actual effect of exposure with a desired degree of confidence. For example, the 95% confidence interval for the risk associated with an occupational exposure is an interval in which the true relative risk will be included 95% of the time. A 95% confidence interval that includes 1.0 implies that a value of 1.0 for the relative risk is plausible, and the null hypothesis of no exposure effect is consistent with the data.

- The simplest statistical technique, the 2×2 table, is useful when occupationally exposed and unexposed individuals are followed for equal amounts of time for disease incidence.
- The most commonly used epidemiologic method that accounts for variable follow-up is the calculation of the disease incidence rate. It is calculated by dividing the observed number of cases of disease by the total person-years of follow-up.
- Sometimes, a study base or internal control group is not available. In these situations, it is necessary to rely on external comparisons. The observed number of cases in an exposed cohort is compared to the expected number using a set of known, standard disease rates. This estimate of relative risk is called the SMR.
- <u>Bias</u> or systematic error is usually a result of flaws in the study design or data collection. <u>Confounding</u> refers to the effect of an extraneous variable that may partially or completely account for an apparent association between a study exposure and disease.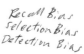
- A set of criteria or principles has been developed that is used when confronted with a possible causal relationship between exposure and disease. These include the strength of association, the presence of a dose-response relationship, the time sequence between exposure and disease, the consistency of the report with other studies, and the biologic coherence.

QUESTIONS

1. Which of the following is a significant shortcoming of epidemiologic studies?

A. Very small observed increases in disease rates for exposed compared with unexposed groups are likely to be accounted for by bias, confounding, or chance occurrence.
B. Reliance on animal studies
C. Inability to consider routes of exposure
D. Cannot estimate risk from observational studies
E. The exposures are more representative of laboratory conditions rather than real world conditions.

*2. Advantages of the cohort study include all of the following **except***

A. Information on exposure is recorded before the development of disease.
B. The cohort study provides a fuller picture of the health effects of the study factor because of the ability to look at more than one disease.
C. Recall bias is generally not a problem.
D. The cohort study is efficient for evaluating rare diseases.
E. The relative risk can be calculated directly from the cohort study.

3. Which one of the following statements reflects a cross-sectional study design?

A. Residents of Framingham are divided into smoking and nonsmoking groups. Thirty years later, the smoking group has an increased incidence of lung cancer and heart disease.

B. The work history of patients diagnosed with angiosarcoma of the liver is compared with the work history of persons with similar demographic characteristics who do not have this disease.
C. Americans have a high prevalence of heart disease. They also eat a high-fat diet.
D. Patients are randomly assigned to one of three treatment groups for high cholesterol. Drug A turns out to be the most effective treatment for lowering cholesterol.
E. Advanced diagnostic testing reveals a unique illness in a single patient. The illness has never before been described in the medical literature.

4. *What is the significance of having "1" in the confidence interval?*

A. The value of 1.0 means the null hypothesis (i.e., no exposure effect) is consistent with the data.
B. If the confidence interval is sufficiently large, the inclusion of "1" is not significant.
C. The risk of disease in the exposed group is much greater than risk of disease in the nonexposed group.
D. It means the null hypothesis can be rejected and chance ruled out as a likely explanation.
E. It means that the *p* value must have been set at 0.05.

5. *Which of the following is an example of confounding factor?*

A. The results of a study were significant but occurred by chance. Other studies have failed to duplicate the results.
B. A case-control study of a blue-collar occupation and bladder cancer fails to take account of cigarette smoking.
C. A study includes only current employees, excluding those who quit, died, or retired.
D. Patients who had a miscarriage recall environmental and occupational exposures in detail, whereas the control patients who had healthy infants tend to forget about their prenatal exposures.
E. Workers who had annual chest radiographs seem to have more lung disease than the comparison population, but the comparison population did not see the doctor as often.

6. *All of the following represent evidence of cigarette smoking causing lung cancer except*

(Note: These are hypothetical examples and may not reflect true numbers in the medical literature).
A. The relative risk of lung cancer in smokers is 9.0.
B. The risk of lung cancer increases with the number of years and number of packs smoked in a linear fashion.
C. The longest study of cigarette smoking was 50 years in duration.
D. Studies in China, Africa, and the United States have yielded similar results.
E. Cigarette smoke contains many chemicals that are known carcinogens.

=41=
Occupational Medical Surveillance

OBJECTIVES

- Explain the primary purpose of medical surveillance
- Identify factors used to assess the needs of a medical surveillance program
- List the characteristics of effective screening programs
- Explain the attributes of each of the phases associated with screening programs

OUTLINE

       1. Example of records based surveillance: ergonomics surveillance
    H. Cancer risk screening
  V. Collection of data
  VI. Interpretation of data
  VII. Interpretation of data to benefit the individual
    A. Example: nonspecific testing (e.g., liver function testing)
  VIII. Individual intervention based on results
  IX. Interpretation of aggregate data for the benefit of groups of workers
    A. Example: identification of overexposures and disease patterns
  X. Communication of results
  XI. Program evaluation

KEY POINTS

- Medical surveillance is the systematic collection, analysis, and dissemination of disease data on groups of workers designed to detect early signs of work-related disease. The primary purpose of medical surveillance is to prevent disease.
- To assess the needs of a medical surveillance program, factors involving the worksite, toxicity of materials, and program goals must be considered. Screening employees to identify work-related disease at an early stage involves a search for previously unrecognized disease or abnormal physiologic or pathologic conditions at a stage at which intervention can slow, halt, or reverse the progression of the disorder. Screening is a secondary preventive measure for the control of occupational illness. The screening test should be valid and reliable, treatment should be available, and the benefits of testing should outweigh the costs. Screening for noise-induced hearing loss is an example.
- In some settings, medical surveillance is designed to detect exposure rather than disease, such as after exposure to some heavy metals. Medical surveillance can also be used to determine a baseline with which future examinations are compared. Regulatory agencies such as OSHA require screening for certain exposure levels such as asbestos fiber exposure.
- Decisions about tests used for medical surveillance should be based on the relative toxicity of the substance, the extent of control measures, sampling results, work practices, and the usefulness of the tests themselves. Medical surveillance is not a substitute for primary control measures. The inclusion of unnecessary tests may lead to difficulties in assessing false-positive results, cause alarm among the well population, and needlessly increase health care costs.
- In biologic monitoring, tests are used to measure the extent of environmental exposures. A biologic specimen (e.g., blood, urine, exhaled air) is analyzed for the quantity of an environmental chemical or one of its metabolites to provide an estimate of a worker's chemical exposure. Biologic monitoring is more helpful in evaluating a hazardous exposure that a person may have experienced than in making a clinical diagnosis.
- OSHA regulates biologic monitoring for lead. Lead encephalopathy in children and peripheral nervous system effects (e.g., motor weakness) in adults may occur with lead toxicity. Lead inhibits hemoglobin synthesis and can cause anemia and renal disease. OSHA mandates that workers with blood lead levels (BLLs) at or above 60 μg/100 mL or whose 6-month average BLL is at or above 50 μg/100 mL be removed from exposure until the BLL is at or below 40 μg/100 mL. Biologic monitoring may be useful in mercury and arsenic exposures.

- Sentinel health events in occupational settings may trigger investigation into disease causality.
- In the occupational setting, a number of techniques have been attempted to screen for cancer. These include assessment of exposure to carcinogens, determination of onco-gene activation, cytogenetic monitoring, immunologic studies for cell surface antigens, cytologic morphologic studies, and clinical testing methods. These tests, however, have not been shown to be effective in evaluating individual patients.
- Minor abnormalities of tests that may be normal variants or may be due to nonoccupa-tional factors can be perplexing.
- The intensity of intervention for risk factors must be chosen based on the gravity of the disease and the ability of the intervention to be effective. The implications for worker's compensation and employer liability should be addressed. The reporting of some diag-noses may be mandatory. The physician's ethical responsibility to the worker must be the foremost consideration, and a physician (no matter in whose employ) must never withhold any information for fear of adverse effects on the employer.
- Analysis of aggregate data may reveal information that is useful for preventing occu-pational disease. There are several ways by which analysis of medical surveillance data can provide beneficial information to groups of workers, rather than just the person tested. These include investigation of the index case or case clusters, the recognition of temporal or geographic trends, and an association of clinical and laboratory results with exposure status. Medical surveillance analysis ideally includes observation of absence patterns that may represent an occupational hazard.
- Information about medical surveillance data may be directed to several targets: work-ers, management, worker representatives (e.g., unions), and government. Such results should be distributed in a timely manner and in an understandable fashion.
- Detection of a medical condition that makes work unsafe for the individual, the pub-lic, or coworkers cannot be ignored. Management is not entitled to specific medical information about an individual, but only the clinician's opinion about its implica-tions.
- Program evaluation includes structural analysis, performance audit, quality control, cost analysis, and outcome measurement.

QUESTIONS

*1. Which one of the following is **not** true of medical surveillance?*

A. It is the systematic collection, analysis and dissemination of disease data on workers.
B. It is designed to detect early signs of work-related disease.
C. It may be designed to detect exposure rather than disease.
D. It may substitute for primary control measures.
E. It can be used to determine an individual's baseline.

2. Which of the following statements about biologic monitoring is correct?

A. Tests are used to measure the extent of environmental exposures.
B. Blood, urine, or exhaled air is analyzed for the quantity of an environmental chemi-cal or its metabolites.
C. Data are not used to make a clinical diagnosis.
D. Blood lead testing is one example of biologic monitoring.
E. All of the above

3. *Which of the following is **incorrect** about lead surveillance?*

A. Workers with a BLL at or above 60 μcg/100 mL must be removed from lead exposure.
B. Lead may affect the peripheral nervous system of adults, causing motor weakness, and may affect the brain in children, causing encephalopathy.
C. Lead may cause anemia.
D. Individuals removed from lead work because of overexposure can be returned to the job after blood levels drop to 45 μg/100 mL.
E. Lead can cause renal disease.

4. *Techniques that show promise in screening for cancer in the occupational setting include the following:*

A. Detection of urinary mutagens
B. Cell-surface antigen detection
C. Cytologic morphology studies
D. Oncogene activation determination
E. All of the above

5. *Medical surveillance data can be used for all of the following **except***

A. Preventing occupational disease by analyzing aggregate data
B. Investigation of case clusters
C. Benefiting individual workers
D. Informing management about specific medical information about an individual
E. Detection of new hazards

=42=

Risk Assessment in the Workplace

KEY POINTS

- The workplace and the environment have always contained risks. Although accidents have traditionally been the most important risks, the vast numbers of chemicals now used in the workplace and found in the environment have increased the complexity of assessing risk. Risks associated with exposure to chemicals may be hidden and hard to detect. The effects of some chemicals may have long latent periods.
- By understanding the elements of the risk assessment calculation, the practicing physician can appreciate those parameters that can increase or decrease risk and provide appropriate guidance to individuals exposed to a variety of occupational and environmental hazards.
- The three-step approach to an individual risk assessment should include (a) an understanding of current and past exposure based on actual dose, if available; (b) modification of risk factors in the workplace through counseling, personal protective equipment, and engineering controls; and (c) a reassessment of the risks to provide the worker with input for determining acceptability of the risk.

- It is recognized that a physician rarely has the information or the time to perform a calculation-based (quantitative) risk assessment. Even so, there are numerous uncertainties in the assumptions involved in risk assessment, making it, at best, a rough estimate.
- A physician can use a table to explain the numerical results of a risk assessment to patients. This is based on comparing risks of death for one situation to the risk of death in another situation. The patient must evaluate the acceptability of a certain risk.
- Several strategies can be used to reduce the risk related to a certain exposure. As shown in Table 42.1, some reduce the concentration of the chemical and some reduce duration of exposure (per day and lifetime). Personal hygiene, personal protective equipment, and work practices may contribute to reducing the current hazard.
- Risk assessment is a statistical procedure employed by various regulatory agencies in an attempt to define an acceptable level of risk for exposure to a hazardous substance. The process uses scientific evidence from human (i.e., epidemiology) and animal studies to develop models to predict toxicity of various substances at low levels of exposure. Formulas for calculating daily exposure for different routes of absorption are listed in Table 42.3.
- NOEL is an acronym used to indicate a level of exposure at which there is no observed effect level.

QUESTIONS

*1. Which one of the following statements about risk assessment is **incorrect**?*

A. It is a statistical procedure employed by various regulatory agencies to define an acceptable level of risk for exposure to a hazardous substance.
B. It uses scientific evidence from human and animal studies to develop models to predict the toxicity of a substance at low levels.
C. Limitations include the reliability of data, extrapolating results from animals to humans, and the legitimacy of assuming a linear relationship between low doses of a substance and adverse health effects.
D. Regulatory agencies, such as the Environmental Protection Agency (EPA), generally assume that potential human carcinogens have a threshold of exposure below which no increased risk of cancer is predicted.
E. The classic dose-response curve is an S-shaped curve.

2. A worker is exposed to a volatile organic compound for 8 hours per day, 5 days per week. The work is characterized as moderate physical activity with an inspiratory rate of 2 m³ per hour. The airborne concentration is 150 mg per 1 m³. You may assume 100% absorption. What is the daily exposure for this worker?

A. 150 mg
B. 300 mg
C. 300 mg/m³
D. 1,200 mg/m³
E. 2,400 mg

$$\frac{8\ hr}{day} \times \frac{2\ m^3}{hr} \times \frac{150\ mg}{m^3} = 2400\ mg$$

3. What factors increase the risk of adverse health effects from a hazard?

A. Duration of exposure
B. Concentration of exposure

C. Body weight
D. Only A and B
E. A, B, and C

4. *For which route is occupational exposure the easiest to quantitate?*

A. Oral
B. Dermal
C. Inhalational
D. Either A, B, or C when personal protection equipment is recommended
E. All routes combined

5. *Concerning chemicals that are identified as human carcinogens, the risk of a particular exposure*

A. Has a direct correlation between animal data on a particular carcinogen (chemical) and the resulting cancer
B. Depends on the target organ
C. Depends on the genetic susceptibility of the individual
D. Both A and B are correct.
E. Both B and C are correct.

=43=

Ergonomics

OBJECTIVES

- Explain the fundamental principles related to ergonomics
- List risk factors and recognize limitations to their application
- Discuss the fundamental principles related to low back ergonomics (i.e., epidemiology, psychophysics, physiology, and biomechanics)
- Explain the basic principles of the revised National Institute for Occupational Safety and Health (NIOSH) guide and recognize its limitations

OUTLINE

KEY POINTS

- Ergonomics is a broad field encompassing biomechanics, work physiology, anthropometry, and man-machine interfaces.
- The field of ergonomics is evolving, and it may be necessary to reexamine theories and beliefs, so that current models used to analyze musculoskeletal disorders (MSD) are consistent with valid observations.
- Occupational physicians may need to understand ergonomic theories when treating musculoskeletal disorders, determining fitness for duty, performing plant walkthrough visits, or serving on an ergonomics team.
- External sources of stress on a worker are called stressors. The effect of such stresses on or inside the worker's body is called *strain*.
- Ergonomists characterize stressors and identify hazardous conditions by using a variety of tools to estimate exposure.
- Disorders of the upper extremity can be grouped into proximal and distal upper extremity disorders, which differ in epidemiology and pathogenesis.
- Rotator cuff injuries and glenohumeral joint abnormalities are the most common proximal upper extremity disorders. Although there are multiple theories of pathogenesis (e.g., impaired healing, ischemia, impingement, static tensile loading), there are no exposure assessment tools with demonstrated ability to identify jobs that are or are not associated with increased risk of proximal upper extremity disorders.
- Complaints in the upper extremity can be categorized as muscle-tendon disorders (e.g., tendon entrapment, peritendinitis, epicondylitis) or disorders of the nervous system (e.g., CTS, cervical spondylosis).
- In general, disorders of the muscle-tendon unit are much more common than CTS. When CTS is suspected to be work related, it is almost always associated with muscle-tendon unit disorders in the same individual or among other workers performing the same job.
- Tendon entrapments in the dorsal wrist compartment (e.g., de Quervain's tenosynovitis) present with pain localized to the affected compartment worsened with firm palpation or loading (i.e., stretching or contraction) of the affected tendons.
- Lateral epicondylitis (i.e., tennis elbow) is associated with collagen degeneration within the tendon and disorganized repair, which may be due microscopic tears of the extensor carpi radialis brevis.
- Peritendinitis presents as an acute inflammatory condition with pain, redness, swelling, tenderness, and dysfunction of the extensor side of the distal forearm.

- CTS produces numbness or tingling (i.e., paresthesia) in the thumb, index, middle, and part of the ring finger due to compression of the median nerve.
- Proposed models to assess exposure from distal upper extremity musculoskeletal hazards include (a) generic risk factors, (b) the TLV for the HAL, and (c) the SI.
- Generic risk factors (i.e., repetitiveness, forcefulness, pinch grasp, awkward posture, localized mechanical compression, vibration, gloves, and cold temperature), when studied, demonstrate marginal to no predictive validity for the identification of jobs with or without a history of workers with distal upper extremity morbidity.
- The TLV for the HAL is based on epidemiologic, psychophysical, and biomechanical studies. It has two components: average HAL and peak hand force. The predictive validity of this method has not been reported.
- The SI relies of the measurement of six task variables (i.e., magnitude or intensity, duration, and frequency of hand exertions; hand-wrist posture, speed of work, and duration of tasks per day) to provide an SI score. The predictive validity of the SI has been established for some industries.
- Low back pain is a common condition. Annually, approximately 10% to 17% of adults have an episode, and 2% of all employees will have a compensable back injury. This problem accounts for 21% of all workplace injuries and illnesses, and 33% of workers' compensation payments.
- Overexertion is considered the most common cause of low back pain, but the exact anatomic cause and underlying pathophysiology of most forms is unclear.
- Most studies of the biomechanical basis for low back pain examine characteristics of lumbar motion segments (i.e., two vertebral bodies and the intervening disk, with or without intact posterior elements).
- The biomechanical models related to the lower back are primarily used to estimate compressive force on the lumbar intervertebral disks. At high levels of disk compression, cartilage end-plate fractures occur that, if accumulated, impair hydration of the disk and lead to a permanent loss of disk height. This is the beginning of disk degeneration.
- Psychophysical criteria refer to strength requirements in relation to strength capability. When requirements exceed capability, the worker is at risk for an overexertion injury. There are several ways to measure back or lifting strength: isometrics, isokinetics, maximum acceptable weight, etc. Maximum acceptable weight may be especially useful for job design.
- A physiologic model related to the lower back is called the energy expenditure model. It estimates the aerobic demand of a job that can be compared to consensus levels of acceptable aerobic demands.
- The NIOSH guide (or equation) for manual lifting is a job analysis tool that is based on the principle that there is an acceptable weight limit for a standard lifting location. The recommended weight limit for a job or task is calculated by multiplying the numeric values of six task variables (i.e., horizontal, vertical, distance, frequency, asymmetry, and coupling multipliers).
- Postural stress is another risk factor for low back pain. It refers to prolonged awkward postures, which lead to localized muscle fatigue.
- Strength demands may be assessed in terms of static strength with a two- or three-dimensional model and in terms of maximum acceptable weight using the Liberty Mutual tables.
- Workplace ergonomic programs should include six elements: hazard information and reporting, management leadership and employee participation, job hazard analysis and control, training, MSD management, and program evaluation.

- OSHA implemented an Ergonomics Program Standard in 2001, but it was rescinded within 2 months. Currently, OSHA is pursuing industry-specific ergonomic guidelines.

QUESTIONS

*1. Which one of the following statements regarding ergonomics is **incorrect**?*

A. Ergonomic theories are useful to the occupational physician when treating musculoskeletal disorders or determining fitness for duty.

B. Disorders of the muscle-tendon unit are more common than CTS.

C. Several exposure assessment tools have the demonstrated ability to identify jobs that are or are not associated with increased risk of proximal upper extremity disorders, such as rotator cuff injury.

D. Complaints in the upper extremity can be categorized as muscle-tendon disorders (e.g., tendon entrapment, peritendinitis, epicondylitis) or disorders of the nervous system (e.g., CTS, cervical spondylosis).

*2. Which one of the following is **incorrect** regarding upper extremity cumulative trauma disorders?*

A. Generic risk factors demonstrate marginal to no predictive validity for the identification of jobs with or without a history of workers with distal upper extremity morbidity.

B. The predictive validity of the TLV for the HAL, based on epidemiologic, psychophysical, and biomechanical studies, has not been reported.

C. Components of the TLV for the HAL include average HAL and peak hand force.

D. Work-related CTS is rarely associated with muscle-tendon unit disorders in the same individual.

*3. Which one of the following statements is **incorrect**?*

A. Complaints in the upper extremity can be categorized as muscle-tendon disorders (e.g., tendon entrapment, peritendinitis, epicondylitis) or disorders of the nervous system (e.g., CTS, cervical spondylitis).

B. Peritendinitis of the distal upper extremity presents as an acute inflammatory condition with pain, redness, swelling, tenderness, and dysfunction of the extensor side of the distal forearm.

C. Symptoms of CTS include numbness or tingling (i.e., paresthesia) in the thumb, index, middle, and part of the ring finger due to compression of the radial nerve.

D. Tendon entrapments in the dorsal wrist compartment (e.g., de Quervain's tenosynovitis) manifest with pain localized to the affected compartment worsened with firm palpation or loading (i.e., stretching or contraction) of the affected tendons.

*4. Which one of the following statements regarding low back pain is **incorrect**?*

A. Low back pain is a common condition that afflicts 10% to 17% of adults each year.

B. An estimated 20% of all employees will have a compensable back injury each year.

C. Lumbar motion segments refer to two vertebral bodies and the intervening disk, with or without intact posterior elements.

D. A physiologic model related to the lower back (i.e., energy expenditure model) estimates the aerobic demand of a job.

5. *Which one of the following regarding low back pain is **incorrect?***

A. The NIOSH guide (or equation) for manual lifting is a job analysis tool that is based on the principle that there is an acceptable weight limit for a standard lifting location.

B. Overexertion is considered the most common cause of low back pain, but the exact anatomic cause and underlying pathophysiology of most forms is unclear.

C. Strength demands may be assessed in terms of static strength with a two- or three-dimensional model and in terms of maximum acceptable weight using the Liberty Mutual tables.

D. Studies have demonstrated that postural stress is unrelated to low back pain.

═══44═══

Medical Center Occupational Health

OBJECTIVES

- Explain how the structure of the medical center environment shapes the scope of Occupational Health Services (OHS) and the risks of health care workers
- List the major components of a medical center occupational health program
- Discuss common physical, chemical, and biologic hazards in a medical center
- Explain common psychosocial hazards associated with a medical center

OUTLINE

2. TB exposure control program
3. Blood-borne pathogens
C. Prevention
   1. Human immunodeficiency virus (HIV)
   2. Hepatitis B virus (HBV)
   3. Hepatitis C virus (HCV)
   4. Infected health care workers
VIII. Conclusions
 IX. Additional sources of information

KEY POINTS

- Medical centers pose a variety of safety and health hazards for workers. Jobs have great diversity (i.e., those who provide direct patient care, administrative support staff, housekeepers, food service, plant operations, pharmacy, maintenance, and security). The employer must provide a safe and healthy workplace and, under the workers' compensation system, provide care for work-related injury or illness.
- When medical centers perform teaching and research, occupational exposures include animals, microbiological laboratory specimens, zoonoses, and a broader range of chemicals.
- OHS in the medical center are geared toward risk management, exposure reduction, and compliance with regulatory requirements. The Joint Commission on Accreditation of Health Care Organizations covers all facets of medical center operations and approval is essential. National Institute for Occupational Safety and Health (NIOSH) makes recommendations related to worker safety and health. Occupational Safety and Health Administration (OSHA) regulates medical center exposures through a range of workplace standards.
- Policies addressing human resource issues, confidentiality, infection control, and safety should clearly delineate the role of the OHS, which often serves as a liaison between administration and employee in legal and ethical matters. Physical inspection of the worksite and attention to work-related incidents helps with identifying hazards and overall risk reduction.
- Postoffer, preplacement examinations identify individuals with disabilities and, according to the Americans with Disabilities Act (ADA), may prevent an employee from beginning a job in which he or she is unsuited or allow for appropriate job accommodation. Screening for preexisting conditions, latex allergy, ongoing illness, or injury is a vital part of these exams. The OHS may evaluate measles, mumps, rubella, HBV infection, and chicken pox infection, for which effective immunizations are available. OSHA requires hepatitis B vaccine at no charge to at-risk employees according to the Bloodborne Pathogen Standard. OSHA also requires postvaccination hepatitis B titers for all at-risk employees.
- Periodic medical surveillance is necessary whenever there is a change in process or personnel. OSHA standards are followed for surveillance of employees exposed to TB, noise, waste anesthetic gases, chemotherapeutic agents, ethylene oxide, latex, lasers, radiation, heavy metals, plastics, and solvents. OHS can be helpful in disability management, reduction of lost work time, modified duty, and managing workers' compensation cases.
- Physical hazards in the workplace are numerous and include musculoskeletal injuries (e.g., back strains, repetitive trauma), noise that may contribute to hearing loss, and the stress of shift work. Heat stress may occur in some areas. Laser exposure in operating

rooms may damage the eye from radiation or expose the worker to smoke plumes containing potential infectious organisms or toxic by-products of tissue combustion. Ionizing radiation from radioisotopes in diagnostic imaging and oncology treatments may cause health problems. There is a high incidence of violence in the health setting with aggressive behavior, assault injuries, and the physical and emotional consequences for patients, family members, and staff. OSHA guidelines suggest written policies to provide clear strategies about violence and to establish a task force of safety, security, and management personnel. Most OHS include Employee Assistance Programs to help employees and their families manage challenging circumstances.

- Chemical hazards in the medical center include anesthetic gases (e.g., nitrous oxide, halogenated agents) that are regulated by OSHA standards. Many different jobs (i.e., physicians, nurses, housekeeping, and maintenance) allow potential for exposure to hazardous drugs, such as antineoplastic agents. Glutaraldehyde is an effective microbiocide used for instrument sterilization. NIOSH has a recommended exposure limit and the American Conference of Governmental Industrial Hygienists a threshold limit value for glutaraldehyde. The American National Standards Institute (ANSI) and the Association for the Advancement of Medical Instrumentation provide detailed recommendations for worker protection. Formaldehyde (an animal carcinogen) and ethylene oxide (a human carcinogen) are two other OSHA-regulated hazardous chemicals used in medical centers. Elemental mercury is a component in dental amalgam, thermometers, and propulsive weights in dilators. Because of a multitude of nervous system and urinary tract effects, OSHA regulates exposure to elemental mercury.
- The use of laboratory animals in large medical centers poses unique risks from allergy and zoonoses. Allergy to latex products has escalated in the workplace. Allergic contact dermatitis involving the hands is most common, but systemic reactions such as asthma or anaphylaxis can also occur.
- A reduction of biological hazards depends on effective infection control and immunization of health care workers. An increase in TB during the 1980s has been attributed to the HIV epidemic, the homeless, prison inmates, immigration, residents of long-term care facilities, and intravenous drug users. It is complicated by emergence of multidrug-resistant pathogens. Foremost among biologic hazards are those associated with HBV and HIV. The OSHA Bloodborne Pathogen Standard provides strict guidelines for surveillance and management. The Centers for Disease Control and Prevention (CDC) provides a wealth of information on prevention, detection, and management of HBV, HIV, and HCV.
- Health care workers infected by HBV, HIV, or HCV also suffer from job discrimination, the potential threat of transmitting the virus to family or patients, the potential loss of their career, discrimination by insurance companies, and the stigma related to the disease.

QUESTIONS

*1. Which of the following is an **incorrect** statement regarding medical center occupational health programs?*

A. Hazard assessment involves physical inspection of patient and nonpatient care areas.
B. Certain work needs to be periodically evaluated as part of a medical surveillance program.
C. Monitoring of airborne contaminants is usually unnecessary.

D. Hazard assessment is an important step in program development.

E. Hazard control strategies include engineering and work practice controls and the use of personal protective equipment.

2. *Which of the following statements is **incorrect** concerning biologic hazards in a medical center?*

A. OSHA's Bloodborne Pathogens Standard specifically targets the prevention of HBV and HIV infection in health care workers.

B. Effective immunization programs for health care workers can help to prevent adverse reproductive outcomes.

C. A suspicion of latex allergy can be assessed by measurement of immunoglobulin E (IgE) antibodies or radioallergosorbent test (RAST).

D. A major component of a tuberculosis control program is the TB skin test.

E. OSHA has no standards for biologic hazards for health care workers.

3. *Which of the following is a true statement about OHS management of TB?*

A. Every medical center should develop a TB exposure control plan based on traditional principles.

B. Employees who have previously had a positive TB skin test should receive a skin test at the time of hire and at least at 12-month intervals.

C. Employees with a history of negative skin test results should not be skin tested.

D. People who have been immunized with BCG should not be skin tested.

E. TB skin testing should not be done more frequently than once per year.

4. *Which one of the following is most correct regarding chemical and physical hazards in a medical center?*

A. Exposure of operating room personnel to waste anesthetic gases is readily controlled by use of proper respirators.

B. Because the duration and degree of exposure to antineoplastic agents are short and relatively low, medical surveillance is not indicated.

C. Good work practice is the most efficient way to control ethylene oxide exposure.

D. Manual lifting of patients is a significant hazard to some medical center employees.

E. The therapeutic application of lasers poses a minimal threat to worker health.

5. *Which of the following statements is/are correct?*

A. Risks of exposure to chemicals in a medical center setting are limited to skin irritation, chemical burns, splashes into the eyes, and allergic reactions.

B. Large medical centers that provide research and academic services are exempt from OSHA regulations.

C. Preplacement examinations for new hires are performed in order to educate workers about safety and administrative practices but may not prevent an individual being accepted for the offered the job.

D. Vaccination is the single most effective step for prevention of HBV infection.

E. Employees with type I latex allergies are excluded from qualification under the ADA.

45

Fitness for Duty in the Transportation Industry

OBJECTIVES

- Recognize the importance of transportation fitness evaluations in protecting the driver, coworkers, and the general public
- Discuss federal and state regulations that impact fitness evaluations
- Describe the jurisdiction of the Department of Transportation (DOT), Federal Highway Administration (FHA), Coast Guard, Federal Railroad Administration (FRA), Federal Aviation Administration (FAA), Federal Transit Administration (FTA), and Federal Motor Carrier Safety Administration (FMCSA)
- Illustrate the physical requirements of the DOT and for a commercial driver's license (CDL), and criteria involving interstate and intrastate licenses
- Provide guidelines for the medical qualification of drivers with various health problems

OUTLINE

I. Highway: FMCSA physical requirements for commercial drivers
   A. Vision
   B. Hearing
   C. Diabetes
   D. Epilepsy
   E. Loss of arm, foot or leg or impairment of hand, finger, arm, foot or leg or other limb defect
   F. Cardiac disease
   G. Pulmonary and allergic disease
   H. Hypertension
   I. Arthritic, rheumatic, orthopedic, muscular, neuromuscular, or vascular diseases
   J. Psychiatric disorders
   K. Drug use or alcoholism
II. Maritime: Coast Guard
III. Railroad: FRA
IV. Aviation: FAA
V. Transit: FTA
VI. Other concerns

KEY POINTS

- A fitness for duty evaluation in the transportation industry is designed to protect not only the examinee or employee, but also coworkers and the general public. Safety-sensitive positions have clearly defined federally mandated medical standards (i.e., hearing, vision, blood pressure, blood sugar, seizure disorders, stroke, and medication use).
- Fitness evaluations are subject to the Americans with Disabilities Act (ADA), but where regulated standards exist, these are not overridden by the ADA. Ensuring public safety is key consideration in court decisions and upheld in the Supreme Court for a company's right to have more stringent standards than the federal requirements.
- The DOT examination encompasses railroad, aviation, pipeline, transit, maritime, and other agencies. The commonly called DOT medical examination performed in many occupational medicine practices is for commercial driver medical fitness. The FMSCA was created in 1999 to oversee highway safety and reports directly to the secretary of the DOT.
- To determine an individual's ability to safely perform a job, the physician must first identify the key tasks. These include but are not limited to entering or exiting the cab, loading or unloading freight, and working with "securement"' devices (i.e., hookups, hitches, and tiedowns). A driver's ability to work with the stress of adverse weather conditions, noise, vibration, hazardous materials, long absences from home, and irregular schedules are major considerations for the medical examiner. Such factors may cause an acute deterioration of a driver's underlying medical status and increase accident risk.
- Certification for a CDL is for no more than a 24-month period. The use of hearing aids and corrective lenses are the only restrictions examiners are allowed to place on drivers.
- The examination for a CDL is required if the driver operates a vehicle in interstate commerce with a gross vehicle combination weight or weight rating of greater than 10,000 pounds; the vehicle is designed to transport 15 or more passengers including the driver; or the vehicle is used to transport quantities of hazardous materials that require the use of placards.
- Testing for controlled substances is required to obtain a CDL for drivers of vehicles with a gross vehicle weight rating of greater than 26,001 pounds that is designed to transport 16 or more passengers, including the driver, or regardless of size is used to transport hazardous materials that require the use of placards based on Hazardous Materials Regulations.
- Most states have adopted federal standards for intrastate commercial driving, but they may have different criteria for medical certification. Carriers are responsible for ensuring a driver is reexamined if any health concerns arise during the 24-month certification period.
- Federal law permits a "licensed, certified and/or registered health care professional" to perform the CDL examination. Doctors of medicine, osteopathy, chiropractic medicine, and depending on the state, physician assistants and advanced practice nurses may perform these examinations.
- The 13 requirements a commercial driver must meet to be medically certified intentionally leave a great deal of discretion to the examiner. The FHA Medical Advisory Criteria of 1977 provided guidance to examiners to help clarify factors in determining driver fitness. In 1997, additional information was outlined in the Federal Register as Regulatory Guidance in response to specific questions to the agency. This outlined

questions concerning drivers with pulmonary, cardiac, neurologic, or psychiatric disorders.

- *The DOT Medical Examination: A guide to Commercial Driver Medical Certification* (Hartenbaum, refer to the textbook) is a current resource. Information is also on the internet at *www.fmcsa.dot.gov/rulesregs/medreports.htm.*
- Physical requirements for CDL where standards leave no discretion are vision, hearing, epilepsy, and diabetes, which requires insulin. Drivers must have central visual acuity of at least 20/40 in each eye and both, with or without corrective lenses. Monovision contact lenses are not acceptable. The driver must be able to identify the color of traffic signals (i.e., red, green, or amber) and must have horizontal field of vision of at least 70 degrees. Exemptions have been granted.
- The ability to hear a forced whisper at 5 feet can be used to screen for significant deficits. If a driver is unable to pass this test, audiometry should be performed. The range of interest is 500, 1,000, and 2,000 Hz, which are frequencies for speech recognition. A driver is qualified *only* if there is no average hearing loss greater than 40 dB in the *better* ear with or without a hearing aid.
- A driver may not be qualified if they require use of insulin to control their diabetes. There are no exemptions for insulin-dependent diabetic drivers. A driver not requiring insulin must be evaluated for blood sugar control; episodes of hypoglycemia; and any other effects of the disease on the nervous system, heart, or kidneys.
- Medical examiners may not qualify drivers taking antiseizure medication or to those with a seizure disorder that may cause loss of consciousness. The advisory committee recommends a 6-month waiting period and a complete neurologic evaluation before qualification. It is recommended that, after a single seizure episode requiring medication, the driver should not be medically qualified until he or she has been seizure free and off medication for 5 years. With a chronic seizure history, a 10-year seizure and medication-free period is advised.
- If the driver has a medical condition that is stable at the time of examination but may deteriorate or need maintenance, the examiner may certify the driver for less than a 2-year period.
- Drivers with limb impairments may be eligible for exemption if they obtain a Skill Performance Evaluation Certificate in addition to the Medical Certificate. The driver, with or without the carrier, must obtain this certificate by applying with their state's office of the FMCSA. An orthopedist's or physiatrist's assessment and a road test are also required.
- Drivers who have had myocardial infarctions should have a normal resting electrocardiogram and stress test before returning to vocational driving. Medications should be reviewed to ensure no impairing side effects. It is important to assess the current status and the natural history of the disease. Valvular disease and coexistent coronary artery disease are considered in the determination as to the risk of arrhythmias. Arrhythmias are the most likely cardiac disorder to cause sudden incapacity. Qualification of drivers with pacemakers is controversial. In general, implantable cardiac defibrillators are not compatible with commercial driving.
- Drivers on Coumadin therapy were not qualified according to the cardiac conference recommendations, whereas pulmonary specialists felt anticoagulants were not a disqualifying treatment. The FHA details recommendations on the use of Coumadin in a recent guidance report.
- Sleep apnea is becoming more recognized as a cause of motor vehicle accidents, and drivers should be disqualified unless this is well controlled and monitored. Cough syn-

cope should be disqualifying. Adverse effects of medications used to treat allergic and pulmonary diseases should be addressed for sedation.

- Qualification of drivers with hypertension requires their blood pressure is less than 160/90 mm Hg without the aid of medication. Drivers with a systolic measurement over 180 or diastolic measurement over 104 mm Hg should not be qualified. The advisory criteria for those with a diagnosis of hypertension and taking medication are subject to more frequent evaluation (annually if the blood pressure was in the mild to moderate range at the time of diagnosis). End-organ damage and side effects of medications are considered on an individual basis.

- Range of motion, strength, and coordination are examined routinely and used to qualify drivers with musculoskeletal abnormalities or complaints.

- To assess psychiatric disorders, the physician must consider whether judgment is impaired and the driver is able to maintain alertness, react appropriately, and if taking medication, is stable and compliant. If instability occurs, such as with schizophrenia and other psychoses, disqualification may be appropriate.

- The examiner may gather through history or by observation if the driver has a clinical "current" diagnosis of alcoholism or substance abuse. If so, the driver should be disqualified. If a controlled substance has been prescribed by a licensed health care professional, the examiner should alert their health care professional about to the nature of the driver's responsibilities and ask for a written waiver of the driver's ability to safely operate the commercial vehicle.

- Maritime or Coast Guard drivers follow medical standards specified in Title 46, Code of Federal Regulations Parts 10, 12, and 14, requiring individuals to be physically fit. Specific requirements for visual acuity and color vision for all and drug and alcohol testing for certain positions apply. Understanding the tasks and environment of the driver in the Coast Guard are important. Workspaces are cramped and often hazardous. The tasks may require heavy physical labor, emergency response, fire fighting, and launching life rafts.

- The FRA oversees numerous transportation jobs in the rail industry. Drug testing is required for all railroad employees. Only engineers are covered with specific federal medical standards. The Ishihara Pseudoisochromatic Plates or similar color vision tests are required as screening tools for engineers. If the engineer does not pass, further evaluation is considered. Employees with safety-sensitive positions may not require the use of medications (i.e., prescription or over-the-counter drugs) that may interfere with safety.

- The FAA requires designated Aviation Medical Examiners (AMEs) to conduct pilot medical examinations. These physicians (i.e., MDs or DOs) are selected based on their professional credentials. The Civil Aeromedical Institute's Certification and Educational Divisions provide guidance for AMEs and conducts ongoing research and training in aviation safety. Pilots may appeal disqualification through the Aeromedical Certification Division and the Federal Air Surgeon.

- The FAA also oversees the 20,000 Air Traffic Control Specialists (ATCS) who work with radar in airport terminals and flight service stations. They must meet the medical standards of FAA Order 3092.3A and the ATCS Health Program requiring examiners be senior AMEs designated by the FAA to examine traffic controllers.

- The FTA regulates public transportation. Bus operators require a CDL, and in general, they must meet the medical standards of the FMCSA. Subway and trolley operators are not covered by federal medical standards. The FRA regulates engineers of regional rail lines.

- The Department of Labor Report of Workplace Injuries and Illnesses in 1999 reported that transportation (specifically, air transportation) had the highest incidence rate within the service-producing sector. Highway crashes were the largest cause of fatal on-the-job injuries, and two fifths of the 898 fatalities in 1999 were truck drivers. Operator fatigue has been identified as a problem, but the National Transportation and Safety Board (NTSB) reports that this problem has only been partially addressed.
- Six major areas to address worker fatigue in 24-hour operations were outlined by Rosekind et al. and include (a) education and training, (b) hours of service, (c) scheduling practice, (d) countermeasures, (e) design and technology, and (f) research.
- Musculoskeletal disorders are a safety concern due to loading or unloading freight, repairing heavy equipment, and increased risk due to vibration and frequent lifting. Newer designs and engineering controls have been implemented.
- Transporting hazardous materials increases risks for spills, fires, and other chemical exposures. The risk of lung cancer has been studied in workers in the rail and trucking industry due to exposure while handling diesel fuel. Studies have revealed an increased risk of cancer among pilots and flight attendants. Cosmic radiation has been suggested as a cause, but the exposure relationship is controversial.

QUESTIONS

1. Which of the following statements concerning ADA is correct?

A. Fitness evaluations in most transportation industry employment settings are subject to the ADA.
B. These regulations override more stringent federal and state standards.
C. The Supreme Court has denied a company's right to have standards that are more stringent than federal requirements if the person has a disability that impairs activities of daily living.
D. There are no circumstances that allow job accommodations if a driver cannot pass a qualifying examination.
E. A driver may be qualified by the ADA if he or she has insulin-dependent diabetes.

2. Which of the following is/are correct concerning the DOT examination?

A. It is regulated by the FHA.
B. It is performed to determine driver fitness and encompasses railroad, aviation, pipeline, transit, and Coast Guard.
C. It has strict, well-defined guidelines, and to perform a qualifying examination, every professional must be aware of local, state, and federal regulations.
D. It requires carriers and employers apply with the Federal Motor Carrier Safety Board for certification.
E. All of the above are true.

*3. Which of the following statements about the commercial driver medical examination is **incorrect**?*

A. The examiner must base the determination on the driver's status at the time of the examination.
B. Examiners may not place restrictions other than use of hearing aid or corrective lenses.

C. Qualification for a CDL requires drug testing if the driver operates vehicles with a gross weight of greater than 26,001 pounds.

D. Federal regulations define a commercial vehicle as one that transports merchandise or paying passengers.

E. The driver must obtain a CDL if the vehicle is used for interstate commerce, is designed to transport 15 or more passengers, including the driver, or requires the use of placards for hazardous cargo.

4. *Which of the following is correct about the four areas that leave the examiner no discretion in the qualification of commercial drivers?*

A. The driver must have central visual acuity of at least 20/40 in each and both eyes, with or without corrective lenses, not including monovision contact lenses.

B. The driver must have a horizontal field of vision of at least 70 degrees in the horizontal plane unless they had a waiver before 1994.

C. A forced whisper at 5 feet can be used to screen for hearing deficits; if failed, the driver must pass an audiometric test.

D. A driver cannot be qualified if he or she uses insulin for control of his or her diabetes.

E. All of the above are true.

5. *Which of the following is **incorrect** about qualification for fitness for duty?*

A. To qualify, a driver with a history of a single seizure that required medication should have a waiting period of 5 years, during which there were no subsequent seizures and he or she is off all antiseizure medication.

B. Drivers with limb impairment may apply for exemption if they obtain a Skilled Performance Evaluation Certificate, an assessment by a physiatrist or orthopedist, and pass a road test.

C. Cardiac and pulmonary consultants agree that drivers taking Coumadin should not be qualified.

D. The American Heart Association and a recent review suggest disqualification of drivers with ventricular fibrillation, ventricular tachycardia, type II second-degree atrioventricular block, and third-degree blocks.

E. Sleep apnea is becoming more recognized as a cause of motor vehicle accidents, and drivers should not be qualified unless the sleep apnea is well monitored and controlled.

46

The Construction Industry: Its Occupational Health and Safety Experience and Needs

OBJECTIVES

- Recognize health and safety aspects of the construction industry
- Identify unique occupational exposures in the construction trades
- Review injury statistics of the construction trade
- Discuss a construction worker's education about workplace hazards
- Examine the morbidity (comorbidity) and mortality among the construction workers
- Explore how factors such as age, behavior, and the construction "culture" affect injuries and illnesses sustained by these workers
- Recognize the need for written injury prevention programs and the physician's role in this process

OUTLINE

KEY POINTS

- The construction industry, because of the admixture of trades, the frequent change of worksites, the variability in duration of employment, and the variety of tasks—maintenance, repair, and creation—differs vastly from other historic organizational undertakings.
- Age considerations are of interest because construction workers, as a group, are slightly younger that those of other industries.
- Injuries sustained on the job are more readily categorized because their occurrence related to place and time is much more obvious. However, the designation of an illness as occupational is less exact because such illnesses may take years to manifest and may be influenced in their development by nonoccupational factors.
- The construction trades account for 6% of total employment yet contribute 20% of the fatalities for this relatively small workforce. The incidence for nonfatal injuries per 100 workers is also higher than other industries when considering the relatively small size of the companies involved.
- Injuries sustained in construction do not differ clinically from many sustained in other industrial divisions, although certain body traumas are more prevalent.
- The identification of work-related illness is difficult because of the mobility of the construction craftsman from job to job, the late appearance of symptoms specific to particular toxic exposure, the lack of knowledge of the poisonous content of building materials by the contract employer and the worker, the transient nature of the workforce, and the constant pressure toward completion of the project.
- Construction workplaces are mobile, with the various craft members moving from job to job, having to adapt to new worksites and to different building contractors whose attitudes toward safety may vary widely.
- Construction workers are highly likely to bring contaminating materials to their homes by means of labor-soiled clothing, inadequate end-of-the-workday cleansing, and vehicular transport.

- Quality educational programs emphasizing work without injury or disease are sorely needed. A single training program is not adequate, because working conditions change as a structure evolves, requiring new materials, new heights, and the addition of different crafts personnel.
- Job satisfaction may be the only significant predictive factor for lost-time injuries due to low back disorders. This points up the necessity for occupational health professionals to systematically address *all* the causative factors that may be associated with back injuries in the construction industry, including lifestyle and psychosocial factors.
- Work assignments in construction require special preventive measures, and the employees so engaged should be involved in the design of the intervention mode, the determination of its use, and its field testing and evaluation.

QUESTIONS

1. Construction workers, as a group, require special consideration because

A. They are older than their industry component.
B. Work-related illnesses may take years to manifest and may be influenced in their development by nonoccupational factors.
C. The incidence for nonfatal injuries per 100 workers is much lower than other industries.
D. Regulatory compliance requires accepting older employees.
E. Construction workers are rarely exposed to chemicals.

2. Which federal government agency is responsible for tracking construction injuries and illnesses?

A. Occupational Safety and Health Administration
B. National Institute of Occupational Safety and Health
C. American Builders and Contractors Association
D. Bureau of Labor Statistics
E. None of the above

3. What is the most prevalent lost time injury among workers in the construction industry?

A. Amputations
B. Bruises and contusions
C. Fractures
D. Cuts and lacerations.
E. Strains and sprains

4. Work-relatedness of illnesses in the construction trades are difficult to associate because of

A. The late appearance of the symptoms specific to a particular exposure
B. The mobility of the construction workforce
C. Uncertainty about the toxicity of selected trade materials
D. All of the above
E. None of the above

5. *What is the most elusive consideration that must be made during the investigation of injuries on the construction worksite?*

A. Psychosocial
B. Ergonomic
C. Age-appropriate assignments
D. Failures in safety procedures
E. Contributions of weather to the incident.

47

Health Risk Communication

OBJECTIVES

- Describe the requirements and advantages of effective hazard communication and training to workers and employers
- Explain general types of training mandated by the Occupational Safety and Health Administration (OSHA)
- Describe the Hazard Communication Standard (HazCom) and its application in hospitals and workplaces
- Explain revisions in the Bloodborne Pathogen Standard and its implementation
- Explain the use and limitations of the Material Safety Data Sheet (MSDS)
- Describe the community right to know standard and role of the physician in the implementation of that standard
- Evaluate the effectiveness of health risk communication programs

OUTLINE

  I. Basis of health risk communication
 II. Health risk communication and regulatory requirements
    A. Mandatory and nonmandatory OSHA training
    B. HazCom
    C. Bloodborne Pathogen Standard
    D. MSDS
    E. Emergency planning and Community Right to Know Act
    F. Process safety management of highly hazardous chemicals
III. Health risk communication with OSHA programs
    A. OSHA posters
    B. OSHA partnerships
    C. Employee involvement in OSHA worksite consultations
 IV. Health risk communication and effective presentations
  V. Health risk communication and concerns with health and safety training
 VI. Evaluation the adequacy of warnings and hazard communications
VII. Necessary skills for risk communication
VIII. Summary of health risk communication

KEY POINTS

- An effective program of safety and health training for workers can result in fewer accidents and illnesses, better morale, and lower insurance premiums, among other benefits.
- The *HazCom*, or the Worker Right to Know Law, is a performance-based standard that requires MSDS, a written hazardous materials program, and training of workers on the specific hazards of chemicals found at their workplace.
- The revised Bloodborne Pathogen Standard includes provisions to control blood-borne diseases such as those caused by hepatitis B virus (HBV) and human immunodeficiency virus (HIV). New provisions require development of safer needle devices and a needle stick injury log.
- MSDSs are generally written for the worker and often omit medically important information required for a treating physician. Accurate information may require a telephone call to the manufacturer.
- The Emergency Planning and Community Right to Know Act of 1986, known as Title III of the Superfund Amendments and Reauthorization Act, mandates that every facility using, storing, or manufacturing hazardous chemicals make public its inventory and report every release of a hazardous chemical to public officials and health personnel. Every facility must also cooperate with physicians who are treating victims of hazardous chemical exposure.
- OSHA has issued a Process Safety Management of Highly Hazardous Chemicals regulation that requires every employee involved in operating processes to receive initial and refresher training on specific safety and health hazards emergency operations.
- Health risk communication programs, to be compliant with regulations, must be appropriate in content, language, and credibility to effectively motivate employees on the importance of compliance, both to the worker and the company. There must be time for meaningful questions and answers. (It is not appropriate to place a videotape in the VCR, leave the room, and come back at the end of the employees' nap.)

QUESTIONS

*1. Which one of the following provisions of HazCom is **incorrect**?*

A. It applies to all companies and employers that handle any hazardous substance in any form or amount.
B. It requires physician review of all medical aspects of the training programs and written procedures.
C. It requires MSDS to be provided by manufacturers to all users of hazardous chemicals.
D. It requires a written plan and a periodic comprehensive training program addressing hazards, health effects, safe work practices, first aid, emergency response, worker rights, labeling systems, and MSDS systems.

*2. Which one of the following provisions of the Bloodborne Pathogen Standard are **incorrect**?*

A. The employer must document exposures to blood-borne pathogens.
B. The employer is required to develop a needlestick safety program to reduce needlestick injuries.

C. Employees who are at highest risk are required to have hepatitis B vaccinations.
D. Employee training must cover epidemiology and symptoms of blood-borne diseases, modes of transmission, methods of recognizing high risk tasks, use of personal protective equipment, incident reporting requirements, and information on the hepatitis B vaccine.

3. *Which one of the following components of an MSDS is often **incomplete**?*

A. Long-term health effects such as cancer and reproductive outcomes
B. Listing of physical and chemical properties of the product
C. Listing of acute health effects
D. Listing of personal protective equipment and emergency procedures

4. *Select the most important aspect of risk communication.*

A. Content and vocabulary of the information must be appropriate for the educational, literacy, and language background of the employees
B. Employees must perceive the educator as credible
C. Educators must effectively motivate the employees regarding the importance of the information to protect their health and safety
D. There must be time for questions and answers
E. All of the above

48

Reproductive Hazards

OBJECTIVES

- List pathophysiologic mechanisms of interference with the reproductive process
- Evaluate human and animal studies on reproductive health effects
- List guidelines for continuation of work during pregnancy

OUTLINE

KEY POINTS

- Concerns about reproductive health are not limited to the pregnant employee in the workplace. Although adverse reproductive outcomes may occur as a result of exposure of the fetus *in utero*, they may also result from toxic exposures experienced by the male or female parent before conception occurs. Consequently, concern about the effects of exposures at the workplace on reproductive health is appropriate for pregnant women, for women of childbearing age, and for men.

- In 1991, the Supreme Court prohibited employers from restricting pregnant or fertile women from working in jobs that might injure a fetus and cause an adverse reproductive outcome. Instead, the Court placed the responsibility on the pregnant employee to decide whether to perform duties that might be potentially hazardous to the fetus. The Court placed the responsibility on the company to inform the employee adequately about potential health risks of the work activities.

- The response to concerns about reproductive hazards should cover four areas: the scientific literature on the substance in question, levels of exposure, safety control measures, and the specific concerns of the individual.

- In the male worker, interference with the reproductive process may occur during sperm production. In the female worker, interference may occur during the production or release of ova, the passage of a fertilized egg through the fallopian tube, or the implantation in the uterus. The embryo may be adversely affected during tissue differentiation or organogenesis. The fetus may not grow normally, resulting in malformations, spontaneous abortion, stillbirth, or premature birth. In childhood, subtle developmental effects may become apparent, sometimes years after birth.

- An agent or factor that causes physical birth defects or malformation of the embryo without producing toxicity in the mother is called a *teratogen*.

- Principles of teratology include the following: An embryo's susceptibility to teratogenesis depends on its genotype and on its stage of development; teratogens act on developing cells, causing abnormal embryogenesis; the outcomes of teratogenesis may be malformation, growth retardation, functional disorder, or death; the access of teratogenic agents to the target fetal tissues depends on the nature of the teratogenic agents; and the amount of teratogenic effect is related to the dose of the teratogen.

- There is a high background rate of adverse reproductive outcomes in humans. About 10% to 20% of normal conceptions result in spontaneous abortions or stillbirths. Birth defects are recognized in about 3% of live births, of which about two thirds have no known cause. Only 3% of birth defects have been associated with chemicals or drugs.

- In exploring the medical literature for guidance on a reproductive outcome question, the following are major points to consider: exposure levels, selection of controls, background incidence of events, reliability of ascertainment, multiple exposures, and the interpretation of the findings.

- Animal data can suggest possible human effects, although extrapolation to the human experience is problematic.

- Lists of chemicals associated with various adverse reproductive health effects may be found in the medical literature. Guidelines such as those from the American Medical Association Council of Scientific Affairs are available to assist the physician to determine the length of time into a pregnancy that an employee may continue to work performing various activities.

QUESTIONS

1. *Which of the following actions would be prohibited under a 1991 Supreme Court decision (International Union v Johnson Controls)?*

A. A company excludes all pregnant women from working in jobs that may involve exposure to lead.
B. An child who was injured as a result of parental exposure to a toxic agent in the workplace files a lawsuit against the parent's employer.
C. A pregnant woman is excluded from her job requiring use of a respirator because she failed the respirator clearance examination by her physician.
D. An employer implements a reproductive surveillance program to determine the rate of adverse reproductive outcomes among the employees.
E. An employer provides annual training on reproductive hazards in the workplace, including some general education about the reproductive process.

2. *A 25-year-old male worker comes to you with concerns about the effects of exposure to toxic substances on his current fertility. Which of the following would be of greatest concern?*

A. As a teenager, he applied arsenic-containing pesticides on his farm.
B. While he was working as a truck driver 4 years ago, some hazardous waste spilled on his pants.
C. Two years ago, he sterilized medical equipment using ethylene oxide.
D. Last month, he applied some pesticides around commercial buildings.
E. He might have had indirect exposure to solvents during his wife's pregnancy.

3. *Which of the following potential reproductive effects is **incorrectly** paired with the potential cause?*

A. Ionizing radiation/Decreased number of sperm
B. Lack of estrogen/Failure of the fertilized ovum to pass through the fallopian tube
C. Damaged blastocyst/Failure of the fertilized ovum to implant
D. Thalidomide during organogenesis/Congenital malformations
E. Ethyl alcohol during pregnancy/Impaired growth and development after birth

4. *What percentage birth defects are known to be caused by drugs and chemicals?*

A. 99%
B. 75%
C. 50%
D. 25%
E. 3%

5. *Which of the following would be most likely to cause you to question the scientific merit of an epidemiologic study on spontaneous abortions?*

A. The exposure level was determined from industrial hygiene monitoring.
B. Controls were matched for age, parity, socioeconomic status, smoking, and alcohol habits.
C. Cases were ascertained by self-report.
D. Workers were exposed to a single chemical hazard.

E. A personal medical history, including previous spontaneous abortions and presence of diabetes, was provided by each study participant

6. *Which of the following statements is true regarding animal data?*

A. Most compounds that produce reproductive toxicity do so at doses that are close to the dose that produces toxicity in nonpregnant adults of the species.
B. Because the concentration of the chemical in feed or water is precisely controlled in an animal study, the actual dose ingested is also precisely known.
C. The usual indicator for maternal toxicity is the dosage producing 10% maternal deaths.
D. The fact that experimental animals and humans may metabolize the chemical differently is irrelevant because the concern is reproductive outcome from exposure to the chemical, not to its metabolites.
E. In a well-designed animal study, any adverse effect on the fetus that reaches statistical significance is also necessarily biologically significant.

7. *Which of the following pregnancy-related conditions and workplace actions is **least** advisable?*

A. Backache responsive to postural change: Woman may continue working, modification desirable.
B. Working in extreme heat exacerbates a pregnant woman's heart condition: Woman may continue working only with job modification.
C. Pregnancy at term (40 weeks): Woman should stop work, regardless of job duties.
D. Woman has preeclampsia controllable by medical therapy and not exacerbated by work: Woman may continue working.
E. Job requires climbing ladders, woman is in her 29th week of pregnancy, and job modifications or job transfer are not possible: Woman may not work.

8. *Which of the following characteristics is most typical of an examination to determine the work-relatedness of an adverse outcome, as opposed to an examination to initiate treatment?*

A. A lesser degree of certainty is required than when initiating treatment.
B. The primary responsibility is the patient's welfare.
C. Total objectivity and a legal requirement of truth
D. Establishing a nonspecific, working diagnosis
E. Communication only with the patient, not with the employer

Answers to Chapters 37–48

CHAPTER 37 ANSWERS

1. The answer is C. (Ref: pp. 530–531)

The profession of industrial hygiene has as its main goals the recognition, evaluation, and control of workplace health hazards. Recognition of a hazard requires knowledge of the processes and the hazards of the materials used in the processes. A thorough grasp of these matters is essential as the foundation for a health hazard investigation. Reviewing the various hazardous materials used can reveal potential air contaminants. Reviewing the process can also uncover air contaminants that may be released as an intermediate or as a decomposition product in the chemical reaction. The decomposition products sometimes may be more hazardous than the raw materials.

After the type of air contaminant that may be released is determined, a sampling strategy can be developed that provides the information needed to evaluate the hazards. This approach determines whether the person is overexposed to any air contaminants and by how much.

If an overexposure exists or if there is a desire to reduce employee exposure, a control measure is then determined to bring the air contaminant concentration below the exposure guideline or to the desired level. Control can be implemented by controlling the contaminant at the source, the pathway, or the person.

2. The answer is D. (Ref: p. 531)

Gases are substances that are normally in the gaseous state at room temperature; in contrast, vapors are the gaseous state of substances that are normally in the liquid state at room temperature.

A fume is a solid that has been vaporized and subsequently condenses. In the process of welding steel, for example, iron oxide fume is produced.

A mist is a liquid that has been dispersed into the air as fine droplets.

3. The answer is D. (Ref: pp. 540–544)

Monitoring employee exposure to air contaminants is the most visible aspect of the industrial hygienist's job. After the sampling strategy is determined, monitoring is performed to assess the extent of exposure to an air contaminant. Monitoring can be done by obtaining personal or area samples. In personal sampling, the sampling device or equipment, or both, is placed on the worker to ensure the most accurate exposure determination. For area sampling, the sampling apparatus is placed in the vicinity of the worker performing the job.

Organic gases and vapors can usually be collected with an absorbing material, such as activated charcoal or silica gal. The absorbing material is contained in a small glass tube that is attached to a sampling pump, which draws a known volume of air.

Gases and vapors are usually reported in parts per million (ppm) units, a volume per volume measurement.

Dusts, including asbestos, coal, wood, and silica, can be monitored using a variety of instruments. The method used depends on the type of dust, the size of the dust, the permissible exposure limit (PEL) or threshold limit value (TLV), and the cost of the method (Table 37.1). The most common method is to collect the dust on a preweighed filter medium using an air-sampling pump.

The type of dust may determine the sampling method. Asbestos, for example, can be sampled with the filter method mentioned previously. The filter medium is not weighed,

TABLE 37.1. *Recognized exposure guidelines*

American Conference of Governmental Industrial Hygienists (ACGIH) threshold limit values (TLVs)
ACGIH biologic exposure indices (BEIs)
Americal Industrial Hygiene Association (AIHA) workplace environment exposure limit (WELL)
National Institute for Occupational Safety and Health (NIOSH) recommended exposure limits (RELs)
Occupational Safety and Health Administration (OSHA) permissible exposure limits (PELs)

as it is for nuisance dusts, but undergoes a microscopic analysis to determine the fiber count, rather than weight.

Respirable dusts, those of 10 μm or less in diameter, are monitored differently. In addition to an air-sampling pump, a cyclone is used to separate the respirable from the larger dusts. This method is used to monitor respirable dusts such as silica that affect the terminal parts of the lungs.

4. The answer is C. (Ref: pp. 540–541)

The permissible exposure limits are found in the Occupational Safety and Health Administration (OSHA) regulations in 29CFR1910.1000 and is defined as the concentration in air of a substance to which nearly all workers may be repeatedly exposed 8 hours per day, 40 hours per week, for 30 years without adverse effects.

5. The answer is D. (Ref: p. 543)

The concentration that should not be exceeded during any part of the working exposure period. Conventional industrial hygiene is practiced; if instantaneous monitoring is not feasible, a ceiling can be assessed by sampling over a 15-minute period, except for chemicals that may present an immediate irritation for even short durations of exposure.

6. The answer is D. (Ref: pp. 530–531)

The industrial hygienist, in particular, can offer valuable assistance to the physician who is asked to consider the health risks associated with certain work settings. The industrial hygienist, usually a graduate-level professional, can help in many areas but most often in the following:

1. Determining the need for medical surveillance or special examinations of workers exposed to particular materials
2. Evaluating whether exposure to an occupational or environmental hazard may have contributed to the development of an occupational illness
3. Determining the presence of potential offending agents and the adequacy of ventilation systems in outbreaks of illness, such as indoor air pollution
4. Complementing the efforts of a physician who has completed a preliminary plant walkthrough

7. The answer is E. (Ref: pp. 530–531)

Any of these methods can control or limit the exposure because the contaminant does not reach the person or its concentration is reduced. The most desirable approach would be to eliminate the hazard altogether, such as by replacing the material with a nonhazardous material. Controlling the hazard at the person by using respiratory protection is the least desirable approach because depends on the person's work habits. An enclosure, however, is desirable because it is independent of the worker's habits.

8. The answer is A. (Ref: p. 541)

The biologic exposure indices (BEIs), also published by the American Conference of Governmental Industrial Hygienists (ACGIH), are warning levels of biologic response to a chemical or its metabolite. These values may be of use to a physician in determining a dose to a worker because routes of entry other than inhalation may be involved. For example, blood lead analysis reflects the relative dose that the worker receives from all routes of exposure, including ingestion.

All guidelines refer to airborne exposures except for the BEI, which refer to safe biologic levels of the substance or its metabolite in body fluids or in expired air. Exposure guidelines can suggest to the occupational health professional how bad or good, in simplistic terms, a workplace exposure is. The TLVs developed by the ACGIH are updated annually and are meant to protect nearly all workers from adverse effects when they are repeatedly exposed to an agent.

9. The answer is B. (Ref: p. 543)

Equivalent exposure is calculated by summing the ratios of each individual contaminant concentration to its respective permissible exposure limit found in the Code of Federal Regulations (CFR) Part 1910.1000. The calculation is provided in (1910.1000(d) (2)(i) that in case of a mixture of air contaminants an employer shall compute the equivalent exposure as follows:

$$E_m = \frac{C_1}{L_1} + \frac{C_2}{L_2} + \dots \frac{C_n}{L_n}$$

$$E_m = \frac{C_{alc}}{L_{alc}} + \frac{C_{acet}}{L_{acet}} = \frac{600}{1000} + \frac{280}{400} = 1.3$$

In which E_m is the equivalent exposure for the mixture, C is the concentration of a particular contaminant, and L is the exposure limit for that substance specified in Subpart Z of 29 CFR Part 1910. The value of E_m shall not exceed unity (1).

10. The answer is A. (Ref: p. 532)

The objectives of the particle size selective (PSS) TLV is to identify the size fraction associated with the health effects of interest and to focus on the mass concentration within that size fraction in establishing a TLV. The potential hazard caused by chemical substances present in air as suspensions of particles or droplets (aerosols) depends on the particle size and mass concentration. This is important to worker health because the effects may vary on the level at which the particle deposits and the association of specific occupational diseases or conditions with specific regions of the lung.

CHAPTER 38 ANSWERS

1. The answer is B. (Ref: pp. 546–547)

However the role is organized, the purpose of safety programs is to assist management in reducing the risk of work-related injury and illness. Specific responsibilities include advice to management on ways to reduce injuries, illnesses, and accidents; coordination of interdepartmental activities, training, and collection and analysis of performance statistics; conducting research; and participating in health and safety committees.

2. The answer is C. (Ref: p. 548)

In the early 1980s, Occupational Safety and Health Administration (OSHA) began to evaluate voluntary compliance programs as an alternative to a chronically understaffed inspection and enforcement approach. One result was the Voluntary Protection Programs (VPPs), which are designed to recognize and promote effective safety and health management. In the VPPs, management, labor, and OSHA establish a cooperative relationship at a workplace that has implemented a strong program.

3. The answer is D. (Ref: p. 549)

Few employers have the internal resources to investigate unexplained clusters of illness or exposures to new or previously unstudied hazards. Health Hazard Evaluations (HHEs) are investigations conducted by National Institute for Occupational Safety and Health (NIOSH) epidemiologists and industrial hygienists in response to a written request to determine whether a substance normally found in the place of employment poses a risk to health. It is an option that a physician can suggest to management if there are unexplained patterns of disease that may be work related.

A typical HHE involves studying a specific operation or work area. The HHE also may evaluate other potentially hazardous working conditions, such as exposures to heat, noise, radiation, or musculoskeletal stresses. Based on the subject matter, NIOSH determines whether it is more appropriate for some other group to respond to the request. Sometimes, these requests are referred to state-administered programs that are available to perform workplace hazard assessments.

4. The answer is E. (Ref: p. 549)

If the injury or illness is work related, OSHA recordability will be triggered if an employee loses a day of work or has significant restriction of duties because of a work-related injury or illness.

5. The answer is D. (Ref: pp. 550–551)

The situation arises infrequently because individuals in safety-sensitive jobs usually recognize the risk created by their impairment (substance abuse excluded). The appropriate medical restriction is simply "cannot work in safety-sensitive jobs." The challenge is to ensure that the physician, the patient, and the employer all agree on the correct definition of a safety-sensitive job. As an example, the presence of frequent, heavy lifting in a job, although it may create an increased risk of back injury, does not make a job safety sensitive.

CHAPTER 39 ANSWERS

1. The answer is C. (Ref: pp. 554–555)

Toxicology is the scientific study of the mechanisms of action and effects of exposure caused by chemical agents in living organisms. The objectives of toxicology are to characterize the potential hazards of exposure to specific agents and to estimate the probability that such effects will follow anticipated types and levels of exposure.

For predicting human health effects, animal and *in vitro* testing are of uncertain value. Although many chemicals cause similar effects in laboratory animals and humans, there are also others for which animal testing failed to predict human toxicity. One example is arsenic, a known human carcinogen for which there is essentially no animal model. (Some studies have reported increased cancer in hamsters after instillation into the lungs.) A second example is thalidomide, a potent human teratogen with toxic activity not detected in standard rodent tests.

The First Law, formulated by the medieval physician and alchemist Paracelsus, states that the dose makes the poison: "What is there that is not poison? All things are poison. . . . Solely the dose determines that a thing is not a poison." The Second Law, attributed to the French surgeon Ambroise Paré (1510–1590), states that the effects of individual chemicals are specific, not general.

2. The answer is C. (Ref: p. 560)

Lipid solubility is of major concern because body membranes are high in lipid content; lipid-soluble molecules cross those membranes much more rapidly and efficiently than do lipid-insoluble molecules. Nonionized and less polar molecules are generally more lipid soluble and therefore more likely to penetrate lipid membrane barriers than are water-soluble molecules. The lipid solubility of chemicals is a useful predictor of molecules likely to be well absorbed.

Intact skin, for example, is an effective barrier to penetration because it consists of multiple layers, each with different physical characteristics. The outer layer is the corneum stratum, a superficial membrane of keratinized cells that prevents foreign materials from contacting living cells and serves as the principal rate-limiting step for skin absorption. Lipid-soluble agents can penetrate the corneum stratum, but water-soluble chemicals penetrate slowly and incompletely.

At the other extreme, fetuses can be more susceptible to toxicants than their mothers. The placenta is a relatively ineffective barrier to many types of chemicals, and many workplace and environmental chemicals are readily transported from maternal to fetal circulation. Simple diffusion appears to be the mechanism by which most toxicants pass across the placenta, but some chemicals actually concentrate in the fetus. For example, carbon monoxide binds more tightly to fetal than adult hemoglobin; after carbon monoxide exposure by pregnant women, fetal levels exceed those of their mothers. Fetuses are also more susceptible because the blood-brain barrier is not completely developed until after birth, and some chemicals can more readily gain entrance into the fetal central nervous system (CNS).

In general, uptake is most rapid and efficient after inhalation exposure, less so after ingestion, and least rapid and efficient after dermal contact.

3. The answer is D. (Ref: p. 564)

Acute toxicity studies are performed by administering a test material to animals on one occasion and evaluating any resulting toxicity over the following hours, days, and even weeks. These studies can determine the median lethal dose for a chemical (LD_{50}). An LD_{50} is defined as the dose that would predictably kill one half of the animal population experimentally exposed.

With appropriate modifications, the basic subchronic test can be used to evaluate mutagenesis, teratogenesis, and effects on reproductive capacity. Except for carcinogenesis and some forms of cytotoxicity, the subchronic test usually reveals most forms of toxicity to adult animals.

Chronic toxicity studies, used to evaluate a chemical's cumulative toxicity, often allow simultaneous consideration of cancer and noncancer end points. The bioassay is designed to assess whether test chemicals produce carcinogenic effects, which are often defined as any of the following changes:

1. The development of types of neoplasia not seen in controls
2. An increased incidence of the types of neoplasia occurring in controls
3. The occurrence of neoplasia earlier than in controls
4. An increased multiplicity of neoplasia in an individual animal

As a first approximation, it is assumed that chemicals capable of causing cancer in animals can also cause cancer in humans. *In vitro* assays provide a rapid and relatively inexpensive means of characterizing certain toxic effects, especially mutagenicity and DNA reactivity.

4. The answer is A. (Ref: pp. 558–559)

Most toxic chemicals cause multiple effects, some more harmful than others, and these effects may develop at different dose levels. For each, there may be different dose-response relationships. For example, chlorinated solvents at high doses may cause CNS depression, cardiac dysrhythmias, and hepatitis, whereas lower doses cause only reversible effects, such as induction of hepatic enzyme systems and liver cell hypertrophy.

A key aspect of dose-response curves is their shape. For many agents, response varies as a normally distributed function of the dose. A second key aspect of dose-response curves is their slope, calculated as the rate that adverse effects increase as dose increases. As a general rule, chemicals with steep dose-response curves require greater caution and controls than those that have shallow curves. A third key aspect of dose-response curves is whether responses occur at all levels of dose or only above some minimum level (i.e., the threshold).

5. The answer is B. (Ref: pp. 558, 562)

For inhalation exposures, dose is most simply calculated as the product: (air concentration) × (exposure duration) × (ventilation rate).

After systemic absorption, many chemicals are metabolically transformed by enzyme-mediated reactions occurring mainly in the liver and to a lesser extent in other metabolically active tissues such as the kidneys and lungs. The metabolic processes increase the water solubility of transformed compounds, which facilitates their excretion and elimination. It seems that such metabolic transformations serve an important detoxification role. However, not all transformations diminish the risks of toxicity. To the contrary, there are many examples in which specific enzymatic processes generate active metabolic intermediates that are more toxic than their parent compounds. Biotransformation of absorbed chemicals can lead to detoxification or to activation and greater toxicity, or both. The enzymatic reactions contributing to these chemical transformations are sometimes referred to as phase I and phase II reactions.

A variety of physiologic disturbances can alter the excretion of toxic materials. For many agents, urinary excretion is affected by urine pH and the sufficiency of blood flow to the kidneys. Diseases that alter normal function of renal tubules can increase or decrease urinary excretion of specific compounds, depending on whether those compounds are normally reabsorbed or secreted by the tubules.

Understanding toxicologic principles and testing methods can assist the physician in evaluating patients with symptoms or illness suspected to be the result of toxic exposures. In evaluating such patients, a detailed and comprehensive exposure history, both occupational and otherwise, is of primary importance.

CHAPTER 40 ANSWERS

1. The answer is A. (Ref: pp. 571–572)

The use of human populations, consideration of various routes of exposure, calculation of risk estimates, and studies using real world conditions are strengths of epidemiologic studies.

2. The answer is D. (Ref: pp. 572–573)

The case-control study is more efficient for addressing rare diseases. The odds ratio can be calculated from the case-control study, and relative risk can be calculated from the cohort study. The odds ratio estimates the relative risk if the disease under study is uncommon in the population.

3. The answer is C. (Ref: pp. 575–576)

Answer A describes a cohort study. B is not a cross-sectional study. C is cross-sectional; it includes simultaneous estimates of the prevalence of two conditions. It cannot provide a risk estimate but can be used to generate hypotheses. D is a randomized study. E is a case report.

4. The answer is A. (Ref: p. 579)

If the confidence interval excludes "1," we can assume that chance is an unlikely explanation for the results. Answers B through E are nonsense.

5. The answer is B. (Ref: pp. 578–579)

Answer A is an example of chance. C is an example of selection bias. D is an example of recall bias. E is an example of detection bias.

6. The answer is C. (Ref: pp. 579–580)

Key principles in interpreting epidemiologic studies:

1. Strength of the association. In general, the higher the risk estimate, the less likely the finding is a result of confounding or bias.
2. Dose-response effect. If the risk of the disease rises with increasing exposure, a causal interpretation of the association is more plausible.
3. Time sequence. The exposure or risk factor must precede the disease.
4. Consistency. Results from other epidemiologic studies of the exposure-disease association should be similar.
5. Biologic coherence. Does the exposure-disease association make biologic sense given what is known of the natural history of the disease?

The length of studies is not of particular importance, although prospective cohort studies are generally the most powerful in detecting an effect from exposure.

CHAPTER 41 ANSWERS

1. The answer is D (Ref: p. 582)

Surveillance should not substitute for primary control measures. Medical surveillance is the systematic collection, analysis, and dissemination of disease data on groups of workers designed to detect early signs of work-related disease. The primary purpose of medical surveillance is to prevent disease.

2. The answer is E (Ref: p. 589)

In biologic monitoring, tests are used to measure the extent of environmental exposures. A biologic specimen (e.g., blood, urine, exhaled air) is analyzed for the quantity of an environmental chemical or one of its metabolites to provide an estimate of the worker's chemical exposure. Mere detection of a chemical, however, does not imply the presence of a disease or of toxicity. Biologic monitoring data does not provide a clinical diagnosis but assesses exposure to a hazard.

3. The answer is D (Ref: pp. 590–591)

According to the Occupational Safety and Health Administration (OSHA) standard, individuals can be returned to work when blood levels drop to 40 μg/100 mL or lower. The OSHA lead standard requires blood lead level (BLL) determination and zinc protoporphyrin (ZPP) testing. ZPP levels are nonspecific, but may reflect long-term exposure to lead. OSHA mandates that workers with BLLs at or greater than 60 μg/100 mL on one test or whose 6-month average BLL is at or greater than 50 μg/100 mL be removed from exposure until the lead concentration returns to legally acceptable levels of at least 40 μg/100 mL.

4. The answer is E (Ref: pp. 592–593)

Although techniques such as oncogene activation determination, cell-surface antigen studies, cytologic morphology of cells, and application of spiral chest computed tomography (CT) have shown promise for cancer screening, other techniques such as cytogenetic monitoring have not proved valuable in the evaluation of individual risk of developing malignancy. Detection of urinary mutagens is the only assay that has shown reliability in following groups of workers. The measurement of adducts created by binding of carcinogens or their metabolites to body chemicals can provide a measure of exposure. Clinical testing methods such as colonoscopy and cytoscopy remain useful in detecting malignancies, although the stage is usually advanced.

5. The answer is D (Ref: p. 596)

Management is not entitled to specific medical information about an individual but only the clinician's opinion about its implications. The primary purpose of medical surveillance is to prevent disease. Medical surveillance is not limited to screening (in which the participant will on the average benefit). In some settings, medical surveillance is designed to detect exposure rather than disease. For example, biologic monitoring measures concentrations of chemical agents or their metabolites in biologic specimens. This type of testing may be useful for determining if exposure is occurring even at levels that do not imply the presence of disease.

CHAPTER 42 ANSWERS

1. The answer is D (Ref: pp. 602–604)

Risk assessment is a statistical procedure employed by various regulatory agencies in an attempt to define an acceptable level of risk for exposure to a hazardous substance. Risk assessment uses available scientific evidence from human (i.e., epidemiology) and animal studies to develop models to predict toxicity of the various substances at low levels of exposure. Limitations inherent in this process include the reliability of the data, the accuracy of extrapolating results from animals to humans, and the legitimacy of assuming a linear relationship between low doses of a substance and the adverse health effect. The latter problem manifests primarily in the evaluation of carcinogenic substances using information generated by U.S. governmental agencies, which do not recognize the presence of a threshold dose below which exposure to a substance is not a health risk.

2. The answer is E (Ref: p. 605, Figs. 42.2 and 42.3)

To perform relevant measurements and estimate an exposure, it is first necessary to assess the routes and conditions by which a worker may be exposed. Such exposure scenarios are usually specific to an absorption route, which may be oral, dermal, or inhalation. Inhalation estimates are the easiest to perform; by knowing the airborne level, one can calculate the exposure, as shown in Fig. 42.3. The air concentration is usually measured in milligrams or micrograms per cubic meter (mg/m^3 or $\mu g/m^3$). For the respiratory route, it is often assumed that there is total absorption of the inspired toxic vapors, although this is not the case for most substances. For an adult, air is inhaled at a rate of

Inhalation:

Daily exposure $=$ air level $\times$ $\dfrac{1-2m^3}{hour}$ $\times$ $\dfrac{hours}{day}$

Oral (Soil):

Daily exposure $=$ soil level $\times$ 25 mg soil/day $\times$ % absorption

Dermal (Surfaces):

Daily exposure $=$ surface level $\times$ 1500 cm² $\times$

fraction of day exposed $\times$ % absorption

(The simplifying assumption of concentration equivalence between of one-half the area of the arms and environment surface levels will generally lead to an overestimation of exposure.)

All Routes:

Lifetime Average Daily Dose $=$

$\dfrac{\text{Daily exposure} \times \text{days exposure/year} \times \text{years exposure}}{25,550 \text{ days/lifetime} \times 70 \text{ kg}}$

FIGURE 42.3.

TABLE 42.2. *Exposure factors that proportionally increase the calculated risk of cancer, assuming a linear-at-low-dose relationship*

For all routes
  Years of exposure
  Hours of exposure per day
  Concentration of toxic substance[a]
For dermal exposure
  Surface area of skin exposed[a]
  Length of time substance remains on skin[a]
For oral exposure
  Mouthing episodes from contaminated hands, cigarettes, food, and other sources[b]

[a]Reduced by personal protective equipment and work practices
[b]Reduced by hygiene.

1 m^3 per hour at rest and 2 m^3 per hour for moderately vigorous activity. An exposure estimate (i.e., dose) can be calculated by simply taking the product of the measured concentration and the air volume inhaled over a specified time interval.

3. The answer is E. (Ref: p. 602)

See Table 42.2.

4. The answer is C. (Ref: p. 604)

To perform relevant measurements and estimate an exposure, it is first necessary to assess the routes and conditions by which a worker may be exposed. Such exposure scenarios are usually specific to an absorption route, which may be oral, dermal, or inhalational. Inhalation estimates are the easiest to perform.

5. The answer is E. (Ref: p. 605)

Animal carcinogen risk assessment does not tell us the site or type of cancer that could be produced in humans, and we do not know if any cancer risk will be present.

CHAPTER 43 ANSWERS

1. The answer is C. (Ref: p. 609)

Rotator cuff injuries and glenohumeral joint abnormalities are the most common proximal upper extremity disorders. Although there are multiple theories of pathogenesis (e.g., impaired healing, ischemia, impingement, static tensile loading), there are no exposure assessment tools with demonstrated ability to identify jobs that are or are not associated with increased risk of proximal upper extremity disorders.

2. The answer is D. (Ref: pp. 611–612)

Carpal tunnel syndrome (CTS) produces numbness or tingling (i.e., paresthesia) in the thumb, index, middle, and part of the ring finger due to compression of the median nerve. In general, disorders of the muscle-tendon unit are much more common than CTS. When CTS is suspected to be work related, it is almost always associated with muscle-tendon unit disorders in the same individual or among other workers performing the same job.

3. The answer is C. (Ref: pp. 610–612)

See question 2. CTS is a disorder of the median nerve, not the radial nerve.

4. The answer is B. (Ref: pp. 614–616)

Low back pain is a common condition. Annually, approximately 10% to 17% of adults have an episode, and 2% of all employees will have a compensable back injury. This problem accounts for 21% of all workplace injuries and illnesses and 33% of workers' compensation payments.

Overexertion is considered the most common cause of low back pain, but the exact anatomic cause and underlying pathophysiology of most forms are unclear.

5. The answer is D. (Ref: pp. 617–620)

Postural stress is another risk factor for low back pain. It refers to prolonged awkward postures, which lead to localized muscle fatigue.

The National Institute for Occupational Health and Safety (NIOSH) guide (or equation) for manual lifting is a job analysis tool that is based on the principle that there is an acceptable weight limit for a standard lifting location. The recommended weight limit for a job or task is calculated by multiplying the numerical values of six task variables: horizontal, vertical, distance, frequency, asymmetry, and coupling multipliers.

CHAPTER 44 ANSWERS

1. The answer is C (Ref: pp. 625, 631)

Occupational Safety and Health Administration (OSHA) regulations exist for airborne contaminants. Environmental monitoring, as well as personal or breathing zone monitoring for airborne contaminants, should be performed where appropriate as part of the medical center's ongoing hazard assessment program.

2. The answer is E (Ref: pp. 636–641)

In 1991, OSHA published a new occupational health standard designed to prevent exposure to hepatitis B virus (HBV), human immunodeficiency virus (HIV), and other agents transmitted by contact with blood and other body fluids. The Bloodborne Pathogens Standard requires that employees with occupational exposure to blood or other potentially infectious materials be protected through a variety of measures as specified in a written exposure control plan.

3. The answer is A (Ref: p. 637)

Health care workers employed in urban medical centers that care for large numbers of tuberculosis patients are at risk of acquiring occupational tuberculosis infection. Every medical center should develop an exposure control plan based on traditional principles of tuberculosis control.

4. The answer is D (Ref: p. 627)

Manual lifting tasks are responsible for a high rate of acute and chronic back and musculoskeletal complaints. Studies have consistently showed that nurses aides rank in the top 10 occupations at risk for back injury as measured by the numbers of workers' compensation claims.

5. The answer is D (Ref: pp. 630–635)

Chemical hazards in the medical center setting include agents that may cause skin and respiratory problems, allergy, infection, and cancer. Ethylene oxide is a known human carcinogen, and formaldehyde is suspected of causing cancer in humans. Glutaraldehyde causes a multitude of health effects and has a potential risk of exposure by dermal, respiratory, and gastrointestinal routes of exposure. OSHA does not exempt research and academic centers. Employees with type I latex allergies may be considered qualified individuals under the Americans with Disabilities Act (ADA), although this question has not been fully tested in the courts.

CHAPTER 45 ANSWERS

1. The answer is A. (Ref: p. 649)

Industry and carrier standards may be more stringent than federal and state criteria if performing the job presents an unsafe condition to themselves, coworkers, or the general public. These standards do not change the Americans with Disabilities Act (ADA) regulations. These statutes have been challenged in the Supreme Court. Other than vision and hearing restrictions, the examinee may not be permitted to include restrictions on the commercial driver's license (CDL). However, there are occasions when waivers have been issued for close monitoring of blood pressure, medications, and other health problems that do not directly affect the driver's abilities to perform the job (i.e., fitness for duty). A driver may not be qualified for a CDL if he or she uses insulin to control diabetes.

2. The answer is B (Ref: p. 649)

The Federal Highway Administration (FHA) no longer regulates the Department of Transportation (DOT) examination. Since 1999, DOT has been under the authority of the Federal Motor Carrier Safety Administration (FMCSA), which answers directly to the Secretary of Labor. The guidelines provide some discretion for the examiner. Unfortunately, the health care professionals performing the examinations are not always aware of local, state, and federal regulations concerning specific health-related problems with which the driver may be afflicted.

3. The answer is D (Ref: pp. 650–651, Table 45.1, Fig. 45.1)

A commercial vehicle is strictly defined as having a gross weight or rating greater than 10,000 pounds; transporting 15 or more passengers, including the driver; and transporting hazardous material requiring placards.

Statement A is true; qualification of a driver is based on the health status at the time of examination. A history of stroke, epilepsy, or medications is considered. If the driver has a history of hypertension or non–insulin-dependent diabetes that is stable at the time of the examination, the examiner may choose to qualify him or her for a shorter amount of time to monitor the condition.

4. The answer is E (Ref: p. 651, Fig. 45.1)

All statements are correct.

5. The answer is C (Ref: pp. 653–655)

Cardiac and pulmonary specialists do not agree on the controversial subject of qualifying drivers taking the anticoagulant medication known as Coumadin.

CHAPTER 46 ANSWERS

1. The answer is B. (Ref: p. 664)

Injuries sustained on the job are more readily categorized because their occurrence as to place and time is much more obvious. However, the designation of an illness as occupational is less exact because such illnesses may take years to manifest and may be influenced in their development by nonoccupational factors. Age considerations are of interest, and construction workers as a group are slightly younger than those of other industries. The average age in 1996 was 37.0 years, in contrast to 38.0 years of wage-and-salary workers in all industries.

2. The answer is D. (Ref: p. 665)

Although the standard statistical base in the United States is the Bureau of Labor Statistics (BLS) of the Department of Labor, other sources may vary in the elements used in epidemiologic approach, rendering comparisons not always feasible. Work-related fatal illnesses are not included in this particular BLS census because the delay in the development of symptoms – or the latency of linking illnesses to work "make identification of a universe problematic."

3. The answer is E. (Ref: p. 667)

The 193,800 lost-time injuries were divided in the construction industry in this order:

Sprains, strains: 72,400
Cuts, lacerations: 19,700
Fractures: 19,100
Bruises, contusions: 13,900
Multiple injuries: 8,500
Heat burns: 2,400
Chemical burns: 1,900
Amputations: 1,400
Carpal tunnel syndrome: 1,200
Tendonitis: 800

Because the numbers shown in the breakdowns do not always approach the totals results from "the inability to obtain detailed information about all cases in the sample, mistakes in recording or coding the data, and definitional difficulties," nonsampling error results. Although the numbers of injuries shown are presented with some inexactitude, they still depict great losses in wages, health care costs, productivity, and personal hurt. Factors that influence the number shown are the level of economic activity, working conditions and practices, worker experience and training, and the actual number of hours worked.

4. The answer is D. (Ref: p. 672)

The difficulties with the identification of work-related illness include the mobility of the construction craftsman from job to job, the late appearance of symptoms specific to particular toxic exposure, the lack of knowledge of the poisonous content of building materials on the parts of the contract employer and the worker, and the constant pressure toward completion of the project.

5. The answer is A. (Ref: p. 674)

Although most physical and ergonomic causes of injury can be identified through adequate investigation and study, the identification of psychosocial causes is more elusive. Certain psychosocial elements or deficits in the lifestyle of construction workers have been explored in an attempt to explain the many injuries and illnesses among this group. It has been found that in the construction trades, there is a need for preventive measures directed toward alcoholism, respiratory tuberculosis among laborers and drywall workers, and accidental drug or alcohol poisoning among painters and drywall workers.

A 1998 study revealed a positive dose-response relationship between smoking and the rate of early retirement due to permanent disability in the construction industry. This finding describes the premature and avoidable loss of skilled personnel and points to the undue burden for society. A Chinese review found that a large proportion of workers who were injured in construction were smokers and beer drinkers. Although it was not demonstrated that smoking was the immediate cause of the sustained trauma, it was thought to have exerted an indirect effect by reducing workers' concentration, in addition to presenting a real risk of fire. Smokers, the investigators believed, risk their own health by smoking and have a general tendency toward risky behavior at work.

CHAPTER 47 ANSWERS

1. The answer is B. (Ref: p. 690)

This standard contains specific provisions regarding the evaluation of health hazards, labeling of containers, use of chemical information sheets (MSDSs), and training of employees. Also known as Hazard Communication Standard (HazCom), the standard originally applied only to chemical manufacturers, importers and distributors, but it was later expanded to cover many additional employers. All companies and employers that handle any hazardous substance in any form are required to comply with the standard. The following list outlines the basic components of the standard:

Manufacturers must produce a MSDS for all hazardous chemicals that they produce and sell.

MSDSs must be shipped to all downstream users of the hazardous chemicals.

In all workplaces in which hazardous chemicals are present, the employer is responsible for the following:
- Labeling all hazardous chemicals in the workplace
- A written hazardous chemicals program that is accessible to employees who ask for it
- A system for managing MSDSs with worker access to them
- A training program for all employees who may experience an exposure to a potentially hazardous chemical

The training program must include information on the following:
- Location and identity of hazardous chemicals
- Physical hazards
- Health effects (acute and long term)
- Proper work practices and personal protection
- First aid
- Emergency response (including fire, leak, and spill)
- Workers' rights under HazCom
- Labeling systems
- MSDS systems

2. The answer is C. (Ref: p. 691)

To achieve compliance, the employer must determine and document exposure. A written exposure control plan also must be available. The Bloodborne Pathogens Standard includes requirements for employee hazard communication and training, as well as management of regulated waste, contaminated laundry, and proper housekeeping procedures. Occupational Safety and Health Administration (OSHA) recognizes the benefits of prophylactic hepatitis B vaccine and therefore requires that the vaccine be available at no charge to employees at risk (i.e., those with occupational exposure to blood or other potentially infectious materials). The main points that relate to employee training include the following: (a) epidemiology and symptoms of blood-borne diseases, (b) modes of transmission of blood-borne pathogens, (c) methods of recognizing tasks that involve exposure to blood or other potentially infectious materials, (d) methods to prevent exposure including personal protective equipment, (e) information on appropriate action after an exposure incident, and (f) information on the hepatitis B vaccine.

On November 6, 2000, Congress passed the Needlestick Safety and Prevention Act directing OSHA to revise its Bloodborne Pathogens Standard to describe in greater detail its requirement for employers to identify and make use of effective and safer medical devices.

3. The answer is A. (Ref: p. 692)

The MSDSs provide workers with enough information about a specific chemical substance to understand (a) potential acute and chronic health effects; (b) recommended personal protective equipment; (c) proper work practices; (d) first aid treatment after exposure; (e) spill, leak, and fire precautions and appropriate responses; and (f) other information that may be necessary to work safely with the potentially hazardous substance (4). The physician treating a patient with an exposure identified on the MSDS should realize that the information contained in the document may be incomplete. Some chemicals may not be listed at all, and the broad class of materials to which they belong may identify others. In some cases, it is necessary to contact the manufacturer listed on the MSDS to obtain additional information. An example of MSDS variability is highlighted in a study that analyzed reproductive health hazard descriptions on almost 700 MSDSs for lead- or ethylene glycol ether–containing products submitted by Massachusetts companies to the Department of Environmental Protection under provisions of the Massachusetts Right to Know Law. More than 60% of the MSDSs made no mention of potential effects of these chemicals on the human reproductive system. Those that did mention these adverse effects were much more likely to address fetal development risks and omit any male reproductive effects.

4. The answer is E. (Ref: p. 695)

OSHA is concerned that training information presented be understood by the employee; otherwise, the training will not be effective. Employers must include training material that is appropriate in content and vocabulary to the educational, literacy, and language background of employees. This ensures that all employees, regardless of their cultural or education backgrounds, will receive adequate training on how to eliminate or minimize their occupational exposure.

Training sessions should be designed so that sufficient time is allocated to present the information and to allow for questions and review of materials as needed. The trainer needs to provide an environment in which participants feel sufficiently comfortable to ask questions and make comments. Asking questions and discussing aspects of a training program can clarify information and reinforce important learning objectives. The effectiveness of warnings and risk communications is dependent on the source. Sources must be credible in order for warnings and risk communications to be effective. Physicians are often viewed as credible because of their special expertise and because they are believed to be trustworthy.

One of the greatest challenges in risk communications is understanding the recipient's attitudes and beliefs that will influence his response to and interaction with a hazardous situation or a warning. The recipient must have expectations about adverse consequences of exposure and be motivated to avoid in order for warnings to be effective. Risk communicators should consider the audience's perception of the magnitude of the hazard, the costs of compliance to the recipient, the perceived effectiveness of the precautionary action, and the audience's competence (e.g., reading ability, language skills, educational background).

CHAPTER 48 ANSWERS

1. The answer is A. (Ref: p. 699)

A 1991 Supreme Court decision (International Union *v* Johnson Controls, 1991) does not allow employers to keep pregnant or fertile women from working in jobs that may injure a fetus and cause an adverse reproductive outcome. Rather, employees decide as individuals whether they will perform potentially hazardous jobs after receiving information on potential risks. The employer has an obligation under Occupational Safety and Health Administration's (OSHA) "general duty clause" to provide all employees with a working environment free from recognized hazards that are likely to cause serious harm.

Answer B is not prohibited, although establishing a causal relationship may prove difficult. Answer C is allowed. An employee may be excluded from specific work activities if he or she is unable to perform the activities in a safe manner. Answers C and D are not prohibited, but rather encouraged. An employee educational and monitoring program for adverse reproductive outcomes may be prudent.

2. The answer is D. (Ref: pp. 700–701)

Sperm cells are most vulnerable during spermatogenesis, the 70- to 80-day period of rapid cell division when sperm are formed from spermatogonia. The 70- to 80-day period before conception occurs (or fails to occur) is most relevant.

Regarding answer A, a new cycle of spermatogenesis is initiated more than 40 times between the ages of 15 and 25 years, and remote exposure to arsenic is therefore less relevant. Arsenic exposure to a pregnant woman during the pregnancy is known to have potential adverse effects on the fetus.

Similar logic applies for answer B. Dermal absorption generally results in less systemic toxicity than inhalation.

Regarding answer C, the exposure is still relatively remote, and the hazards of ethylene oxide are more relevant for pregnant women.

Regarding answer E, the father's exposure during pregnancy is irrelevant, unless he brings the toxic chemicals home to his pregnant wife.

3. The answer is B. (Ref: pp. 700, 701)

Scar tissue from pelvic inflammatory disease may prevent passage through the fallopian tubes. Lack of estrogen is associated with decreased ovulation. The other answer choices are listed in the text.

4. The answer is E (Ref: p. 701, Table 48.3)

Most congenital anomalies, or birth defects, are caused by unknown factors. Few are caused by known teratogens.

5. The answer is C. (Ref: p. 701)

An early spontaneous abortion may be mistaken as normal menses or a late, heavy menses. A pregnancy test on the first day of each cycle would provide a more objective measure than self-report.

For answer A, industrial hygiene data is ideal but often unavailable. For answer B, these are the most important variables that affect reproductive outcome. For answer D, single exposures are easier to interpret than multiple exposures. For answer E, these are potential confounding factors affecting pregnancy outcomes.

6. The answer is A. (Ref: pp. 707–709)

Regarding answer B, it can be difficult to determine how much food or water the animal has ingested. Regarding answer C, the maximum tolerated dosage is defined as the dosage producing a 10% rate of maternal death. The usual indicator for maternal toxicity is inadequate weight gain during pregnancy. Regarding answer D, the metabolites, rather than the unchanged chemical, usually produce toxicity. Metabolites vary widely between species and also may differ between different age groups within a single species. Regarding answer E, statistical significance does not equal biologic significance. Scientific judgment should be applied to the interpretation.

7. The answer is C. (Ref: p. 710, Fig. 48.2, Table 48.2)

If there are no complicating conditions, a pregnant woman may perform professional, managerial, secretarial, and sedentary or light work throughout her pregnancy. See the reference under Table 48.6. The other answer options are supported by Fig. 48.2.

8. The answer is C. (Ref: p. 711)

Total objectivity and a legal requirement of truth that may, at times, conflict with the patient's interest characterize the examination for work-relatedness. Answer A is incorrect because a greater degree of certainty is required. The cause should be established to a "reasonable degree of medical certainty." Answer B is incorrect because the physician has an increased responsibility to society in addition to the patient's welfare. Answer D is incorrect because a specific, accurate diagnosis is essential to determine the cause. Answer E is incorrect because the employer and other third parties are often involved in the determination of work-relatedness.

49

Environmental Health

OBJECTIVES

- Discuss approach to environmental health issues
- Review management of water resources including control of microbiologic hazards and chemical contamination
- List methods of solid and municipal waste disposal
- Discuss issues related to hazardous waste disposal
- Explain the implications of the greenhouse effect, stratospheric ozone depletion, and acid rain

OUTLINE

   I. Introduction
  II. Water quality
      A. Water resources management
      B. Microbiologic hazards
      C. Chemical contamination
 III. Solid and municipal waste disposal
  IV. Hazardous chemicals
      A. Hazardous properties of chemicals
      B. Groundwater contamination
   V. Global ecologic change
      A. Enhanced greenhouse effect
      B. Stratospheric ozone depletion
      C. Other global and regional environmental problems
  VI. Further preparation for environmental issues

KEY POINTS

- Occupational health issues most often affect small populations of healthy adults under circumstances of greater exposure of limited duration occurring in a small area. Environmental health issues concern the general population, including the very young, the very old, the ill, and other vulnerable populations under circumstances of less exposure over longer periods in a larger area. Environmental exposures may often be multiple, continuous in nature, and penetrating through several routes of entry.
- Water resources must be suitable in quality and access to protect human health. All water resources are part of the hydrologic cycle in which water flows from the oceans to the atmosphere, falling from the atmosphere as rain onto the ocean, land, or fresh

water, including lakes, rivers, and underground cavities. It then returns to the oceans as runoff or to the atmosphere by evaporation. Underground water is usually cleaner than surface water because it has been effectively filtered. Natural filtering systems composed of soil and rocks clean the water, trapping disease-causing microorganisms and particulates containing toxic elements. However, once polluted, groundwater is much more difficult to decontaminate than surface water.

- On a global scale, there is no shortage of total water resources. However, the problem is water's availability in the right place at the right time in the right form. Because of waste and pollution of water resources, the secure fresh water available for human use is not sufficient. Water resources are often polluted by human activities such as domestic sewage and by industrial and agricultural waste. In general, protection of water resources from pollution is urgent and important for sustainable development.

- Water resources management involves three fundamental issues: (a) assurance of a secure and reliable supply of water; (b) treatment of drinking water to ensure safety from microbiologic and chemical hazards and to ensure acceptability by the public; and (c) handling and treatment of wastewater, so that it can be safely discharged and will not come into contact with drinking water supplies.

- Purification of drinking water can be accomplished in many different ways (e.g., coagulation, flocculation, settling, filtration, and chlorination). Filtration and chlorination are used on a large scale. These techniques, especially chlorination, have drastically reduced the incidence of water-borne diseases to present negligible levels, except for incidents where there is a break in the system resulting in downstream contamination. Although there are adverse health effects from the by-products of chlorination, it is by far the cheapest and most effective method of disinfection. The reason for this is that the chlorine continues to act downstream, providing a margin of safety all the way to the tap. Alternative technologies, such as ozonation, irradiation, or ultraviolet (UV) treatment, do not disinfect water beyond the point of treatment.

- Conventional methods of wastewater management include disposal and treatment of household wastewater by way of septic tank disposal systems in rural areas and centralized water treatment plants that collect wastewater in cities from sewer systems. The principal causes of water-borne diseases are that (a) polluted water is provided for drinking without proper purification and disinfection; (b) the treated, secure water is repolluted by pathogens in the process of transportation or storage; and (c) the water supply is inadequate, forcing people to use unsafe water sources. By far the most important water-borne illness in the United States is diarrhea. In the United States, outbreaks of water-borne disease are usually limited to enteritis associated with any of a number of viruses or, less commonly, giardiasis. Dysentery and diarrhea are ranked among the main avoidable causes of death for children in China.

- Chemical contamination of drinking water mainly comes from two sources: (a) contamination of ground and surface water sources by chemicals, solvents, pesticides, and metals and (b) the process of drinking water treatment creating by-products of chlorination. Sources of water pollution can be divided into point source and nonpoint sources (i.e., runoff and seepage).

- The amount of waste produced by human society is increasing. Commercial and domestic solid waste is a great practical problem for many local governments. Industrial wastes are usually much smaller in volume but are more likely to contain hazardous materials, such as toxic chemicals, flammable liquids, and asbestos.

- The composition of solid waste is very complex. Because plastic is hard to degrade or decompose in a general environment and its half-life in soil spans several decades, plastic disposal becomes an important environmental issue. Most municipal solid waste systems do not allow chemical and other hazardous wastes so that they do not contaminate the solid waste stream.

- The basic strategies for disposal of solid waste are as follows: (a) reduction of waste sources, (b) recycling and resource recovery, (c) incineration, and (d) sanitary landfill.
- Although the total amount is less, the disposal of hazardous industrial waste has been a greater concern than of domestic waste because of the perceived hazard to health and the risk of environmental contamination. Incineration at high temperatures is an effective means of disposing of much hazardous waste, but it is very expensive. Because of population distribution, land use restrictions, transportation costs, and concerns from society over environmental effects (i.e., *NIMBY—not in my back yard—syndrome*), there is intense pressure to find a solution to the problem of economical disposal of hazardous waste. This has led to increased interest in proven methods *such as source reduction, recycling, chemical neutralization, and secure hazardous waste disposal sites*. Once chemicals permeate the liner of a waste site, they enter the ground and migrate downward because of the effect of gravity, creating a *plume*.
- The greenhouse effect results from the accumulation of heat stored as radiant energy and retained predominantly in the oceans. It is the direct result of accumulation of carbon dioxide and some other gases in the atmosphere. Carbon dioxide effectively traps or absorbs long-wave radiation emitted from the Earth's surface, and this trapped radiation heats the atmosphere. As the amount of carbon dioxide in the atmosphere increases, the atmosphere has a corresponding increase in temperature. This increase is a result of the combustion of fossil fuels and significant deforestation. The greenhouse effect is necessary to create a temperature suitable for life on Earth, but the expected exaggeration of the effect from emissions of carbon dioxide from human activity is expected to lead to numerous adverse consequences.
- Depletion of the stratospheric ozone layer by released chlorofluorocarbons (CFCs) (including medical products containing CFCs), bromofluorocarbon, and some other chemicals such as nitrogen dioxide will result in increased UV radiation reaching the Earth's surface. The predominant health effects associated with depletion of the stratospheric ozone layer are caused by UV-B (289–320 nm) radiation. One of the implications is skin cancer, including malignant melanoma. Other health implications include cataracts, accelerated actinic changes (i.e., skin aging), and possible immunologic responses. The principal strategy for controlling depletion of the stratospheric ozone layer is to reduce or to restrict the production and use of CFCs. Viable substitutes have been found. Unfortunately, some CFCs have half-lives of 75 years or longer, and the effect will continue for many years.
- Depletion of primary resources, reduction of cultivatable land, and disruption of economic activity may lead to social disruptions resulting in civil unrest and large-scale migration (i.e., ecorefugees). This is particularly likely in developing countries.

QUESTIONS

1. Which bodies of water are most difficult to decontaminate once chemicals or microbiological pathogens infiltrate them?

A. Lakes and ponds
B. Oceans
C. Rivers

D. Groundwater
E. Aqueducts

2. *Water resources management involves each of the following **except***

A. Assurance of a secure and reliable supply of water
B. Treatment of drinking water to ensure safety from microbiologic and chemical hazards
C. Handling and treatment of wastewater, so that it can be safely discharged
D. Monitoring the use of water in bathing and personal hygiene to reduce consumption
E. Separation of wastewater streams from drinking water

3. *The only technology for disinfection of drinking water that extends protection downstream in the distribution system, as it leaves the supply system and moves toward the household tap, is which of the following?*

A. Ozonation
B. Chlorination
C. Filtration
D. Ultraviolet radiation
E. Settling of solid compounds

4. *The leading cause of diarrhea as a water-borne illness in the United States is which of the following?*

A. Viruses
B. Giardiasis
C. Typhoid
D. Fecal coliform bacteria
E. Cholera

5. *Which of the following has **not** been demonstrated to be effective in reducing the risk of hazardous waste?*

A. Source reduction
B. Recycling of materials
C. Chemical neutralization
D. Hazardous waste transport to a distant site
E. Incineration

6. *Which of the following health effects is **not** predicted as a consequence of the enhanced greenhouse effect?*

A. Increased frequency of extreme weather conditions
B. Change in distribution of vector-borne disease
C. Increase in the cancer rate
D. Increased incidence of heat stress
E. Occasional locally severe cooling episodes

7. *Which of the following effects is **not** predicted as a consequence of stratospheric ozone depletion?*

A. Accelerated "aging" of skin due to damage in people who spend much time outdoors
B. Increased incidence of melanoma
C. Increased incidence of cataracts
D. Increased frequency of allergies
E. Increased frequency of squamous cell carcinoma of the skin

50

Environmental Medicine: Regulatory Issues

OBJECTIVES

- List and explain the major environmental regulatory acts and agencies of the federal government
- Discuss the relationship between environmental regulation and the practice of environmental medicine
- Discuss the various reporting requirements of the Toxic Substances Control Act (TSCA) and how they impact the practicing environmental physician

OUTLINE

    I. Framework of environmental regulations
   II. Chronology of environmental laws in the United States
      A. Table 50.1: Major U.S. environmental regulatory statues
  III. Environmental regulation and its interface with environmental medicine
  IV. Air pollution control
   V. Clean water standards
  VI. Regulation of storage and disposal of toxics: the Resource Conservation and Recovery Act (RCRA)
 VII. Superfund: the Comprehensive Environmental Response Compensation and Liability Act
VIII. Superfund Amendments and Reauthorization Act: the Emergency Planning and Community Right to Know Act (EPCRA)
  IX. TSCA
      A. Premanufacture notification
      B. Reporting requirements
      C. Testing requirements and regulation of existing chemicals
   X. The occupational and environmental physician's role
  XI. Summary

KEY POINTS

- Environmental protection policies and laws create an expansive set of regulations to control pollution. Many of these regulations are oriented to minimize exposure by controlling emissions of categories of pollutants according to the medium of exposure.

- Environmental regulations mirror public concern and its reflection of actual risk. As a result, regulations in the United States and other countries have been driven by a series of environmental issues, many of which arose from catastrophic situations.
- The Environmental Protection Agency (EPA) was established in 1970 and unified federal regulation of the environment. The EPA's charter included all media (i.e., air, water, and solid and hazardous waste).
- In 1970, the National Environmental Policy Act (NEPA) was established to promote concern for the environment by all federal agencies, and the Council of Environmental Quality was instituted.
- Other regulations that were passed included the Clean Air Act (CAA) and the Federal Water Pollution Control Act or Clean Water Act (CWA).
- In 1976, the TSCA was passed in response to growing public concerns about the hazards of certain chemicals such as polychlorinated biphenyls (PCBs) and insecticides. In the same year, the RCRA was passed to regulate the disposal of solid and liquid hazardous waste.
- In 1980, the Comprehensive Environmental Response, Compensation, and Liability Act (CERCLA) was passed. This regulation addresses existing hazardous waste sites in the United States. It created the Superfund to address issues of adverse health effects from hazardous waste sites.
- The potential interfaces between environmental medicine and these regulations include (a) recognition of the database for correlating exposure to disease, (b) reporting requirements generated by environmental exposures, (c) knowledge of the regulatory system for environmental pollution, and (d) intervention strategies in environmentally induced disease or risk of disease.
- RCRA addresses the management of solid and liquid hazardous waste and is designed to minimize such waste by regulation of its transportation, storage, treatment, and disposal. It also addresses underground storage tanks by establishing design, monitoring, reporting, and removal requirements.
- CERCLA (i.e., the Superfund) is designed to cover past hazardous waste activities, but it also has reporting requirements for spills or other releases.
- In 1986, an amendment of the Superfund created the EPCRA. It is designed to make emergency planning entities aware of the presence of potentially hazardous substances through reporting requirements to state and local authorities.
- The TSCA addresses the need to fully evaluate the potential toxicity and environmental impact of existing and new chemicals. A manufacturer (or importer) must notify the Office of Toxic Substances 90 days before producing or importing a new chemical substance. Such notification may prompt the need for additional testing. For existing chemicals, the act requires reporting of any significant adverse effects from animal or human studies or clinical cases that are not already known or reported.

QUESTIONS

1. Environmental regulations are

A. All federally mandated
B. Designed to prevent human disease
C. Designed to protect animals and plants
D. Only based in civil law
E. Pollutant specific

2. *The review of testing of new commercial chemicals for potential toxicity primarily comes under the jurisdiction of the*

A. The NEPA from the EPA
B. The TSCA from the EPA
C. The EPCRA under provisions of the Superfund Amendments and Re-Authorization Act (SARA) administered by the EPA
D. The Resource Conservation and Recovery Act (RCRA) under EPA
E. The Occupational Safety and Health Act from the Department of Labor

3. *Environmental legislation frequently follows major catastrophic events. Community Right to Know legislation came in the aftermath of*

A. Bhopal
B. Love Canal
C. Kepone spill
D. Three Mile Island
E. Valdez oil spill

4. *Public access to air pollution information data is primarily mandated by the*

A. CERCLA
B. CAA under EPCRA
C. RCRA
D. TSCA
E. NAAQS

5. *Which of the following is **not** regulated by the CWA?*

A. Discharge permit programs
B. Grants for treatment facilities
C. Minimal effluent guidelines
D. Storage tank holdings
E. Storm water runoff

=51=

International Environmental Health

OBJECTIVES

- Identify sources of international pollution
- Distinguish between sources of pollution in developing and developed nations
- Recognize primary air pollutants of concern
- Understand causes of water pollution

OUTLINE

  I. Introduction
 II. Global air pollution
     A. Sources of pollution
     B. Global monitoring of air pollution
     C. Health effects of primary pollutants: SO_x, NO_x, CO, particulate material (PM), ozone, lead
     D. Air pollution in major cities
     E. Asthma and air pollution
     F. Overview
III. Global water pollution
     A. Water and disease
     B. Water supply and quality standards
     C. Sanitation
 IV. Global solid and hazardous waste
     A. Waste disposal systems
     B. Special programs for chemical and hazardous wastes
  V. Global environmental issues

KEY POINTS

- Most countries base pollution regulations on the involved medium—air, water, and solid and hazardous waste.
- Air pollution is a prominent global issue because of industrialization and the use of motor vehicles. The World Health Organization (WHO) plays a major role in reporting air pollution and in providing guidelines for acceptable exposure levels.
- Emphasis on indoor and outdoor air pollution became a focus of environmental research and regulation in the 1970s.

- On a global basis, lignite is still a significant pollutant; electric power generation has been a significant source of atmospheric air pollution. The primary pollutants have been SO_x, PM (e.g., fly ash), and NO_x.
- Motor vehicle emissions, a major source of air pollution, have replaced coal smoke as the major concern in developed countries. Control of air pollution from motor vehicles may include (a) limitation of use and (b) the use of postcombustion technology (e.g., tailpipe controls).
- Indoor air pollutants are generated by combustion sources, off-gassing of chemicals, dust, allergens, and many other compounds.
- Air pollution is commonly divided into primary pollutants (e.g., PM, SO_x, NO_x, CO) and air toxics. Ambient target levels are commonly set for primary pollutants, whereas point-source permitting (for smokestacks and tailpipes) or engine certification processes regulate air toxics.
- SO_x effects are related to the formation of acid and the secondary formation of sulfur-containing particles. Acid rain is primarily a product of sulfur-based acid formation. NO_x can also form nitric or nitrous acid and acidic fogs, but it is regulated because of its ability to produce ozone through a photochemical reaction. Ozone can have acute effects on the upper and lower airways, and it has been associated with fibrosis in animal models. The acute effects of CO are well known, although chronic effects from environmental levels are controversial.
- Daily increases in PM concentration have been associated with several indices of ill health, including daily death rates, hospital admissions, emergency department visits, antiasthma drug use, and lung function measures.
- Water pollution issues can generally be divided into ensuring safe drinking water and good sanitation. There are biologic and chemical agents that cause water pollution, and sources of pollution include runoff water and treated sewage. The cities of industrializing countries have been areas with the highest risk of water-borne infectious contamination. The pollution from upstream industrial and nonindustrial sites has had a major public-health impact on downstream communities.
- Chemical pollution has become a major issue for industrialized countries. Particular concern developed about contamination with potentially carcinogenic chemicals and the formation of mutagenic compounds from the interactions of chlorine with organic materials.
- Health concerns from water pollution go beyond ingestion. *Water-borne diseases*, caused by ingestion of human or animal wastes, include typhoid, cholera, giardiasis, cryptosporidiosis, amebiasis, and a wide range of bacterial diseases. *Water-contact diseases* are caused by vectors that usually penetrate the skin during contact with water or with moist, contaminated soil (e.g., schistosomiasis, ascariasis, hookworm). *Water hygiene* diseases are caused by lack of water for personal hygiene (e.g., louse-borne disease). *Water-habitat* diseases are associated with standing water, which allows breeding of insects (e.g., mosquito-borne diseases such as malaria, dengue, and yellow fever).
- Water supply and sanitation (WS&S) interventions are required to protect public health, but water supply is a much more common focus in developing countries. The quantity of water required varies directly with the size of the community, its location and climate, and its economic status.
- Although previous regulation focused on assuring safe levels in water sources (e.g. rivers, lakes) groundwater and point-source permitting control emissions better. Such permitting prohibits contaminants from entering industrial and community facilities.

Runoff water from industrial agriculture and mining creates significant pollution if it is not held (e.g., in holding ponds) and treated before discharge.

- Sanitation is highly variable in developing countries. Untreated wastewater may be used for watering and fertilizing crops. Treatment of wastewater is often ineffective or includes only primary (sedimentation) and not secondary (biologic) treatment. Treatment facilities are often poorly maintained.
- Solid waste is nonhazardous waste produced by homes, industries, institutions, markets, and commercial establishments. Lower-income-country waste contains little packaging and is not recyclable.
- Sanitary landfills in developed countries predominately use materials recovery and incineration. Developing countries burn solid waste, use home or neighborhood landfills, or transport waste to local landfills.
- Developing countries have limited management programs for chemical waste (and often have limited generation of hazardous waste). However, the country of generation is often not the country of disposal, and transportation of hazardous waste from developed to developing countries for disposal is a global health risk.
- There are three primary systems of toxic waste management in developed countries. First, chemicals must be evaluated for toxicity by regulations such as the Toxic Substances Control Act (TSCA). Second, regulation-listed chemicals must be tracked from the manufacturing process through the storage, transportation, and disposal or recycling processes. Third, some countries, such as Germany and the United States, have active programs to clean up hazardous waste buried in past years (e.g., Superfund).

QUESTIONS

*1. Which of the following statements is **incorrect** regarding pollution?*

A. Pollution regulations are usually based on the involved medium (e.g., air, water, solids).
B. Air pollution is a global issue because of industrialization and the use of motor vehicles.
C. WHO reports on air pollution.
D. Electric power generation has been a significant source of atmospheric air pollution.
E. Coal smoke has replaced motor vehicle emissions as a major source of air pollution in developed countries.

*2. Which of the following statements about air pollution is **least** correct?*

A. Acid rain is primarily a product of carbon monoxide pollution.
B. NO_x can also form nitric or nitrous acid and acidic fogs.
C. Ozone can have acute effects on the upper and lower airways
D. Chronic effects from environmental levels of CO are controversial.
E. PM concentration has been associated with hospital admissions, emergency department visits, and antiasthma drug use.

3. Which of the following statements about water pollution is most correct?

A. Chlorination is ineffective at reducing waterborne infectious diseases.
B. Chemical pollution not an important issue in industrialized countries.
C. Water-borne diseases include diseases caused by ingestion of human or animal wastes.

D. Water-contact diseases are caused by lack of water for personal hygiene.

E. Sanitation is of more importance than is water supply in developing countries.

4. Which of the following statements is most correct about international environmental pollution?

A. The exposure levels to pollutants are lowest in the major cities of Asia, Mexico, and South America.

B. In developing countries, untreated wastewater may be used for watering and fertilizing crops.

C. In developing countries, sanitary landfills predominately use materials recovery and incineration.

D. Developed nations face challenges preventing the transportation of hazardous or sanitary waste from less affluent countries.

E. The nation that generates hazardous waste is always the country where disposal occurs.

=52=

Clinical Environmental Medicine

OBJECTIVES

- Discuss the relationship between epidemiology, toxicology, and the practice of environmental medicine
- Explain approaches used in the evaluation of the patient with suspected environmentally related disease

OUTLINE

KEY POINTS

- Environmental medicine can be considered to be the study of effects upon human beings of external physical, chemical, and biologic factors in the general environment. The discipline of environmental medicine combines clinical, epidemiologic, and toxicologic approaches. It uniquely seeks to understand causation and then to adopt policy, engineering, or human factor interventions to prevent or mitigate the caused outcomes.

- We can prevent environmental disease far more effectively and still more cost effectively than we can treat it.
- Assignment of clinical or laboratory findings to environmental causes necessitates repeatability of those findings and clear epidemiologic linkage. Accuracy of diagnostic testing, in relation to exposures and efficacy of therapeutic intervention, needs to be tested by recognizable scientific means.
- The physician who practices environmental medicine is likely to encounter patients who have a variety of concerns about the potential health implications of exposure to environmental hazards. Patients rely on their physician to provide them with advice concerning sources of toxins, exposure prevention, and related public health interventions.
- In most cases, the extent of the exposures are considerably less than in the traditional occupational setting.
- Environmental health physicians may be involved directly in episodic or periodic health evaluations, diagnosis and treatment; patient and community education; implementation of public health protection; planned abatement of source stressors; exposure and outcome assessments; and disaster preparedness.
- The key to treating lead poisoning is preventing exposure through good public health measures.
- Sources of lead include lead paint, outdoor soil, water, proximity to lead smelters, Mexican products, and other unique sources
- When lead is discovered in paint, moving the family to a home without lead is ideal; if this is not practical, families may abate the lead in the contaminated home or at least carefully supervise the child and clean the contaminated home. The latter approach is often ineffective.
- The recommended action level considering the child's environment is 10 mg/dL; this is not a safe or desirable level because less is better.
- In managing patients with disabling, multiorgan symptoms with no detectable disease, conservative management with frequent physician visits and reassurance is ideal. Avoid treatments involving isolation or avoidance.

QUESTIONS

1. The most effective approach to lead poisoning is

A. Use of succimer as a chelating agent
B. Meticulous housecleaning and hand washing in homes with lead-based paint
C. Lowering the action level
D. Testing buildings for lead before a case of lead poisoning is reported and abatement of lead before a home is occupied
E. Following lead-poisoned children with neuropsychiatric testing to ensure early detection of developmental disabilities

2. Typical office encounters in environmental medicine include which of the following?

A. Pulmonary disease (e.g., asthma, colds, bronchitis) in residents living near power plants or other industry
B. Environmental cancer concerns in residents of asbestos-containing buildings

C. Dietary concerns related to fish, meat, hormones in meat, or irradiated food
D. Lead exposure in children, home renovators, or painters
E. All of the above

*3. Typical sources of lead poisoning include all of the following **except***

A. Soil near a lead smelter
B. Inappropriately constructed cookware
C. Latex paint in a new home
D. Older metal plumbing
E. Mexican pottery

*4. Which is the **least** important skill for environmental physicians?*

A. Obtaining an accurate clinical diagnosis
B. Expertise in administration of chelating agents
C. Understanding the toxicology of chemical environmental hazards
D. Application of epidemiologic principles to environmental illness
E. Familiarity with the medical surveillance and disease outbreak literature

=53=

Indoor Environmental Quality

OBJECTIVES

- Discuss the relationship between indoor environmental quality (IEQ) and health effects
- List sources that contribute to IEQ
- Identify categories of pollutants and factors that may impact IEQ
- Distinguish between building-related illness (BRI) and building-related occupant complaint syndrome (BROCS)
- Explain various causes of chronic building-related disease
- List steps in the clinical evaluation of building-associated illness
- List steps involved in the evaluation of problem buildings

OUTLINE

I. Historical perspective
II. The indoor environment
  A. Sources of indoor environmental contamination
    1. Table 53.1: Common sources and types of indoor contaminants
    2. External sources
    3. Building structure and interior furnishings
    4. Mechanical systems
    5. Occupant-generated pollution
  B. Characterizing the indoor environment
    1. Biologic agents
    2. Combustion products
    3. Ozone
    4. Particulates
    5. Pesticides
    6. Radon
    7. Volatile organic chemicals
    8. Physical factors
    9. The problem building
  C. Health effects of indoor pollution: acute BRIs
    1. Definitions
      a. BRI
      b. BROCS
    2. Hypersensitivity diseases
    3. Infectious diseases

KEY POINTS

- IEQ is a significant and expensive health concern.
- Poor IEQ is not simply a matter of comfort, but may be associated with illness and death. Many toxins are present at higher levels indoors than outdoors. Lifestyle changes have led the average citizen in the United States to spend 90% of his or her life indoors. The most vulnerable segments of the population (i.e., the infirm, the very young, or the very old) are also the most exposed.
- There are five general sources of indoor environmental contamination: (a) the external environment, (b) building structure, (c) building furnishings and finishing, (d) mechanical systems, and (e) occupant-generated pollution.
- The key factors involved in IEQ include (a) biologic agents, (b) combustion products, (c) ozone, (d) particulates, (e) pesticides, (f) radon, (g) volatile organic chemicals, and (h) physical factors.
- A "problem building" is one in which more than 20% of the occupants have building-related health complaints or specific environmental contaminants have been linked with BRIs. A "crisis building" is one in which complaints and public concern has reached a point where normal activities have been disrupted.
- A BRI is a disease with a defined pathophysiology attributable to a specific building contaminant.
- BROCS refers to a group of transient, nonspecific symptoms, affected by entering and leaving a particular building. The case definition of BROCS remains vague and its causes speculative.
- Indoor environmental contaminants have the potential for causing chronic diseases. Those of chief concern include cancer, cardiovascular disease, neurobehavioral syndromes, and pulmonary disorders.

- IEI, formerly called multiple chemical sensitivity, is a clinically recognized syndrome without well-defined cause. *(BRI)*
- The clinical evaluation of building-associated illness begins with an interview aimed at recognizing symptoms and the temporal sequence to specific environments or activities. Complaints of other building occupants may be relevant.
- The evaluation of a problem building should be staged. The first step involves the collection of information about the building and the complaints of occupants. Subsequently, specific environmental or medical hypotheses should be generated. "Shotgun" attempts to measure every possible pollutant should be avoided. (Timing of industrial hygiene measurements may be critical.)

QUESTIONS

*1. All of the following are true **except***

A. Americans typically spend 90% of their lives indoors.
B. Indoor environmental quality problems are a top priority of the Environmental Protection Agency (EPA).
C. Indoor levels of pollutants of concern rarely exceed outdoor levels.
D. Poor indoor environmental quality has been associated with illness and death.
E. Those most vulnerable to indoor environmental contaminants—the infirm, the very young, and the elderly—are often those most exposed.

*2. Each of the following contributes to workplace indoor environmental quality problems **except***

A. Building structure
B. Mechanical systems
C. Occupant-generated contaminants
D. Outdoor air
E. Water-purification systems

3. Complaints about indoor environmental quality decrease with

A. Increased ventilation
B. Increased occupant density
C. Increased density of office equipment
D. Recent renovation and new carpeting
E. All of the above

*4. The following statements relate to BRI. Which statement is **false**?*

A. The clinical evaluation of a patient should begin with an interview to elicit symptoms and the temporal relationship of these symptoms with specific events or activities.
B. Patients presenting with BRI should be assessed with a comprehensive series of tests focusing on the immune and respiratory systems.
C. In the evaluation of a suspect building, the first step is to gather information on the building, as well as the patients and any temporal relationship.
D. In the evaluation of a suspect building, the second step should be a comprehensive industrial hygiene evaluation, to include bioaerosols, of the entire building with a focus on the heating, ventilation, and air conditioning (HVAC) system.
E. To minimize microbial contamination in a building, water leaks must be repaired promptly, and humidity and temperature must be carefully controlled.

=54=
Medical Aspects of Environmental Emergencies

OBJECTIVES

- List components of the worksite emergency response that are relevant to physicians
- Review government regulations that are related to emergency responders

OUTLINE

   I. First aid and emergency medical care
  II. Protection of emergency response personnel
 III. Provision of emergency medical information
 IV. Medical surveillance
  V. Emergency response planning guidelines for chemical releases
 VI. Further information

KEY POINTS

- Environmental emergencies may result from forces and processes that are "natural," such as storms, geologic disturbances, and epidemics. Others emergencies are man-made, such as industrial accidents.
- Emergency response planning is required at most worksites under a variety of federal and state regulations.
- Occupational physicians are likely to be involved in the development and implementation of worksite emergency response plans.
- Most worksite emergency planning requirements are found within the standards and regulations of Occupational Safety and Health Act (OSHA) and the Environmental Protection Agency (EPA).
- Worksite emergency response requirements of relevance include (a) first aid and emergency medical care, (b) protection of emergency response personnel, (c) provision of emergency medical information, (d) medical surveillance, (e) coordination with community health care providers, and (f) emergency response planning guidelines for chemical releases.
- The most basic requirement for worksite emergency planning is OSHA's requirement that there be ready access to first aid for all injured employees. As a rule of thumb, first aid and cardiopulmonary resuscitation (CPR) must be available to employees within 5 minutes.

- OSHA and EPA require that an emergency response plan be developed and implemented before the start of hazardous waste and emergency response operations at a facility. The employer must develop an emergency response plan for emergencies to address, as a minimum, emergency medical treatment and first aid.
- Emergency response personnel are exposed to greater variety and severity of health risks than are most employees.
- Persons should not be assigned to tasks requiring use of respirators unless it has been determined that they are physically able to perform the work and use the equipment.
- When emergency responders wear personal protective equipment (PPE), especially impervious clothing and encapsulating suits, they lose the temperature control benefits normally derived from sweating. The higher the ambient temperature and the longer the suits are worn, the greater is the risk of dehydration and heat stress.
- Emergency response personnel are also protected by OSHA's Bloodborne Pathogens Standard that requires employers to develop an exposure control plan, including training and the availability of hepatitis B vaccination for employees who, as a result of performing their duties, risk contact exposure of skin, eye, and mucous membranes or parenteral exposure to blood and other potentially infectious materials.
- Worksites at which hazardous substances are processed or stored should have detailed medical information available on the specific health effects of exposure to those substances. Facility emergency response plans should include protocols and procedures for medical treatment of exposure victims.
- The Emergency Notification requirement in Title III of the EPA's Superfund Amendments and Reauthorization Act applies to spills or releases of hazardous substance in excess of their "reporting quantities." In the event of such a spill or release exceeding the reporting quantity, the facility must immediately notify local and state emergency response officials of all local areas and states "likely to be affected by the release" and detailed medical information such as "any known or anticipated acute or chronic health risks associated with the emergency, and, where appropriate, advice regarding medical attention necessary for exposed individuals."
- OSHA and the EPA require employers to develop medical surveillance programs for emergency response personnel and other employees involved in hazardous materials emergencies. Members of "organized and designated HAZMAT teams" and others trained to the OSHA/EPA level of Hazardous Materials Specialist must receive baseline medical examinations, follow-up examinations at least every 12 to 24 months and at termination of employment, or reassignment (if the previous examination was more than 6 months before).
- Important components of facility emergency response plans are explicit agreements between the facility and the surrounding community's emergency response organizations, including emergency medical service (EMS) organizations and hospitals. It is important that occupational physicians correctly understand the abilities and limitations of the hospitals and EMS services that serve the facilities at which they work or to which they provide medical services.
- The accidental release of industrial chemicals can pose emergency hazards far beyond the point of release, most notably when the chemicals become airborne.
- An international program has developed Acute Exposure Guideline Levels (AEGLs). For each chemical considered, AEGLs are developed for exposure durations of 30 minutes, 1 hour, 4 hours, and 8 hours and for each of three levels of toxicity. AEGL-1 is the airborne concentration of a substance above which it is predicted that there might be transient discomfort or irritation but no disabling or persistent effects. AEGL-2 is

the airborne concentration of a substance above which it is predicted that there may be disabling effects or impaired ability to escape. AEGL-3 is the airborne concentration of a substance above which life-threatening effects may occur.

QUESTIONS

*1. Which of the following is **not** a requirement of worksite emergency planning for environmental disasters?*

A. Coordination with community health units
B. First aid services
C. Medical surveillance
D. Mobile testing laboratory or laboratories
E. Provision of emergency medical information

*2. Regarding worksite first aid, which of the following is **incorrect**?*

A. In the absence of infirmary, clinic, or hospital in proximity to the workplace that is used for the treatment of all injured employees, a person or persons shall be adequately trained to render first aid.
B. First aid supplies approved by the consulting physician shall be readily available.
C. It is generally understood that "first aid" includes at least care for victims of trauma, response to corrosive and thermal injuries, and CPR.
D. As a rule of thumb, first aid and CPR must be available to employees within 30 minutes.
E. The need for training and the number of individuals to be trained is determined in part by the proximity of the worksite to other sources of emergency care.

3. Emergency response plans should include coordination with

A. EMS organizations
B. Fire departments
C. Hospitals
D. Police departments
E. All of the above

*4. Protection of emergency response personnel must include all of the above **except***

A. Determination of physical ability to use a respirator
B. Availability of hepatitis B vaccination
C. Provision of a self-contained breathing apparatus (SCBA)
D. Annual chest radiographs and pulmonary function testing
E. Procedures for monitoring vital signs when using impermeable suits and heavy equipment

*5. Which of the following statements is **incorrect** regarding emergency response plans?*

A. Explicit agreements must exist between the facility and the surrounding community's emergency response organizations, including EMS organizations and hospitals.
B. The contingency plan must contain actual letters of agreement signed by these organizations.

C. Many hospital emergency departments lack the equipment, knowledge, and experience to care for patients with toxic chemical exposures.
D. The National Fire Protection Association has established mandatory standards for EMS personnel responding to hazardous materials emergencies.
E. Industrial facilities using quantities of hydrofluoric acid are advised to provide calcium gluconate gel to local EMS services along with appropriate training in its use.

═══ 55 ═══
Emergency Response to Environmental Incidents

OBJECTIVES

- Understand the role of the occupational medicine physician in environmental emergencies
- Identify sources of assistance in chemical emergencies
- Identify the components of an emergency response plan (ERP)
- List the components of a risk inventory from a facility survey
- Explain factors that determine the level of appropriate emergency response
- Discuss importance of debriefing after an ERP is activated

OUTLINE

    J. Containment of incident
    K. Evacuation and site security
    L. Systems of outside notification
    M. Site communications
    N. Role of outside agencies
    O. Public relations
    P. Debriefing: postincident and critical incident stress debriefing
  IV. Training
   V. Role of the occupational medicine physician
  VI. Summary

KEY POINTS

- The emergency response to environmental incidents combines the principles of occupational medicine and emergency medicine.
- Unexpected events that challenge routine capabilities of local and regional emergency response systems are known as *mass casualty incidents*.
- The potential for mishaps with hazardous materials is underscored by the fact that approximately 4 billion tons of regulated materials are transported annually in the United States.
- Physicians must have a firm understanding of the toxicity of materials used at various sites to properly advise the planning for emergencies. A well-developed and rehearsed plan is essential for responding appropriately to incidents.
- A risk inventory can be developed by conducting a facility survey of materials used and their respective processes.
- To deal effectively with unexpected releases of hazardous materials, an ERP should consider the following: (a) exposures may affect a single worker or result in a mass casualty incident, (b) necessary contacts and information sources need to be outlined, and (c) guidelines should be prepared for grading the response.
- The response plan should address issues such as (a) the types of events that will trigger the ERP and the corresponding level of response, (b) the responsibilities of the response team, (c) the relationship with neighboring businesses, and (d) the role and contact mechanisms for government agencies.
- Selection of PPE or chemical protective clothing requires knowledge of substances to which the garment will be exposed and the duration of such exposure.
- The level of response appropriate for a given incident should be determined by the level of technical expertise necessary to control the materials, the presence of fire or explosion hazards, and the potential radius of risk.
- To prevent confusion, a clear chain of command is critical in the event of an incident.
- Decontamination issues must be included in the response plan.
- After activation of the ERP, debriefings are important, with evaluation of events leading up to the incident and attention to prevention of similar events.

QUESTIONS

1. Which of the following should be addressed when developing an ERP?

A. The type of event that will trigger an ERP, including the level of response

B. The responsibilities of the internal emergency response team
C. The relationship with neighboring businesses through mutual aid agreements
D. The role and contact mechanisms for local, state, and federal agencies
E. All of the above

2. *All of the following statements regarding selection of PPE are true **except***

A. It is important to know what chemical substances will be involved in any response.
B. Level D PPE is acceptable for use with a chemical that has respiratory toxicity.
C. PPE should be properly tested in accordance with standardized methods.
D. Duration of exposure to a chemical is important for proper PPE selection.
E. PPE can lose its effectiveness during use, reducing its protective lifetime.

3. *In the absence of a local community hazardous materials (HAZMAT) ERP, which of the following entities is tasked with developing an ERP?*

A. The Environmental Protection Agency (EPA)
B. Occupational Safety and Health Administration (OSHA)
C. The responsible company
D. The Department of Transportation
E. The local community government

4. *The training activity that best correlates with an effective response to an environmental incident is*

A. Teaching responders about how to use PPE
B. Attending a training program sponsored by OSHA
C. Learning about various chemical hazards in a classroom setting
D. Repeated drilling by team members for response to an environmental incident
E. Providing first responders with a copy of the ERP to review

5. *An occupational medicine physician involved in emergency planning and response to environmental incidents should*

A. Be aware of potentially hazardous materials used in relation to the business for which he or she is working
B. Be involved in development of the ERP
C. Understand his or her role in medical surveillance of employees exposed to hazardous substances
D. Be familiar with regulatory agencies and federal statutes that have direct relevance to environmental and HAZMAT incidents
E. All of the above

56

Occupational Medicine Aspects of Terrorism

OBJECTIVES

- Understand the definition of terrorism and how it may impact the workplace
- List the types of threats that may be encountered
- Discuss relevant responses to terrorist attacks
- Understand the importance of protective measures and preparation

OUTLINE

I. Introduction
    A. Figure 56.1: Lethality of terrorist attacks
II. Philosophical position of the occupational physician
III. Risk assessment
    A. Table 56.1: National Safety Council list of errors in emergency response plans
IV. Types of threats and relevant responses
    A. Figure 56.2: The Haddon matrix
    B. Explosive blast
        1. Table 56.2: Delivery mechanisms used by terrorists
        2. Figure 56.3: Vehicle bomb explosion hazard evacuation distance table
    C. Biologic agents
        1. Table 56.3: Airborne infectious disease transmission protection
        2. Table 56.4A: Respirator protection level classifications
        3. Table 56.4B: Nonpowered, air-purifying particulate filter respirator categories
        4. Table 56.4C: Respirator chemical cartridge coding
        5. Anthrax
            a. Table 56.5: Clinical syndromes produced by *Bacillus anthracis*
            b. Table 56.6A, B: National Institute for Occupational Safety and Health (NIOSH) interim recommendations for the selection and use of protective clothing and respirators against biologic agents
            c. Table 56.7: Recommended postexposure prophylaxis for exposure to *B. anthracis*
        6. Smallpox
            a. Table 56.8: Differentiation of smallpox and chickenpox
        7. Brucellosis

KEY POINTS

- The Department of State defines terrorism as "premeditated, politically motivated violence perpetrated against noncombatant targets by subnational groups or clandestine agents."
- Attacks on businesses and their employees represent an area of increasing concern to employers and employees.
- The apparent level of violence and the indiscriminate nature of such violence both increased significantly in the last 20 years of the twentieth century.

- Although most multicasualty aggressions have involved simple explosive devices, increasing attention has been directed at the possibility of aggressive acts involving what are known as weapons of mass destruction (WMD), including nuclear, biologic, and chemical (NBC) agents.
- Events in 2001 brought the concern of terrorist attacks to a higher level of consciousness throughout the occupational medical world.
- Terrorist aggressions can be divided into two distinct classes: immediately apparent and insidious. Immediately apparent incidents include bombs and most of the chemical agents. Insidious aggressions include most of the biologic agents and chemicals that do not have an immediately apparent effect on life or health.
- Explosive devices remain the most common of all terrorist attack tools.
- Armies have employed biologic agents as weapons for many centuries. Most of the biological organisms considered by governments for weaponization depend on dispersal through the air. For effective air dispersion with adequate respiratory tree penetration, particles must generally be in the range of 5 μm of less.
- *B. anthracis* is a gram-positive rod with the capability of forming a spore. It is the spore that gives it the potential to be used as a weapon. Anthrax infection presents as three relatively distinct clinical syndromes: cutaneous, gastrointestinal, and pulmonary.
- Most authorities consider smallpox, caused by the variola virus, to be the next most likely agent to be used for terrorist attacks on larger population groups after anthrax. Smallpox is relatively easily weaponized because it does not lose virulence on drying.
- Other biologic agents that may have potential for terrorist use include those that cause brucellosis and plague. There are a number of other agents as well that could be used in a terrorist attack.
- Chemical agents have also been used as weapons throughout the ages. They are generally divided into several classes (Table 56.11).
- Botulinum toxin is a biologic product derived from *Clostridium botulinum*, an anaerobic, gram-positive bacillus. The toxin inhibits the release of acetylcholine leading to a dose-related flaccid paralysis.
- Nuclear threats are not limited to nuclear explosions. Dispersal of radioactive material through an explosive device or some other mechanism is a possible threat.
- A major goal of any terrorist attack is the elicit a psychologic impact. In the event of any attack, psychological support services are likely to mitigate the dysfunctional responses.
- The medical aspects of planning for and responding to intentional attacks on a business should be viewed as an integral part of the overall business continuity plan. Ensuring a safe work environment involves planning for potential routes of entry of an attack, as well as assuring that the structure is constructed in such a way as to offer maximum protection to the occupants.
- Many threats could arrive through the mail. Mail screening training is essential for any large organization. The U.S. Postal Service has published guidelines for mail evaluation.
- OSHA has put forward a number of regulations governing emergency response (Table 56.14). Any responders to chemical or biological situations would fall under the regulations of 29 CFR 1910.120, which covers hazardous materials emergency response workers.
- Training should include designated safety personnel and those responsible for responses to terrorist incidents. The best way to ensure an optimal response in such sit-

uations is through repeated practice, including tabletop strategic drills combined with mock event drills and subsequent debriefing.

QUESTIONS

*1. All of the following statements regarding terrorism are true **except***

A. It may be defined as premeditated, politically motivated violence perpetrated against noncombatant targets.
B. Intentional, aggressive, indiscriminate attacks on corporate entities have decreased over the last 20 years of the 20th century.
C. Most multicasualty aggressions have involved simple explosive devices.
D. Business interests of employees are sometimes specific targets of terrorist attacks.
E. Attacks on businesses and their employees represent an area of increasing concern.

2. Which of the following are errors found with emergency response plans?

A. Poor or no planning
B. Lack of training and practice
C. Failure to keep the plan up-to-date
D. OSHA regulations are not a part of the plan.
E. All of the above

3. The most common of all terrorist attack tools is

A. Radioactive substances
B. Biologically derived toxins
C. Explosive devices
D. Chemical agent weapons
E. Biologic agent weapons

(vesicles)

4. Which of the following chemical warfare agents is classified as a vesicant?

A. Sarin (GB)
B. VX
C. Nitrogen oxide
D. Nitrogen mustard
E. Chlorine

*5. All of the following are manifestations of pulmonary anthrax **except***

A. A papular lesion that develops into a black eschar
B. Prodrome of flulike symptoms
C. Hemorrhagic mediastinitis
D. Multiorgan failure
E. Incubation for 20 to 60 days

57

The Environmental Health and Safety Audit

OBJECTIVES

- Identify the role of the environmental health and safety audit in compliance assurance
- Describe the environmental health and safety audit process
- Discuss the process of the environmental audit
- Discuss the process of a health and safety audit
- Discuss the role of the occupational and environmental medicine physician in an audit team

OUTLINE

    I. Overview of the environmental and health and safety audit
   II. Role of the environmental and health and safety audit
  III. The legal foundation for the audit
  IV. Timing of the audit
   V. Conducting the environmental audit
  VI. Conducting the health and safety audit
 VII. Comparison of the environmental and the health and safety audits
VIII. Environmental and health and safety management systems
  IX. Role of standards and guidelines
   X. Role of the occupational and environmental physician

KEY POINTS

- An environmental audit is a process that includes the gathering of information on activities at a facility that may impact the environment or human health, especially any activities subject to legal or regulatory requirements.
- The most important role of the environmental audit is to ensure regulatory compliance and prevent violations, fines, public relations problems, and even criminal charges.
- An environmental audit may be appropriate on a regularly scheduled basis, at the time of changing or upgrading facilities, during divestiture or acquisition, and in anticipation of an external audit.
- The first step in an environmental audit is information gathering. Later, a site visit will focus on the entire process from raw materials to final product. At the conclusion of the site visit, an exit interview is usually held. A staged follow-up action plan may also be included.

- Health and safety audits require a significant time commitment but can provide an evaluation of many aspects of a facilities compliance picture.
- It is very important that an audit be conducted properly in order to reduce undue liability.
- Proper organization and implementation of an effective audit program can reduce costs associated with compliance and prepare a facility for long-tern reviews by the regulatory agencies.

QUESTIONS

1. The most important role of the environmental audit is to

A. Anticipate regulatory reform
B. Increase insurance coverage
C. Provide information for occupational physicians
D. Verify regulatory compliance
E. Provide toxic tort reform

2. It is appropriate to conduct environmental audits in which of the following time frames?

A. At time of plant upgrade
B. Divestiture of properties
C. On a 1- to 3-year cycle
D. Before an external audit
E. All of the above

*3. Each of the following is an appropriate role for the environmental physician in regards to audits **except***

A. To assist in report writing
B. To direct laboratory testing
C. To interpret results for management
D. To review audit results
E. To serve as a team member

4. The first step in either environmental or health and safety audit is

A. Sampling the facility
B. Information gathering
C. Interviews with employees and key administrators
D. Review of safety procedures
E. Development of compliance checklists

*5. Considered the international benchmark for environmental management systems, ISO 14001 **does not** include*

A. Worker health and safety objectives
B. Goals to protect the environment
C. Pollution prevention strategies
D. Waste minimization and recycling
E. Energy reduction

=58=
Environmental Risk Assessment

OBJECTIVES

- Explain the usefulness of risk assessment
- List types of information used in the formation of a risk assessment
- Distinguish between the no observable effect level (NOAEL) and lowest observed adverse effect level (LOAEL)
- Recognize levels in the International Agency for Research on Cancer (IARC) cancer classification system

OUTLINE

KEY POINTS

- Low-level exposures that may produce chronic diseases, particularly neoplasms, are often managed through the process of qualitative or quantitative risk assessment. These assessments are also used for policy decisions at local, state, and federal levels and in multiple regulatory settings.
- Qualitative risk assessment is commonly performed by authoritative bodies, including the IARC, the American Conference of Governmental Industry Hygienists (ACGIH), the Environmental Protection Agency (EPA), and others.
- The risk assessment process involves four steps: (a) hazard identification, (b) exposure-dose-response relationship, (c) exposure assessment, and (d) risk characterization.
- Clinical and epidemiologic studies are especially useful in that data are obtained on people. Laboratory animal studies, like controlled human exposure studies, have the advantage of using carefully defined conditions matched to experimental needs. *In vitro* studies that use cells and tissues from people and laboratory animals represent the ultimate "reductionist" approach of defining pollutant effects.
- The approach used by the ACGIH and the EPA for noncancer end points makes use of safety or uncertainty factors to extrapolate from levels of observed effect or absence of effect to levels of exposure that may be viewed as acceptable.
- The LOAEL is the lowest observed adverse effect level, whereas NOAEL is level at which no observable effect is seen.
- The IARC conducts a formalized risk assessment that leads to a qualitative clarification of a compound's carcinogenic potential. The evaluation process considers three types of data: human carcinogenicity data, experimental carcinogenicity data, and supporting evidence of carcinogenicity. The evidence of carcinogenicity is classified into four categories. Group 1 includes chemicals and processes established as human carcinogens. Group 2 includes those that are probably (group 2A) or possibly (group 2B) carcinogenic to humans. Group 3 includes agents that are not classified. Group 4 includes agents that are probably not carcinogenic.
- Risk assessments based on regulatory guidelines always need to be considered as candidates for refinement based on regulatory guidelines knowledge.

QUESTIONS

1. Which of the following organizations conducts carcinogen assessment studies?

A. ACGIH
B. EPA
C. IARC
D. National Toxicology Program (NTP)
E. All of the above

*2. The risk assessment process includes each of the following **except***

A. Exposure assessment
B. Exposure dose-response assessment
C. Hazard identification

   D. Personal exposure measurement
   E. Risk characterization

  3. Risk assessment is best approached with

   A. Experimental data on individual patients
   B. Computer models
   C. Human epidemiologic data, if available
   D. Laboratory animal studies
   E. Laboratory based human group exposures

  4. When assessing the carcinogenic potential of a compound, the most relevant information for regulatory purposes is

   A. Anecdotal data
   B. Chemical composition of the compound
   C. Human epidemiologic and clinical data
   D. Mechanistic data
   E. Threshold level

  5. Which of the following best describes a compound's carcinogenic potential if it is in IARC group 1?

   A. Probably not carcinogenic
   B. Possibly carcinogenic to humans
   C. Agent that has not been classified
   D. Agent that has been established as a human carcinogen
   E. None of the above

=59=

Ambient Particulates and Health Effects

OBJECTIVES

- Identify agencies that regulate exposure to airborne particulate matter (PM) in the workplace and in the ambient environment
- Know the approximate levels (airborne concentrations) of PM that have been determined to be protective of health both for workplace exposures and for the ambient environment
- Identify strengths and weaknesses of the separate lines of health evidence that are used to set workplace and general population exposure limits for PM
- Discuss the separate lines of health, the nature of data obtained, and the exposure-response behavior for PM that has been discovered
- Understand difficulties inherent to using population studies of correlations between PM at central monitors and health end points as a basis for regulatory standards, or emissions-reductions benefit calculations
- Discuss controversies regarding the appropriate interpretation of the PM time-series or cohort studies, and critique assumptions involved when relying on the epidemiology of PM-exposed populations

OUTLINE

- I. Introduction: airborne PM
- II. Agencies that identify PM levels protective of health
- III. Approaches to assessing the toxicity of PM
- IV. Epidemiologic studies of populations on health effects of ambient PM
- V. Health effects of inhaled PM as revealed by the other lines of investigation
  - A. Data on humans (including asthmatics) exposed to elevated levels of PM
  - B. Data from animal and laboratory toxicology
- VI. Attribution of health effects to undifferentiated, "generic" PM
  - A. PM differs in physical, biologic, and chemical nature
  - B. Sulfate as an example of fine PM
- VII. Sources of personal PM exposure
- VIII. Asthma and ambient PM levels
  - A. Variations in asthma hospitalizations by location
  - B. Variations in asthma prevalence by location
  - C. Time trends in asthma and in ambient PM levels
  - D. Clinical evidence on environmental factors in asthma prevalence

    E. Exposure of asthmatic volunteers to PM
  IX. Examining the hypothesis behind the PM associations
    A. Tests of causality
    B. Alternative causal pathways

KEY POINTS

- Serious health effects can result from chronic inhalation of elevated levels of certain classes of PM, as demonstrated by health statistics for cigarette smokers, for workers exposed to elevated levels of specific types of airborne PM, and for populations that experienced historical, elevated air-pollution episodes.
- Standards and guidelines have been developed, aimed at protecting health both for workers exposed occupationally and for the general public exposed to outdoor, ambient PM. Over the past decade, increasing interest has focused on correlations detected between low, ambient PM concentrations and population health statistics, notably mortality. These findings have sparked controversy, because associations with health outcomes are reported for ambient PM concentrations ($10–30 \ \mu g/m^3$).
- Guidelines for health-protective levels in the United States are available from the American Conference of Governmental Industrial Hygienists (ACGIH) for threshold limit values (TLVs) and the Occupational Safety and Health Administration (OSHA) for permissible exposure levels (PELs). For the ambient environment, the 1967 Clean Air Act (modified by the 1970, 1977, and 1990 Clean Air Act Amendments) requires the Environmental Protection Agency (EPA) to set the National Ambient Air Quality Standards (NAAQSs) for sulfur dioxide, carbon monoxide, nitrogen dioxide, lead, photochemical oxidants (later changed to ozone), and PM.
- The original NAAQS for PM, was set for "total suspended particulates" (TSP, which included particles with diameters less than about 40 μm). Subsequently, it was determined that little of the PM with aerodynamic diameter greater than 10 μm was inhaled, and in 1987 the standards were changed to particles with diameters of 10 μm or less (PM-10). Later, it became appreciated that mouth-breathing people allow PM-10 particles to reach the lungs, but for nose breathers, penetration to the lungs is primarily limited to particles less than 2.5 μm aerodynamic diameter (PM-2.5). In 1997, the approved NAAQS for PM retained (reaffirmed) the existing annual and 24-hour standards for PM-10 and established new annual-average and 24-hour standards for PM-2.5. The TSP standard is no longer enforced. The criteria air pollutants include air PM, sulfur dioxide, nitrogen dioxide, carbon monoxide, ozone, and lead.
- Different health effects have been linked with the constituents of ambient air pollution, including PM. Epidemiology of general populations is a crucial component of available evidence, because in these studies the response of sensitive subgroups is included. However, to protect these groups, it is essential to understand which PM emissions may be responsible (i.e., to elucidate the underlying mechanisms).
- Of the several lines of evidence, one, the epidemiologic studies of the general population, provides the most voluminous literature on health effects at ambient pollution levels near to and below the NAAQS. Despite considerable effort, other lines of evidence (i.e., clinical exposures, analysis of smoking populations, occupational studies, studies in animals, and mechanistic toxicology) have not provided strong support for the existence of health effects at low levels of PM. Due to significant increases in funding, the number of studies showing associations of ambient PM and various health outcomes has dramatically increased in recent years. Understanding of the mechanistic basis for

the PM associations has lagged behind the accumulating epidemiology. It remains possible that at least some of the many health outcome associations reported in the epidemiological studies have a non–air-pollution basis.

- Population studies examine differences in mortality and morbidity across time or across different locations. So-called cross-sectional cohort studies correlate geographical differences in monitored air pollution levels over long periods of time with chronic disease rates or mortality rates. The time-series studies exploit short-term (e.g., day-by-day) time heterogeneity in air pollution levels measured at central monitors to look for correlations with day-by-day mortality or morbidity counts. The statistical correlations can arise for a variety of reasons aside from cause and effect and are susceptible to artifactual factors such as coincidence, measurement error, confounding, and bias.

- Other lines of human evidence with better characterization of individual exposure and individual sensitivity or outcome include (a) exposure of normal and asthmatic volunteers to controlled atmospheres (i.e., chamber studies) and (b) health data on smokers (i.e., a population heavily exposed to "combustion" particulate). Although asthmatics were found to be more sensitive to high levels of acid aerosols than normal subjects, neither asthmatics nor normal subjects exhibited decrements in pulmonary function after exposure to PM at levels in the 100 to 200 $\mu g/m^3$ range. Low levels of exposure, typical of the outdoor environment, did not produce a response. Linear extrapolation of studies on the health effects of tobacco smoke in smokers does not provide support for the idea that low levels of ambient PM, with far fewer potentially toxic compounds, can induce significant morbidity and mortality. Data available from workers exposed to elevated PM levels go counter to the idea that PM causes morbidity and mortality at low, outdoor levels. Overall, other lines of research do not adequately support the statistical associations reported in the population studies. PM does cause health effects at sufficiently high concentrations, but the disagreement between the epidemiologic associations and direct-exposure data is substantial.

- Laboratory toxicology and animal exposures have not as yet provided a mechanistic basis for the health-effect associations with low, ambient PM levels. Moreover, if PM produces different adverse health effects at low levels, each effect likely depends on distinctly different, but currently unknown, aspects of PM (i.e., exposure-response functions). An additional significant problem with interpreting the PM associations is that the list of airborne contaminants tested so far in the epidemiological studies is extremely short, omitting many vapors and gases that may also be associated with general air pollution.

- A major fraction of an individual's exposure to PM comes from indoor, nearby sources and personal activities, not general, outdoor PM. For almost all of us, the majority of our time is spent indoors rather than outdoors. Indoor sources generally dominate PM concentrations in the indoor environment and include home heating, air conditioning, cooking, smoking, other combustion sources, dusting, vacuuming, spraying, cleaning, and resuspension of settled dust by human activity. An individual's total dose, whether of PM-10 or of PM-2.5, will be dominated by sources other than regional outdoor PM concentrations. This result poses another difficulty for correctly interpreting the epidemiologic associations.

- A number of lines of reasoning suggest outdoor PM levels are not significant contributors to modern asthma problems. These include geographic variations in asthma hospitalization rates that do not mirror differences in air pollution. The clinical literature on asthma in children does not identify outdoor PM as a key element in asthma prevalence or asthma attacks. The reasons for the rise in asthma are not understood, but suspected factors include improved hygiene (i.e., reduced early-life exposure to soil bacteria, fungi, and parasites is hypothesized to increase asthma risk), changing patterns of childhood illnesses, changing diet, changing exercise patterns, changing housing, changing body mass index, increased vaccinations against childhood respiratory disease, and increased exposure to indoor-air allergens. In summary, clinical data, time-trend data, and prevalence data do not support a causal basis for correlations between outdoor PM levels and frequency or severity of asthma.

• An effective test of whether PM is the direct causal basis of the correlations is through vigorous efforts at disproof. If the PM hypothesis survives such a challenge, it has been strengthened. Although the PM associations are called into question by these alternative causal pathways, a toxicologic role for ambient PM cannot be ruled out, but neither can we rule out the possibility that monitored PM levels are acting as a surrogate measure for fluctuating societal factors linked to mortality or morbidity risk.

QUESTIONS

1. Human exposures to airborne PM are most often given in units of

A. ppm
B. $\mu g/m^3$
C. mg/kg
D. μm MMAD
E. $\mu M/L$

2. Which of the following descriptors refers to airborne PM in the smallest size class?

A. TSP
B. PM-10
C. Ozone
D. Coarse particulate
E. PM-2.5

3. For the smallest PM class identified in the previous question, which region of the respiratory tract are these particles more likely to penetrate on inhalation compared with the particulates in larger size ranges?

A. Oral cavity
B. Pharynx
C. Alveolar region
D. Tracheobronchial region
E. Trachea

4. The time-series studies of PM health effects provide data on

A. Changes over time in the health of animals exposed to concentrated air particulate
B. Correlations of day-by-day variations in PM versus day-by-day variations in health statistics
C. Volunteer exposures to a series of daily PM exposures in chambers
D. Hospital admissions for respiratory causes for workers exposed in dusty occupations

✓ E. Time trends in annual-average PM concentrations and time trends in population health

5. *In most epidemiology studies of population exposure to PM, the surrogate(s) used for measuring the relevant PM exposure is/are*

A. A personal exposure monitor worn by selected members of the target population.
B. A series of indoor air exposure monitors, selected to be where people spend the most time
C. A series of outdoor-air monitors, placed near the residences of the individuals being studied
D. Centrally located air monitors at sites selected by EPA for determining regional compliance
E. Calculated results from air dispersion models that use regional PM emissions as an input

6. *The constituent of PM responsible for the increases in mortality and morbidity reported by the epidemiologic associations for PM at ambient concentrations is*

A. Unknown
B. Sulfate and/or nitrate
C. Polycyclic aromatic hydrocarbons (PAHs)
D. Elemental carbon
E. Crustal materials

7. *Over the past 10 or 20 years, asthma prevalence appears to be increasing in modern, industrialized countries. This increase in asthma prevalence correlates with and may be caused by*

A. Global warming
B. Increasing annual average PM-10 concentrations
C. Increasing PM emissions from vehicles
D. Increasingly improved hygiene, and reduced early-life exposure to soil bacteria
E. Increasing exposure to airborne lead (Pb) particles

8. *Which of the following air pollutants is **not** a "criteria" air pollutant regulated by the National Ambient Air Quality Standards (NAAQSs)?*

A. NO_2 (nitrogen dioxide)
B. HCHO (formaldehyde)
C. SO_2 (sulfur dioxide)
D. O_3 (ozone)
E. PM (particulate matter)

60

Accessing Environmental Data

OBJECTIVES

- Discuss the types and sources of data that may help with diagnosis and management of suspected environmental health problems
- Explain the assessment of the quality of data

OUTLINE

I. Introduction
    A. Table 60.1: Parameters of interest for environmental data
II. Data quality issues
    A. Table 60.2: Key questions in evaluating environmental data
III. Types of environmental data
IV. Commonly asked questions that trigger environmental data searches
V. Agency resources
    A. Agency for Toxic Substances and Disease Registry (ATSDR)
    B. Environmental Protection Agency (EPA)
    C. State health and environmental departments
VI. Other resources
VII. Case studies in environmental medicine
    A. Case 1: Adult diagnosed with acute leukemia
    B. Case 2: Patient concern over proximity to Superfund hazardous waste site
VIII. Emerging and reemerging disease
X. Appendix to Chapter 60: Other inventories of environmental or health databases

KEY POINTS

- A variety of environmental data collection systems exist in the United States. Some exist because of regulatory requirements. Most are not designed to be useful for the clinician and may lack human data and information on dose.
- Data should be assessed for validity, accuracy, and reliability. Data are less useful than information, which represents data in an interpretable and useful form.
- For a true picture of human exposure to emerge, the practitioner must address the cumulative nature of exposure from multiple pathways, including exposure by dermal and respiratory routes, as well as by ingestion. The magnitude, duration, and frequency of exposure must also be considered.

- Two on-line data systems that may provide the practitioner with general information regarding an agent are the Toxicology Information (TOXLINE) and Toxicology Data Network (TOXNET).
- The public may look to physicians as experts on environmental issues covered in the news media.
- Many federal and state agencies are responsible for the collection and dissemination of environmental data. Some of these include the ATSDR, the EPA, and various state departments.
- For questions about cancer etiology, review known causes, request incidence statistics from the state cancer registry, and get a lifetime exposure history from the patient.
- For questions about proximity to a hazardous waste site, inquire about a Public Health Assessment of the site and consider multiple pathways of exposure.

QUESTIONS

1. Which of the following statements is most correct?

A. Data are valid if the method can adequately approach the true result.
B. Data are reliable if they truly measure the desired attribute.
C. Data are accurate if the method demonstrates consistency in the generation of values.
D. Data are raw measurements, such as the concentration of a contaminant.
E. Information, as described in the textbook, consists of raw data that cannot be summarized.

*2. Which of the following is **not** correct?*

A. Monitoring data are routinely collected by government agencies to measure environmental media for contaminants specified by statute or special interest.
B. Surveillance connotes a more encompassing, ambitious research plan for the visualization of a specific environmental agent, such as the NHANES study.
C. Special studies are often conducted during the cleanup and discovery process surrounding specific Superfund sites.
D. IRIS is an electronic database of summary health risk assessment and regulatory information on chemical substances.
E. TRI includes information on agent-specific characteristics, including toxicity in humans and animals.

3. Which of the following agencies is properly paired with its mission or areas of responsibility?

A. ATSDR/Prevent or mitigate human health problems and diminished quality of life resulting from exposure to hazardous substances
B. EPA/Dispense critical clinical information to health practitioners and patients alike regarding exposure to poisonous substances
C. State health departments/Conduct health assessments at hazardous waste storage or destruction facilities with authority under amendments to the Resource Conservation and Recovery Act (RCRA)
D. Poison control centers/Perform health risk assessments of brownfields

E. Local health departments/Administer pollution control programs and environmental monitoring programs for air and water

4. *What is the **least** likely pathway of exposure to the surrounding community emanating from a hazardous waste site?*

A. Airborne contaminants entering the lungs
B. Airborne contaminants irritating the eyes
C. Runoff to ground and surface waters, with human exposure from drinking the water
D. Runoff to ground and surface waters, with human exposure from volatilized chemicals during showering with the contaminated water
E. Direct skin contact with contaminated soil

Answers to Chapters 49–60

CHAPTER 49 ANSWERS

1. The answer is D. (Ref: p. 715)

Water resources must be suitable in quality and access to protect human health. All water resources are part of the hydrologic cycle in which water flows from the oceans to the atmosphere, falling from the atmosphere as rain onto the ocean, land, or fresh water, including lakes, rivers, and underground cavities. It then returns to the oceans as runoff or to the atmosphere by evaporation. Underground water is usually cleaner than surface water because it has been effectively filtered. Natural filtering systems composed of soil and rocks clean the water, trapping disease-causing microorganisms and particulates containing toxic elements. However, once polluted, groundwater is much more difficult to decontaminate than surface water.

2. The answer is D. (Ref: p. 715)

Water resources management involves three fundamental issues: (a) assurance of a secure and reliable supply of water; (b) treatment of drinking water to ensure safety from microbiologic and chemical hazards and to ensure acceptability by the public; and (c) handling and treatment of wastewater, so that it can be safely discharged and will not come into contact with drinking water supplies.

3. The answer is B. (Ref: p. 715)

Purification of drinking water can be accomplished in many different ways, such as coagulation, flocculation, settling, filtration, and chlorination. Filtration and chlorination are used on a large scale. These techniques, especially chlorination, have drastically reduced the incidence of water-borne diseases to present negligible levels, except for incidents in which there is a break in the system resulting in downstream contamination. Although there are adverse health effects from the by-products of chlorination, it is by far the cheapest and most effective method of disinfection. The reason for this is that the chlorine continues to act downstream, providing a margin of safety all the way to the tap. Alternative technologies, such as ozonation, irradiation, or ultraviolet treatment, do not disinfect water beyond the point of treatment.

4. The answer is A. (Ref: p. 716)

By far the most important water-borne illness in the United States is diarrhea. The type and degree of pathogen entry into water depends on the nature of the contamination and the health of the population from which the sewage in wastewater originates. Runoff from a feedlot for cattle, for example, poses much less of a threat to human health than leakage from a sewer line. In the United States, outbreaks of water-borne disease are usually limited to enteritis associated with any of a number of viruses or, less commonly, giardiasis. Typhoid and cholera are rare in the United States and usually are imported cases rather than outbreaks associated with water-related disease.

5. The answer is D. (Ref: p. 719)

Well-designed hazardous waste disposal facilities, using the best available technologies of recycling, dehalogenation, and containment, are urgently needed and have been built in many locations. However, when waste is hauled a tremendous distance at great expense, it may expose drivers and residents along the way to the risk of accidents and leakage. More often, the waste may mysteriously "disappear" by the side of the road, causing exposure of residents and uncontrolled contamination.

Incineration at high temperatures is an effective means of disposing of much hazardous waste, but it is very expensive. Because of population distribution, land use restrictions, transportation costs, and concerns from society over environmental effects, there is intense pressure to find a solution to the problem of economical disposal of hazardous waste. This has led to increased interest in proven methods such as source reduction, recycling, chemical neutralization, and secure hazardous waste disposal sites.

New disposal sites are not a perfect solution because someone inevitably has to live near one. The NIMBY (not in my back yard) syndrome makes it very difficult for governments to find new sites for undesirable developments such as hazardous waste disposal sites. Without such sites, however, society may lose control of the situation entirely. What happens when a hazardous waste disposal site is not available is often worse than the presence of a poorly managed disposal site. Sometimes, hazardous waste is disposed of illegally and in an even more dangerous manner because the owner cannot find a cheap way to get rid of it.

6. The answer is C. (Ref: p. 721)

The greenhouse effect is necessary for there to be a temperature suitable for life on Earth, but the expected exaggeration of the effect from emissions of carbon dioxide from human activity is expected to lead to numerous adverse consequences. These include chaotic weather conditions, rising ocean levels due to ice cap melting, and regional weather disturbances, possibly including local cooling in some areas. It has been predicted that mean global sea level will rise by about one-third to one-half meter by 2100. Health implications may include heat-related illness and deaths; physical and psychologic trauma due to disasters; vector-borne diseases due directly to higher temperatures and indirectly to changes in vector distribution by flooding; decreased food availability and hunger; respiratory effects due to weather disturbances, and related air pollutants and pollens; population displacement; and social disruption. Morbidity and mortality resulting from the greenhouse effect can be estimated but not predicted with any certainty. The speed of carbon dioxide increase can be modified by emission controls and by protection and regrowth of forests. The ultimate consequences and the effects on health are difficult to predict.

7. The answer is D. (Ref: p. 721)

Depletion of the stratospheric ozone layer by released chlorofluorocarbons (CFCs) (including medical products containing CFCs), bromofluorocarbon, and some other chemicals such as nitrogen dioxide results in increased ultraviolet (UV) radiation reaching the Earth's surface. The predominant health effects associated with depletion of the stratospheric ozone layer are caused by UV-B (289–320 nm) radiation.

One of the implications is skin cancer, including malignant melanoma. According to estimates by the Environmental Protection Agency (EPA), with each percentage point of ozone depletion, the incidence of nonmelanoma skin cancer will increase by 2% to 3%. Other health implications include cataracts, accelerated actinic changes (i.e., skin aging), and possible immunologic responses.

CHAPTER 50 ANSWERS

1. The answer is B. (Ref: Section I)

The primary prevention of environmental exposure and disease is implemented by the combination of local, state, and federal regulations. In contrast to human risk-based occupational standards, many environmental regulations are oriented to minimize exposure by controlling emissions of categories of pollutants according to medium of exposure. However, environmental regulations are being carefully scrutinized to determine their impact on human health risk, an area of expertise for occupational and environmental physicians.

To comprehend the current approach to the prevention of environmental disease, the physician must understand the regulatory framework as well as the science that supports these rules. These prevention-based regulations serve as the basis for the control of hazardous exposure and ultimately of the prevention of disease. Exposure control strategies must be recommended with clear knowledge of applicable regulations.

2. The answer is B. (Ref: Section IX)

The Toxic Substances Control Act (TSCA) addresses the need to fully evaluate the potential toxicity and environmental impact of many existing and all new chemicals. There are specific provisions for premanufacture notification of new chemicals before they are made and introduced into commerce.

3. The answer is A. (Ref: Section VIII)

In 1986, Comprehensive Environmental Response, Compensation, and Liability Act (CERCLA) amendments, including another extension of the scope of environmental oversight with Emergency Planning and Community Right to Know Act (EPCRA), were passed. In the aftermath of Bhopal, EPCRA requires industries to notify governmental authorities of the hazardous substances located on a site.

4. The answer is B. (Ref: Section V)

Exceeded limits and unusual emissions must be reported under the Clean Air Act (CAA) and Emergency Right to Know provisions. These publicly available reports can provide excellent exposure data in evaluating an individual case or cluster of cases.

5. The answer is D. (Ref: Section V)

The Clean Water Act (CWA) has the following five major components: (a) a system of minimum national effluent guidelines, (b) water quality standards, (c) discharge permit programs, (d) provisions for special issues such as toxics, and (e) a grant program for publicly owned treatment works (POTWs). Storm water runoff is also regulated by the CWA.

Failures to meet discharge requirements for effluent or storm water must be reported to the EPA, normally at the state level. Significant storage tank regulations also exist under the Resource Conservation and Recovery Act (RCRA).

CHAPTER 51 ANSWERS

1. The answer is E. (Ref: pp. 732–733)

Motor vehicle emissions are a major source of air pollution and have replaced coal smoke as the major concern in developed countries. Air pollution is a prominent global issue because of industrialization and the use of motor vehicles. The World Health Organization (WHO) has plays a major role in reporting air pollution and in providing guidelines for acceptable exposure levels.

2. The answer is A. (Ref: p. 733)

SO_x effects are related to the formation of acid and the secondary formation of sulfur-containing particles. Acid rain is primarily a product of sulfur based acid formation.

NO_x can form nitric or nitrous acid and acidic fogs, but it is regulated because of its ability to produce ozone through a photochemical reaction. Ozone can have acute effects on the upper and lower airways and has been associated with fibrosis in animal models.

The acute effects of carbon monoxide are well known, although chronic effects from environmental levels are controversial.

Daily increases in particulate material (PM) concentration have been associated with several indices of ill health, including daily death rates, hospital admissions, emergency department visits, antiasthma drug use, and lung function measures.

3. The answer is C. (Ref: pp. 734–735)

Water-borne diseases include diseases caused by ingestion of human or animal wastes (e.g., typhoid, cholera, giardiasis, cryptosporidiosis, amebiasis) and a wide range of bacterial diseases.

Water-contact diseases are similar, except the vectors usually penetrate the skin during contact with water or with moist, contaminated soil (e.g., schistosomiasis, ascariasis, hookworm).

Water hygiene diseases are caused by lack of water for personal hygiene (e.g., louse-borne disease). *Water-habitat diseases* are caused by standing water, which allows breeding of insects (e.g., mosquito-borne diseases such as malaria, dengue, and yellow fever).

Both water supply and sanitation interventions are required to protect public health, but water supply is a much more common focus in developing countries.

4. The answer is B. (Ref: pp. 735–736)

Sanitation is highly variable in developing countries. Untreated wastewater may be used for watering and fertilizing crops.

Lower-income-country waste contains little packaging and is not recyclable. Sanitary landfills in developed countries predominately use materials recovery and incineration. Developing countries burn solid waste, use home or neighborhood landfills, or transport waste to local landfills.

The country of generation is often not the country of disposal, and transportation of hazardous waste from developed to developing countries for disposal is a global health risk.

CHAPTER 52 ANSWERS

1. The answer is D. (Ref: pp. 740–741)

Answer D is an example of primary prevention, the ultimate goal in environmental medicine. Answers A and E relate to treatment (i.e., tertiary prevention), and answer B relates to surveillance (i.e., secondary prevention). Answer C could be considered primary prevention but is notoriously ineffective.

2. The answer is E. (Ref: p. 738, Table 52.1)

Answer E is an occupational exposure. Occupational exposures are usually more intense, more specific, and more limited than environmental exposures.

3. The answer is C. (Ref: pp. 740–741)

Latex paint in new homes in the United States typically does not contain lead, which was prohibited from paint for homes in the 1970s. If a new home was painted with very old paint, it is conceivable (but unlikely) that lead-containing paint was used.

4. The answer is B. (Ref: p. 744)

Answers A, C, D, and E are essential to the practice of environmental medicine. A physician with training and experience in chelation therapy should administer chelating agents. Environmental medicine specialists should be familiar with chelating agents, but do not necessarily need to administer them.

CHAPTER 53 ANSWERS

1. The answer is C. (Ref: p. 746–747)

As research progressed through the late 1980s, the federal government recognized indoor environmental quality (IEQ) as a significant and expensive health concern. Investigators found the following:

Poor IEQ was not simply a matter of comfort but was associated with illness and death. Many toxins were present at higher levels indoors than outdoors.

Changes in lifestyle over the past century had led average citizens of the United States to spend 90% of their lives indoors.

The most vulnerable segments of our population, the infirm, the very young, and the very old, were the most exposed.

These revelations led the EPA to place indoor environmental pollution among the top environmental priorities.

2. The answer is E. (Ref: pp. 747–750)

Five sources contribute to IEQ: external environment, building structure, building furnishings and finishing, mechanical systems, and occupant activities.

3. The answer is A. (Ref: pp. 752, 759)

Indoor environmental quality complaints improve with increased ventilation, decreased work area density, and decreased office equipment density but often increase after recent renovation and painting as well as after the installation of new carpeting.

4. The answer is D. (Ref: pp. 760–761)

The clinical evaluation of a patient should begin with an interview to elicit symptoms and the temporal relationship of these symptoms with specific events or activities (Section VII).

Patients presenting with building-related illness should be assessed with a comprehensive series of tests focusing on the immune and respiratory systems. This type of testing is rarely useful for patients with building-related occupant complaint syndrome (BROCS) (Section VII).

In the evaluation of a suspect building, the first step is to gather information on the building, the patients, and any temporal relationship (Section VIII).

In the evaluation of a problem building, the second step should proceed only with specific medical or environmental hypothesis in mind. Shotgun attempts to measure every possible pollutant should be avoided (Section VIII).

To minimize microbial contamination in a building, water leaks must be repaired promptly, and humidity and temperature must be carefully controlled (Section VIII).

CHAPTER 54 ANSWERS

1. The answer is D. (Ref: p. 768)

Worksite emergency response requirements of relevance include (a) first aid and emergency medical care, (b) protection of emergency response personnel, (c) provision of emergency medical information, (d) medical surveillance, (e) coordination with community health care providers, and (f) emergency response planning guidelines for chemical releases.

2. The answer is D. (Ref: pp. 768–769)

As a rule of thumb, first aid and cardiopulmonary resuscitation must be available to employees within 5 minutes. In the absence of infirmary, clinic, or hospital near to the workplace that is used for the treatment of all injured employees, a person or persons must be adequately trained to render first aid. First aid supplies approved by the consulting physician must be readily available.

3. The answer is E. (Ref: p. 771)

Important components of facility emergency response plans are explicit agreements between the facility and the surrounding community's emergency response organizations, including emergency medical services (EMS) organizations and hospitals.

4. The answer is D. (Ref: pp. 770–771)

The content of medical examinations or consultations "shall be determined by the attending physician."

Emergency response personnel are exposed to a greater variety and severity of health risks than most other employees. Employers are obliged by the Occupational Safety and Health Administration (OSHA) and by the Environmental Protection Agency (EPA), in some cases, to provide acceptable levels of protection to those personnel.

Use of respirators is one example. OSHA requires that self-contained breathing apparatus (SCBA) be provided to and used by members of industrial fire brigades and emergency personnel responding to hazardous materials releases. That latter requirement is also found in the EPA's Worker Protection Standards.

Medical concerns also arise when emergency responders wear personal protective equipment (PPE), especially impervious clothing and encapsulating suits. By design, such PPE is impermeable to water, and therefore, the wearer quickly loses the temperature control benefits normally derived from sweating. The higher the ambient temperature and the longer the suits are worn, the greater is the risk of dehydration and heat stress. A protocol to monitor response personnel, including at least some measure of vital signs before donning of PPE and after PPE removal, should be developed, along with criteria for referral for medical evaluation.

OSHA's Bloodborne Pathogens Standard requires employers to develop an exposure control plan, including training and the availability of hepatitis B vaccination for employees who, as a result of performing their duties, risk contact exposure of skin, eye, and mucous membranes or parenteral exposure to blood and other potentially infectious materials.

5. The answer is D. (Ref: pp. 771–772)

Although the National Fire Protection Association has established minimum competencies for EMS personnel responding to hazardous materials emergencies, that standard is voluntary and ignored by many services and states.

Important components of facility emergency response plans are explicit agreements between the facility and the surrounding community's emergency response organizations, including EMS organizations and hospitals. It is important that occupational physicians correctly understand the abilities and limitations of the hospitals and EMS services that serve the facilities at which they work or to which they provide medical services.

Facilities can encourage and assist their EMS neighbors to develop necessary protocols and procedures. For example, industrial facilities using quantities of hydrofluoric acid should provide calcium gluconate gel to local EMS services along with appropriate training in its use for decontamination and burn care.

CHAPTER 55 ANSWERS

1. The answer is E. (Ref: pp. 779–780)

Companies that develop and enact their own response plans should take into account the potential types of exposures, necessary contacts and information sources, mutual aid, and methods of grading the response.

2. Answer is B. (Ref: pp. 781–782, Table 55.10)

Level D personal protective equipment (PPE) is for use with materials that do not have respiratory, skin, or mucous membrane toxicity. When choosing PPE, it is important to consider the chemical substance that will be encountered, the duration of exposure, and risk associated with penetration or permeation of the chemical through the PPE. It also is important to recognize that the effectiveness of the PPE can be degraded with use and may result in exposures. All PPE should be thoroughly tested and certified by standardized methods such as that done by the American Society of Testing Materials.

3. The answer is C. (Ref: p. 779)

If a community hazardous materials (HAZMAT) emergency response plan (ERP) does not exist, the responsible company will take the lead in establishing such a plan.

4. The answer is D. (Ref: p. 786)

Although training for persons responding to environmental incidents is varied based on needs and mandated requirements, repeated drilling is the most important factor in ensuring a high-quality response.

5. The answer is E. (Ref: pp. 786–787)

Physicians working with employers and companies should have an understanding of the regulatory issues that are relevant to environmental and hazardous material incidents. The physician should also be aware of regulatory requirements involving the health and safety of employees, including evaluation for medical fitness for the use of PPE. Physicians should have knowledge of the toxic potential of the hazardous materials that are present at the worksite.

CHAPTER 56 ANSWERS

1. The answer is B. (Ref: pp. 791–792)

The apparent level of terrorism violence and the indiscriminate nature of such violence have increased significantly in the last 20 years of the 20th century.

2. The answer is E. (Ref: p. 793, Table 56.1)

The 10 most common errors found with emergency response plans include no upper management support, lack of employee buy-in, poor or no planning, lack of training and practice, no designated leader, failure to keep the plan up-to-date, no method of communication to alert employees, Occupational Safety and Health Administration (OSHA) regulations that are not a part of the plan, no procedures for shutting down critical equipment, and employees who are not told what actions to take in an emergency.

3. The answer is C. (Ref: p. 792)

Of all the types of weapons and agents available for terrorists to use, explosive devices remain the most common. There has been increasing attention directed at the possibility of aggressive acts involving what have come to be known as weapons of mass destruction. (WMD)

4. The answer is D. (Ref: p. 803, Table 56.11)

Vesicants are chemical warfare agents that cause vesicle formation and burns to the mucosa and skin. In addition to nitrogen mustard, other vesicant agents include sulfur mustard, Lewisite, and phosgene oxime.

5. The answer is A. (Ref: p. 798, Table 56.5)

Anthrax infections are caused by the bacteria *Bacillus anthracis*, a gram-positive rod. Anthrax infection presents as three relatively distinct clinical syndromes: cutaneous, gastrointestinal, and pulmonary. The papular lesion that develops a black eschar is a manifestation of cutaneous anthrax.

CHAPTER 57 ANSWERS

1. The answer is D. (Ref: p. 814)

The most important role of the environmental audit is to ensure regulatory compliance and prevent violations, fines, public-relations problems, and even criminal charges.

2. The answer is E. (Ref: p. 815)

There are several occasions on which environmental audits should be conducted: (a) as an ongoing review of environmental programs—regular review (e.g., 1 to 3 years) is commonly scheduled by major industries, (b) at the time of the decision to invest in new or upgraded existing facilities, (c) during acquisition and divestitures, and (d) in anticipation of an external audit.

3. The answer is B. (Ref: pp. 820–822)

Occupational and environmental medicine (OEM) physicians may be a part of the environmental audit team, review the audit report, or be informed users of it. The OEM physician has a unique understanding of the relationship between human health and environmental exposure. Although the audit commonly focuses on regulatory compliance, protection of human health is the ultimate goal of regulations. Many regulations essentially require an assessment of health risk. As a result, the OEM physician may increasingly become a part of the audit team and participate in report preparation.

A second role for the OEM physician is to review the audit. This activity may focus on the accuracy of the observations and conclusions, especially the implications of the audit on the health of the workforce or community, or both, and the need for preventive actions. Although the audit does not usually include an initial action plan, a plan is commonly generated for each major observation noted in the audit. Implementing and integrating the substance of this plan with ongoing health programs is an important activity that may require the knowledge of an OEM physician. For example, particularly in acquisition audits, the representative sampling of soils and final products must be conducted.

A third interface of the OEM physician with environmental auditing is to use the data, especially exposure sampling findings, modeling results, and risk assessment reports. This information may prove useful in evaluating a clinical case or an illness among groups of individuals or in communicating risk to members of the community. Reliable data should be preferentially used, especially those that document exposure, concentration, biologic dose, and potential health effect.

4. The answer is B. (Ref: pp. 815–817)

The first step in any of the audits is information gathering. This can include collecting the regulatory efforts of the facility in document form and a questionnaire to evaluate the compliance accomplishments made by the company.

5. The answer is A. (Ref: p. 819)

ISO-14001 includes in its framework the development of management systems designed to achieve environmental objectives. These objectives include not only compliance with applicable laws and regulations but also other environmentally protective goals, including pollution prevention, waste minimization, corrective action, recycling, energy reduction, toxic agent reduction, and related goals. To become ISO-14001 certified, a facility must also be committed to a process of continuous improvement and to community outreach. A planning process is required to identify activities that affect the environment or are subject to regulation.

CHAPTER 58 ANSWERS

1. The answer is E. (Ref: p. 823)

Qualitative risk assessment is commonly performed by authoritative bodies, including the International Agency for Research on Cancer (IARC), American Conference of Governmental Industry Hygienists (ACGIH), Environmental Protection Agency (EPA), National Toxicology Program (NTP), and other agencies. These organizations weigh available evidence and categorize carcinogens or safe levels for exposure to toxicants.

2. The answer is D. (Ref: pp. 823–824)

The risk assessment process, as codified by the National Academy of Sciences (NAS), involves four steps. The first, hazard identification, is qualitative; it assesses the toxicant's potential for causing health effects. The second, exposure dose-response assessment, establishes a quantitative relationship between exposure and response. Both of these steps use human data if available. In the absence of comprehensive human data (which is usually the case), information from studies with laboratory animals, cells, or tissues from animals and people must be used. Exposure assessment, the third step, may use actual measurements or, more frequently, results obtained by modeling. The fourth step, risk characterization, involves integration of results from steps 2 and 3 to assess risk for the specific exposure scenario under consideration (Fig. 50.1).

3. The answer is C. (Ref: pp. 824–825)

Multiple sources of information are used in developing guidelines and standards for limiting human risk from toxicants. Clinical and epidemiologic studies are especially useful in that the data are obtained on people.

4. The answer is C. (Ref: pp. 828–829)

The evaluation process considers three types of data: human carcinogenicity data, experimental carcinogenicity data, and supporting evidence of carcinogenicity. Definitive evidence of human carcinogenicity can only be obtained from epidemiologic or clinical studies.

5. The answer is D. (Ref: p. 829, Table 58.2)

The IARC conducts a formalized risk assessment that leads to a qualitative clarification of a compound's carcinogenic potential. The evaluation process considers three types of data: human carcinogenicity data, experimental carcinogenicity data, and supporting evidence of carcinogenicity. The evidence of carcinogenicity is classified into four categories. Group 1 includes chemicals and processes established as human carcinogens. Group 2 includes those that are probably (group 2A) or possibly (group 2B) carcinogenic to humans. Group 3 includes agents that are not classified. Group 4 includes agents that are probably not carcinogenic.

CHAPTER 59 ANSWERS

1. The answer is B. (Ref: p. 835)

During the past decade, increasing interest has focused on correlations detected between low, ambient particulate matter (PM) concentrations and population health statistics, notably mortality. These findings have sparked controversy because associations with health outcomes are reported for ambient PM concentrations (10–30 µg/m³).

2. The answer is E. (Ref: p. 836)

The original National Ambient Air Quality Standard (NAAQS) for PM was set for total suspended particulates (TSP), which included particles with diameters less than about 40 µm). Subsequently, it was determined that little of the PM with aerodynamic diameter greater than 10 µm was inhaled, and in 1987, the standards were changed to particles with diameters of 10 µm or less (PM-10). Later, it became appreciated that mouth-breathing people allow PM-10 particles to reach the lungs, but for nose breathers, penetration to the lungs is primarily limited to particles with an aerodynamic diameter less than 2.5 µm (PM-2.5).

3. The answer is C. (Ref: p. 836)

See question 2. Penetration to the lung alveoli is primarily limited to particles less than 2.5 µm aerodynamic diameter (PM-2.5).

4. The answer is B. (Ref: pp. 838–840)

Population studies examine differences in mortality and morbidity across time or across different locations. So-called cross-sectional, cohort studies correlate geographic differences in monitored air pollution levels over long periods with chronic disease rates or mortality rates. So-called time-series studies exploit short-term (e.g., day-by-day) time heterogeneity in air pollution levels measured at central monitors to look for correlations with day-by-day mortality or morbidity counts.

5. The answer is D. (Ref: p. 838–839)

See question 4. It is important to realize that the population epidemiology used by the Environmental Protection Agency (EPA) in setting the 1997 PM NAAQS did not involve studies of individual PM exposures. In these studies, individual PM exposure is unknown. There is also limited information available on the health history of individuals being hospitalized or dying. The time-series studies use a weak design, called *ecologic*, albeit the population acts as its own control. An ecologic study relies on aggregate, group-level measures of exposure and outcome. The cohort studies are "semiecologic" in that they have data on individual health outcomes but use aggregate data on exposure. Typically, occupational epidemiology (or cigarette-smoker epidemiology) uses a stronger design that compares health outcomes in known individuals whose level of exposure to a specific agent is known with greater accuracy than in the air pollution studies.

In essence, almost all of the air-pollution correlative studies are opportunistic, meaning they use existing, observational data as opposed to data generated specifically for the study. The statistical regression analysis consists of examining the following correlation in a wide variety of settings and with a wide variety of corrections and smoothing: outdoor PM concentrations measured routinely at central locations by monitoring programs *versus* daily morbidity and/or mortality statistics routinely collected by health agencies.

6. The answer is A. (Ref: p. 837)

Several health effects have been linked with the constituents of ambient air pollution, including PM. Epidemiology of general populations is a crucial component of available evidence, because in these studies the response of sensitive subgroups is included. However, to protect these groups, it is essential to understand which PM emissions may be responsible (i.e., to elucidate the underlying mechanisms).

Toxicology researchers are attempting to narrow the possibilities. For example, some studies evaluate insoluble ultrafine particles. Some EPA researchers are focusing on specific transition metals. Others quantify various immunologically active fractions of fine PM or focus on PM rich in specific sets of organic chemicals, such as polycyclic aromatic hydrocarbons (PAHs). Some have suggested that endotoxin may be an important component of PM toxicity. However, the toxicity of ambient levels of sulfate, a PM component that is frequently implicated by the epidemiologic studies, is not supported by experimental studies.

7. The answer is D. (Ref: p. 845)

The clinical literature on asthma in children does not identify outdoor PM as a key element in asthma prevalence or asthma attacks. A commentary on the increase in asthma prevalence gives the following ordered list of possible environmental factors, with no mention of a factor associated with outdoor PM: (a) improved hygiene (i.e., reduced early-life exposure to soil bacteria, fungi, and parasites is hypothesized to increase asthma risk); (b) changes in diet; (c) increased use of antibiotics; (d) altered patterns of infant feeding; (e) greater exposure to allergens; (f) increased obesity in children; (g) reduced physical activity in children; and (h) changes in the prenatal environment.

8. The answer is B. (Ref: p. 837)

The criteria air pollutants include air particulate (PM), sulfur dioxide, nitrogen dioxide, carbon monoxide, ozone, and lead. Typical measures of air pollution that have been consistently monitored over extended periods include the following:

Airborne particles [black smoke (BS), TSP, haze (COH), PM-10, PM-2.5, ultrafines]
Sulfur dioxide (SO_2) and the secondary sulfates (SO_4^{2-}) formed in the atmosphere
Nitrogen dioxide (NO_2) and the secondary nitrates (NO_3^-) formed in the atmosphere
Ozone (O_3)
Carbon monoxide (CO)
M constituents [e.g., crustal, elemental carbon (EC), organic matter (OM), acids]

CHAPTER 60 ANSWERS

1. The answer is D. (Ref: p. 852)

Data are raw measurements of the concentration, distribution, and environmental fate of a given agent or contaminate. Data are valid if it truly measures the desired attribute. Data are reliable if the method demonstrates consistency in the generation of values. Data are accurate if the method can adequately approach the true result. Information, as described by the author, consists of summarized data that is interpretable and useful for decision-making.

2. The answer is E. (Ref: p. 853)

Answers A, B, C, and D are correct statements. Answer E describes the Registry of Toxic Effects of Chemical Substances (RTECS). The TRI database is a compilation on the release of toxic substances by manufacturing facilities.

3. The answer is A. (Ref: pp. 854–855)

Correct pairings for answers B through E are as follows:

The Agency for Toxic Substances and Disease Registry's (ATSDR) mission is to prevent or mitigate human health problems and diminished quality of life resulting from exposure to hazardous substances. They conduct health assessments at hazardous waste storage or destruction facilities with authority under amendments to RCRA.
Poison Control Centers dispense critical clinical information to health practitioners and patients alike regarding exposure to poisonous substances
The Environmental Protection Agency (EPA), with state and local environmental agencies, performs health risk assessments of "brownfields."
State agencies administer pollution control programs and environmental monitoring programs for air and water. These activities generally fall to the state environmental agency, if one exists.

4. The answer is B. (Ref: pp. 854–858)

Although answer B may be conceivable, eye irritation is not usually associated with hazardous waste sites. It is not mentioned in the textbook chapter. Concerns about chronic carcinogenic or reproductive effects usually predominate.

Subject Index

Page numbers followed by "t" denote tables

A

AAAHC. *See* Accreditation Association for Ambulatory Health Care

Abortion, spontaneous, 271, 295

ABPA. *See* Acute bronchopulmonary aspergillosis

ABPM. *See* American Board of Preventive Medicine

Absenteeism, 42, 46

Accreditation, 37–39

Accreditation Association for Ambulatory Health Care
core standards, 38
description of, 37–38, 99
survey, 38

Accreditation Council for Graduate Medical Education, 59, 106

ACGIH. *See* American Conference of Governmental Industrial Hygienists

ACGME. *See* Accreditation Council for Graduate Medical Education

Acid rain, 306, 344

ACOEM. *See* American College of Occupational and Environmental Medicine

Acoustic trauma, 143

Acute barotitis media, 50

Acute bronchopulmonary aspergillosis, 156, 158, 211

Acute exposure guideline levels, 316

Acute intoxication syndromes, 151

Acute mountain sickness, 50

ADA. *See* Americans with Disabilities Act

Adjustment disorders, 151

Administrative controls, 14

AEGLs. *See* Acute exposure guideline levels

Aerobics, 46

Agency for Toxic Substances and Disease Registry, 11, 88, 337, 356

Aggravation, 25, 94

Air contaminants, 228, 277, 289

Air pollution, 305–306, 344, 355

Air Traffic Control Specialists, 260

Airborne particulate matter
asthma and, 333
epidemiologic studies of, 332–333
exposure to, 333
guidelines for, 332
health effects of, 332, 355
indoor levels of, 333
National Ambient Air Quality Standards, 332, 354
outdoor levels of, 333
size of, 354
standards for, 332
studies of, 354
types of, 355

Airborne transmission, of infectious diseases, 163

Alcohol abuse, 47, 98

Alcohol dependence, 153, 209

Alcohol testing, 98

Allergic reactions, 117, 146, 156, 197

Allergy
hypersensitivity reactions, 155
laboratory studies, 155–156
latex, 157, 211, 255
questions regarding, 158–159

Alpha1 antitrypsin, 224t

AMA. *See* American Medical Association

American Board of Preventive Medicine, 59

American College of Occupational and Environmental Medicine
accreditation, 37–38
Code of Ethical Conduct, 7, 85
drug screenings, 35
guidelines of, 2
medical management education, 76, 107
slit lamp examination, 181

American Conference of Governmental Industrial Hygienists, 228, 279, 329

American Medical Association, hearing loss guidelines, 143

American National Standards Institute, 63, 255

Americans with Disabilities Act
definitions, 18
disability under
communicable diseases considered, 19
definition of, 85
determination of, 7, 18
discrimination prohibited by, 90, 193, 222, 225
disorders excluded under, 91
drug testing, 19, 35, 90
Equal Employment Opportunity Commission enforcement of, 11, 90
fitness for duty evaluations, 258
function of, 15, 18, 90
history of, 18
medical examinations, 18, 53, 85
medical records requirement, 18, 86
mental or psychologic disorder definition under, 19–20, 91
occupational health programs, 104
preemployment medical inquiries, 18, 85, 254
prohibitions under, 18
purpose of, 90
record-keeping requirements, 18, 86
strength testing, 18
title I, 18
voluntary examinations under, 18

AMEs. *See* Aviation Medical Examiners

AMS. *See* Acute mountain sickness

Anaphylaxis, 157

Ancillary services, 81

Animal toxicity testing, 235–236, 281–282

ANSI. *See* American National Standards Institute

Anthrax, 167, 324–325, 350

Antigens, 155–156

Anxiety disorders, 150

AOE. *See* Arising out of employment

Apportionment, 25, 94

Arising out of employment, 70, 111

Arm pain, 159–161

Arsenic, 205t

CPSIA information can be obtained at www.ICGtesting.com
Printed in the USA
BVOW061805271112

306609BV00003B/68/P